NOTICE

Medicine is an ever-changing science. As new research and clinical experience broaden our knowledge, changes in treatment and drug therapy are required. The authors and the publisher of this work have checked with sources believed to be reliable in their efforts to provide information that is complete and generally in accord with the standards accepted at the time of publication. However, in view of the possibility of human error or changes in medical sciences, neither the authors nor the publisher nor any other party who has been involved in the preparation or publication of this work warrants that the information contained herein is in every respect accurate or complete, and they disclaim all responsibility for any errors or omissions or for the results obtained from use of the information contained in this work. Readers are encouraged to confirm the information contained herein with other sources. For example and in particular, readers are advised to check the product information sheet included in the package of each drug they plan to administer to be certain that the information contained in this work is accurate and that changes have not been made in the recommended dose or in the contraindications for administration. This recommendation is of particular importance in connection with new or infrequently used drugs.

DEJA REVIEW™

Obstetrics & Gynecology

Second Edition

Emily S. Miller, MD, MPH

Resident, Obstetrics and Gynecology
Northwestern University School of Medicine
Chicago, Illinois

Catherine J. Lee, MD

Fellow, Internal Medicine
Memorial Sloan-Kettering Cancer Center
New York, New York

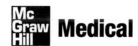 **Medical**

New York   Chicago   San Francisco   Lisbon   London   Madrid   Mexico City
Milan   New Delhi   San Juan   Seoul   Singapore   Sydney   Toronto

Déjà Review™: Obstetrics & Gynecology, Second Edition

Copyright © 2011, 2008 by The McGraw-Hill Companies, Inc. All rights reserved. Printed in the United States of America. Except as permitted under the United States Copyright Act of 1976, no part of this publication may be reproduced or distributed in any form or by any means, or stored in a data base or retrieval system, without the prior written permission of the publisher.

Déjà Review™ is a trademark of The McGraw-Hill Companies, Inc.

1 2 3 4 5 6 7 8 9 0   DOC/DOC   15 14 13 12 11

ISBN 978-0-07-171513-3
MHID 0-07-171513-4

This book was set in Palatino by Glyph International.
The editors were Kirsten Funk and Christine Diedrich.
The production supervisor was Catherine Saggese.
Project management was provided by Manisha Singh, Glyph International.
RR Donnelley was printer and binder.

This book is printed on acid-free paper.

Cataloging-in-Publication data for this title is on file with the Library of Congress.

McGraw-Hill books are available at special quantity discounts to use as premiums and sales promotions, or for use in corporate training programs. To contact a representative please e-mail us at bulksales@mcgraw-hill.com.

To all who have taught me the art of medicine, inspired me to make change, and supported me throughout the process of becoming a physician.
Emily S. Miller

To my family, friends, and mentors—thank you for all of your support, wisdom, and teachings in my journey to become a competent and compassionate physician.
Catherine J. Lee

Contents

Contributors

Jessica Maria Atrio, MD
Mount Sinai School of Medicine
Department of Obstetrics and Gynecology
New York, New York
*Chapter 4: General Gynecology (Contraception
Overview, Sterilization Methods, Barrier
Methods of Contraception, Intrauterine
Devices, Elective Abortion)*

Gilad Filmar, MD
Chief Resident, Department of Obstetrics and
Gynecology
North Shore-Long Island Jewish/Lenox Hill
Hospital
New York, New York
Chapter 6: Urogynecology

Yafit Partouche-Avidan, MD
Department of Obstetrics and Gynecology
Lenox Hill Hospital
New York, New York
*Chapter 7: Reproductive Endocrinology and
Infertility*

Kristi Tough, MD, NCMP
Fellow, Center for Specialized Women's
Health
Staff, Department of Medicine
Cleveland Clinic
*Chapter 4: General Gynecology (STIs of Lower
Genital Tract, STIs Causing Genital
Ulcerations, Cervicitis, Infections of the Upper
Genital Tract, Vaginitis, Other Gynecologic
Infections, Benign Cervical Masses, Benign
Uterine Masses, Sexual Dysfunction)*

Student Reviewers

Barrett Little
Third Year Medical Student
Temple University School of Medicine
Class of 2010

Kevyn To
Fourth Year Medical Student
SUNY Upstate College of Medicine
Class of 2009

Elina Zaretsky
Fourth Year Medical Student
Robert Wood Johnson Medical School -
    UMDNJ
Class of 2011

Acknowledgments

The authors would like to thank all the contributors, artists, and faculty reviewers from the first and second edition for their invaluable time and effort in contributing to this book and making it a useful resource for all medical students.

The authors would like to recognize all the faculty and staff at New York University School of Medicine, Harvard Medical School, Stanford University School of Medicine, Lenox Hill Hospital, Memorial Sloan-Kettering Cancer Center, Cleveland Clinic, Mount Sinai School of Medicine, and Northwestern University Feinberg School of Medicine for their endless commitment and dedication to educating medical students.

We would also like to thank the students who used this text in preparation for the boards and provided essential feedback necessary to write an improved high-yield, comprehensive book.

Finally, a special thanks to the editors and publishers at McGraw-Hill for their extraordinary patience and guidance at each step of the process to see this project through.

Introduction

Thank you for using the second edition of *Deja Review: Obstetrics & Gynecology* to assist you in your preparation for the core clerkship in Obstetrics and Gynecology and for the Ob and Gyn-related questions in Step 2CK of the United States Medical Licensing Exam (USMLE). This book is a compilation of essential facts, organized into an easy-to-read question and answer format, with difficult concepts illustrated by figures and mnemonics. It is intended for rapid-fire review, conducive to studying between patients in clinic or during down-time on labor and delivery. Once you finish each chapter, make sure you are able to answer the sample review questions. As you near the end of your clerkship, take the comprehensive final practice exam at the end of the book to identify where you need to focus your studies.

ORGANIZATION

The *Deja Review* series is a unique resource that has been designed to allow you to review the essential facts and determine your level of knowledge on the subjects tested on your clerkship shelf exams, as well as the United States Medical Licensing Examination (USMLE) Step 2CK. All concepts are presented in a question and answer format that covers key facts on commonly tested topics during the clerkship.

This question and answer format has several important advantages:

- Provides a rapid, straightforward way for you to assess your strengths and weaknesses
- Prepares you for "pimping" on the wards
- Allows you to efficiently review and commit to memory a large body of information
- Serves as a quick, last-minute review of high-yield facts
- Conducive to studying on the go with a compact, condensed design

At the end of each chapter, you will find clinical vignettes. These vignettes are meant to be representative of the types of questions tested on national licensing exams to help you further evaluate your understanding of the material.

HOW TO USE THIS BOOK

This book is intended to serve as a tool during your obstetrics and gynecology clerkship. Remember, this text is not intended to replace comprehensive textbooks, course packs, or lectures. It is simply intended to serve as a supplement to your studies during your obstetrics and gynecology rotation and throughout your preparation for Step 2CK. This text was thoroughly reviewed by a number of medical students and interns to represent the core topics tested on shelf examinations. For this reason, we encourage you to begin using this book early in your clinical years to reinforce topics you encounter while on the wards. You may use the book to quiz yourself or classmates on topics covered in recent lectures and clinical case discussions. A bookmark is included so that you can easily cover up the answers as you work through each chapter. The compact, condensed design of the book is conducive to studying on the go. Carry it in your white coat pocket so that you can access during any downtime throughout your busy day.

It is our hope that this book will supplement topics learned in the clinical setting and will facilitate success on the clerkship shelf exam and the USMLE Step 2CK. We also hope to stimulate interest in the fascinating fields of obstetrics and gynecology through exposure to some of the exciting clinical cases that are typical of this field. Thank you for letting us help you with your medical education!

Emily S. Miller, MD, MPH
Catherine J. Lee, MD

Useful Facts for the Wards

CHAPTER 1

Lab Values

Common Lab Values in the Nonpregnant Woman and Their Change During Pregnancy

Chemistries	Nonpregnant Values	Compared to Nonpregnant Woman
Sodium	135-145 mEq/L	Slightly decreased
Potassium	3.5-5.1 mEq/L	Slightly decreased
Chloride	98-106 mEq/L	Unchanged
Bicarbonate	22-29 mEq/L	Decreased
Blood urea nitrogen (BUN)	7-18 mg/dL	Decreased
Creatinine	0.6-1.2 mg/dL	Decreased
Glucose	70-115 mg/dL	Decreased
Calcium	8.4-10.2 mg/dL	Decreased
Ionized calcium	4.4-5.3 mg/dL	Unchanged
Phosphate	2.7-4.5 mg/dL	Unchanged
Magnesium	1.3-2.1 mg/dL	Decreased
Lipase	10-140 U/dL	Unchanged
Amylase	25-125 U/dL	Unchanged
SGOT/AST	7-40 U/L	Slightly decreased
SGPT/ALT	7-40 U/L	Slightly decreased
GGT	9-50 U/L	Slightly decreased
Bilirubin	0.2-1.2 mg/dL	Slightly decreased
Albumin	3.8-5.2 g/dL	Decreased
Alkaline phosphate	38-126 U/L	Increased
LDH	120-240 U/L	Unchanged
Uric acid	2.0-6.9 mg/dL	Decreased
TSH	0.32-5.00 mIU/mL	Slightly decreased
Free T_4	0.71-1.85 ng/dL	Slightly decreased
Free T_3	0.13-0.55 ng/dL	Slightly decreased
Total thyroxine (T_4)		Increased

(Continued)

Common Lab Values in the Nonpregnant Woman and Their Change During Pregnancy (*Continued*)

Chemistries	Nonpregnant Values	Compared to Nonpregnant Woman
Urinalysis		
Specific gravity	1.003-1.035	Unchanged
pH	4.5-8.0	Unchanged
Ketones	Negative	Unchanged
Protein	Negative	Slightly increased
Blood	Negative	Unchanged
Glucose	Negative	Slightly increased
Nitrite	Negative	Unchanged
Leukocyte esterase	Negative	Unchanged
Hematology		
WBC	4,700-11,000/mm^3	Increased
RBC	$3.8\text{-}5.7 \times 106/\text{mL}$	Increased
Hemoglobin	13.5-17.0 g/dL	Decreased
Hematocrit	39%-50%	Decreased
Mean corpuscular volume (MCV)	80-96 fL	Increased
Platelets	$150\text{-}400 \times 103/\text{mL}$	Decreased
Erythrocyte sedimentation rate (ESR)	0-20 mm/h	Increased
Coagulation		
PT	12.3-14.2 s	Slightly decreased
PTT	25-34 s	Slightly decreased
Fibrinogen	200-400 mg/dL	Increased
D-dimer	0-300 ng/mL	Increased
Bleeding time	2-7 min	
Thrombin time	6.3-11.1 s	
Arterial Blood Gas		
pH	7.35-7.45	Slightly increased
Paco$_2$	35-45 mm Hg	Decreased
Pao$_2$	80-100 mm Hg	Increased
HCO$_3^-$	21-27 mEq/L	Decreased
O$_2$ saturation	95%-98%	Unchanged

CHAPTER 2

Common Procedures

These tables list several of the most common procedures performed in obstetrics and gynecology. Procedures not listed here are reviewed in topic-specific chapters.

Table 2.1 Common Obstetric Procedures

Procedure	Description	Indications/ Contraindications	Benefits/Risks	Comments
Amniocentesis	Transabdominal withdrawal of fluid from the amniotic sac	Determine the presence of genetic abnormalities (eg, Down syndrome), fetal structural anomalies (neural tube defects), fetal lung maturity, or intrauterine infection	Bleeding, chorioamnionitis, preterm labor, fetal injury, or fetal loss (< 0.5%)	Usually performed using ultrasonographic guidance. Amniocentesis for genetic analysis are done between 14-20 weeks
Cerclage	Placement of a suture into and around the cervix to hold it closed	Used either prophylactically in a woman with a history of cervical insufficiency or therapeutically in an abnormally dilated/ effaced cervix	In some clinical circumstances, it reduces the likelihood of a preterm delivery	Prophylactic cerclages are placed between 12-16 weeks. A therapeutic cerclage is placed before 24 weeks
Cesarean section	The delivery of the fetus by making an incision through the abdomen and uterus	Performed when a vaginal delivery would be harmful to the mother or fetus	Complications include bleeding, infection, damage to nearby organs, postoperative adhesions, and problems with the next birth (ie, placenta accreta, uterine rupture)	The incision can be made in two ways: (1) Classical-midline longitudinal incision through uterus (2) Low transverse– transverse cut above the bladder; more commonly used; less bleeding

6

Chorionic villus sampling (CVS)	A small cannula is passed through the cervix or transabdominally, and villus cells are aspirated for genetic analysis	Cells are taken for genetic studies	Slightly higher rates of fetal loss compared with midtrimester amniocentesis	CVS is usually performed between 10-13 weeks to allow earlier decision making regarding possible pregnancy termination
Circumcision	The removal of the foreskin from the penis of a newborn male	It has been performed as part of religious and social customs, and health reasons	Risks are the same as for any surgical operation (bleeding, infection, surgical damage)	There is controversy over the medical value of the procedure
Episiotomy	An incision made through the perineum to facilitate delivery	Used to facilitate passage of the fetal vertex or shoulders	Episiotomy seems to cause more morbidity (3rd/4th degree tears, postpartum pain, dyspareunia) and is not routinely recommended	
External cephalic version	The application of constant gentle pressure (between 36 and 39 weeks) to the abdomen of the mother with a breech fetus to move it to cephalic presentation	To position a breech fetus into cephalic presentation	Risks include rupture of membranes, placental abruption, fetal bradycardia, and the need for an emergent cesarean delivery	Success rates range from 50%-75%. Fetal monitoring is advised after the procedure as well as administration of Rh-immune globulin to Rh-negative women because of risks of fetomaternal hemorrhage

(Continued)

Table 2.1 Common Obstetric Procedures (Continued)

Procedure	Description	Indications/ Contraindications	Benefits/Risks	Comments
Fern test	Vaginal secretion from the posterior vaginal pool is collected with a sterile swab and placed on a clean slide to dry	It detects the leakage of amniotic. It is helpful to diagnose rupture of membranes. If positive, the amniotic fluid will form a fern-like pattern after crystallization of the salt		Used in conjunction with the nitrazine test (pH paper turns blue demonstrating an alkaline pH) and pooling (collection of fluid in the posterior vaginal vault) to diagnose ruptured membranes
Forceps delivery	An instrument applied to the fetal head used for assistance in vaginal delivery	Used to provide traction to augment and/or direct the expulsive forces during the second stage of labor	Maternal complications: GU lacerations, blood loss, and hematomas. Fetal complications: bruising, cephalohematomas, facial lacerations	Four types of forceps are classified as outlet, low, mid, and high depending on the station of the fetal vertex. High forceps are not recommended by American College of Obstetricians and Gynecologists (ACOG)

Pelvimetry	The assessment of the size of the female pelvis in relation to the space needed for a vaginal delivery	Should be done early in prenatal care to assess the potential of a successful vaginal delivery	Can be performed by physical examination Used to be radiologically evaluated
Percutaneous umbilical blood sampling (PUBS)	A needle is placed transabdominally and fetal blood is obtained from the umbilical vein under ultrasonographic guidance	Usually performed for the assessment/treatment of alloimmunization. Fetal blood gas and metabolic status, fetal hemogram, fetal blood chemistries, and fetal genetic studies can be performed	The risks are similar to that of an amniocentesis. There may also be bleeding at the umbilical puncture site or development of a cord hematoma	Also referred to as cordocentesis
Tubal ligation	A permanent form of female sterilization where the fallopian tubes are severed, sealed, or "pinched shut" to prevent fertilization	Used when fertility is no longer desired	The most common risk is regret. There is an increase rate of ectopic pregnancy, **if pregnancy occurs**	Tubal ligation does not affect hormone production, libido, or menstrual cycle

(Continued)

Table 2.1 Common Obstetric Procedures (Continued)

Procedure	Description	Indications/ Contraindications	Benefits/Risks	Comments
Ultrasound imaging	Specific parts of the fetus are exposed to low-energy sound waves which produce images reflective of the structure and movement of the internal organs	Used to establish the presence of a living embryo/fetus, estimate the age of the pregnancy, diagnose congenital abnormalities, evaluate the position of the fetus and placenta, determine if there are multiple pregnancies, determine the amount of amniotic fluid, check for opening or shortening of the cervix	It is a painless procedure and does not involve any ionizing radiation	Doppler ultrasound can be used to evaluate blood flow through a blood vessel
Vacuum extraction	A suction cup device that is applied to the fetal vertex to help in delivery	Indications are similar to that of forceps delivery	Less maternal complications as compared to forceps delivery, but increased rates of scalp hematomas (cephalohematomas)	

Table 2.2 Common Gynecologic Procedures

Procedure	Description	Indications/ Contraindications	Benefits/Risks	Comments
Angiography	It is a medical imaging technique in which a radiographic contrast medium is injected into the blood vessel and an x-ray picture is taken to visualize the blood vascular system	It can be used to locate the source of continued bleeding from postoperative procedures, visualize bleeding from sites infiltrated by cancers, help assist in the embolization of the uterine arteries to reduce the size of uterine myomas		Usually done by interventional radiologists

(*Continued*)

Table 2.2 Common Gynecologic Procedures (Continued)

Procedure	Description	Indications/ Contraindications	Benefits/Risks	Comments
Bimanual pelvic examination	Two fingers are placed in the vagina and the flat of the opposite hand is placed on the lower abdominal wall. Gentle palpation and manipulation should delineate the position, shape, mobility, tenderness, and size of the uterus and adnexal structures. See Fig. 2.1	Part of routine gynecologic examination and part of investigation for gynecologic pathology	Difficult to elicit much information on obese patients	
Cervical conization	It is a surgical procedure that involves excising a cone-shaped sample of tissue that includes the entire cervical transformation zone and a portion of the endocervical canal. The sample is then examined for any signs of malignancy	Used for either diagnostic or therapeutic reasons. The test is done when results of a cervical biopsy indicate precancerous cells in the area or early cervical cancer	An early complication is excessive bleeding. Infrequent complications include cervical stenosis or cervical incompetence (in a future pregnancy)	Conization can be performed using a knife (cold knife cone), laser excision, or electrocautery (loop electrosurgical excision procedure [LEEP])

Colposcopy	A magnified inspection of the surface of the cervix, vagina, and vulva, using a light source and a binocular microscope	Used to facilitate detailed evaluation of a suspect malignancy and to assist in directed biopsies of suspicious areas	Minimal risk	Can be performed in the office and rarely requires any anesthesia
Computed axial tomography (CT)	A form of imaging that uses x-ray information to generate detailed cross-sectional images of internal structures	Can help evaluate for pelvic masses, signs of adenopathy, and plan for radiation therapy CT heavily relies on the use of IV contrast. This contrast can cause kidney damage and so should not be used in patients with renal failure	Superior contrast resolution which provides a significant amount of information. However, it is considered as a moderate to high radiation exposure	CT is best suited to study bone and calcifications in the body, or vessels and bowel which have been enhanced with contrast
Cryotherapy	It is a technique to destroy tissue by freezing with liquid nitrogen or liquid carbon dioxide	Most frequently used to destroy dysplastic sections of the cervix and other benign lesions (ie, condyloma)	Minimal risk. Inexpensive and generally effective, although not as precise as laser ablation	Not as useful for treating changes in the upper cervix; a cone biopsy is recommended instead

(Continued)

13

Table 2.2 Common Gynecologic Procedures (Continued)

Procedure	Description	Indications/ Contraindications	Benefits/Risks	Comments
Culdocentesis	It is the passage of a needle into the cul-de-sac to obtain fluid from the pouch of Douglas	A diagnostic procedure to check for abnormal fluid. Bloody fluid may indicate a ruptured ectopic pregnancy; pus-filled fluid indicates acute infection; ascetic fluid may indicate cancer	There is a slight risk of puncturing a mass, the uterine wall, or the bowel	Not as commonly performed today with advances in ultrasound technology
Dilation and curettage (D&C)	The process of opening and dilating the cervix using a series of graduated dilators followed by curettage, or scraping, of the uterine lining	May be used to take an endometrial sample, remove polyps or excess endometrial lining, or to treat cases of spontaneous abortions	If done roughly, uterine perforation may occur or scarring could develop leading to future infertility	It is generally performed under local anesthesia and/or light sedation

Dilation and evacuation (D&E)	A procedure used in the second trimester to remove the products of conception by first dilating the cervix and then using grasping forceps. Vacuum aspiration may also be used to facilitate the removal	It is used in pregnancy termination	Mild bleeding, cramping. There is also slight risk of uterine perforation and scarring	D&E is the most common and safest procedure used for an abortion in the second trimester
Hysterectomy	The removal of the uterus. It can be performed by entering the abdomen (abdominal hysterectomy), extracting the uterus through the vagina (vaginal hysterectomy), entering laparoscopically, or a combination of the above	It may be indicated for patients with benign or malignant changes in the uterine wall or cavity, menstrual disturbances or abnormal bleeding, endometriosis, uterine prolapse, or chronic pelvic pain. It is not recommended for the sole purpose of sterilization	Advantages include eliminating future pregnancies, ceasing menses, and treating uterine and early stage cervical cancer	There are different types of hysterectomy: *Total*: removal of all of the uterus and cervix *Subtotal or supracervical*: the body of the uterus is removed near the level of the internal cervical os, leaving the cervix in situ *Radical*: is a cancer surgery procedure where the uterus, cervix and adnexa are removed with wide margins of surrounding tissues

(Continued)

15

Table 2.2 Common Gynecologic Procedures (Continued)

Procedure	Description	Indications/ Contraindications	Benefits/Risks	Comments
Hysterosalpingography	It is an x-ray of the uterus, fallopian tubes, and abdominopelvic cavity that involves the injection of dye through the cervix	It is useful to assess the size, shape, and anatomy of the uterine cavity for evaluation of infertility or genital anomalies	There is a risk of infection, bleeding, pain, and allergic reaction to the dye	High risk patients should be given prophylactic antibiotics (eg, doxycycline) to prevent development of PID
Hysteroscopy	A small endoscope which has a built-in viewing camera that allows direct visualization of the endocervix and endometrial cavity	Used for evaluation of bleeding or structural abnormalities which may cause infertility, or location of missing intrauterine devices; it is also used for therapeutic reasons (ie, polypectomy, endometrial ablation, removal of the uterine septum)	Risks include bleeding, cramping, infection, uterine perforation, and electrolyte abnormalities from the loss of too much distension fluid	Fluid is used to distend the uterine cavity. Usually performed as an outpatient procedure under local or general anesthesia

Hysterosonography	Used to visualize the uterine cavity by use of ultrasound during slow infusion of sterile saline into the uterine cavity	Used to evaluate abnormal growths inside the uterus; abnormalities of the tissue lining the uterus (the endometrium); or disorders affecting deeper tissue layers	Does not use ionizing radiation, contrast media, or invasive surgical techniques. Mild bleeding and cramping may occur post procedure	It is useful as a screening test to minimize the use of more invasive diagnostic procedures, such as biopsies and D&C
Laparoscopically assisted vaginal hysterectomy (LAVH)	A procedure using laparoscopic surgical techniques and instruments to remove the uterus and/or tubes and ovaries through the vagina	Indications are similar to that of a hysterectomy	Advantages include avoiding a large abdominal incision, reducing postoperative pain, and minimizing recovery time. Disadvantages include technical difficulty leading to increased operative time and increased anesthesia exposure	

(Continued)

Table 2.2 Common Gynecologic Procedures (Continued)

Procedure	Description	Indications/Contraindications	Benefits/Risks	Comments
Laparoscopy	The inspection and manipulation of tissue within the abdominal cavity using endoscopic instruments (camera)	It is used for diagnostic and therapeutic purposes. It is a minimal access surgical approach	Less morbidity than laparotomy, but injury to the bowel and vessels can occur. Postsurgical infection and bleeding is possible	The abdominal cavity is usually distended with carbon dioxide or nitrous oxide gas to facilitate viewing
Laparotomy	An incision through the abdominal wall to gain access into the abdominal cavity	It is for both diagnostic and therapeutic purposes. Exploratory laparotomy is used to identify the cause of disease	The operative procedure time may be less time consuming compared to laparoscopic technique, but there is more postoperative pain and a longer recovery time	A Pfannenstiel incision is a transverse incision and just above the pubic symphysis. It is the incision of choice for cesarean delivery and for benign gynecologic disease confined to the pelvis.
Laser vaporization	High-energy light waves are used to destroy abnormal cells and dysplastic tissue	Can be used to treat cervical dysplasia	It is expensive	Infrared and CO_2 lasers are commonly used in the office, and can be coupled to colposcopes for treatment of cervical dysplasia

Loop electrosurgical excision procedure (LEEP)	A thin wire loop electrode and an electrosurgical generator used to electro-surgically cut away cervical tissue in the immediate area of the loop wire	It has both diagnostic and therapeutic uses. It is most commonly used to excise vulvar condylomas and cervical dysplasias	Minimal pain, minimal damage to the surrounding tissue, and low morbidity. Can lead to future cervical stenosis or insufficiency	It is an office procedure and usually requires only local anesthetic
Magnetic resonance imaging (MRI)	A form of imaging based on the magnetic characteristics of various atoms and molecules in the body. It uses nonionizing radiofrequency signals	Used to evaluate any soft tissue mass but emerging clinical applications include assessment of breast lesions and staging of cervical cancer	There are no harmful effects to a fetus	MRI is best suited to evaluate soft tissue or noncalcified tissue
Mammography	An x-ray examination of the breasts. The breasts are placed between two plates and pressed flat	Used as a diagnostic and screening modality for breast masses	Lower dose radiation exposure makes this examination safe	Women should receive screening mammograms every 1-2 years when they reach age 40 and annually after 50

(Continued)

Table 2.2 Common Gynecologic Procedures (Continued)

Procedure	Description	Indications/ Contraindications	Benefits/Risks	Comments
Pap smear	A microscopic examination of cells scraped from the ectocervix and endocervix	Mainly used as a screening modality, it can detect cancerous or precancerous conditions of the cervix		ACOG recommends annual Pap smear screenings from 3 years after the start of sexual intercourse but not later than age 21. Women at risk should have annual Pap smears; women who have had three consecutive negative tests can be screened every 2-3 years after the age of 30
Schiller test	Iodine solution is placed on areas of the cervix and vagina that are suspect for dysplasia. Any portion of the tissue that does not absorb the dye is biopsied for signs of cancer	It is performed on areas of the cervical or vaginal mucosa where malignant changes are suspected		Often used in conjunction with colposcopy

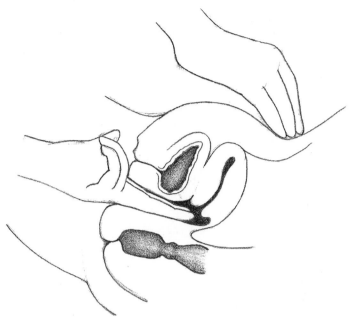

Figure 2.1   Bimanual examination of the uterus and adnexa.

CHAPTER 3

Female Anatomy

BONY PELVIS

What forms the bony pelvis?

Sacrum

Coccyx

Paired hip bones (ilium, ischium, and pubis) (see Fig. 3.1)

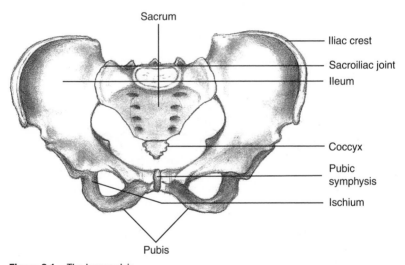

Figure 3.1 The bony pelvis.

What is the sacral promontory and what is its significance?

The most anterior projection of the sacrum, it is a landmark for the insertion of a laparoscope as it demarcates the point of bifurcation of the common iliac arteries.

What is the arcuate line and what is its significance?

Also called the linea semicircularis, it is the line that marks the pelvic brim. It lies between the first two segments of the pelvis and demarcates the site of entry of the inferior epigastric artery into the rectus sheath.

What is the ischial spine and what is its significance?	It is the medial protrusion of the ischium and an important landmark for giving a pudendal nerve block. It also provides a good landmark by which to assess progression of fetal descent during labor.
What are the four pelvic configurations found in females and how common are each?	1. Gynecoid (50%) 2. Anthropoid (25%-50%) 3. Android (16%-33%) 4. Platypelloid (3%)
Describe the shape of a gynecoid pelvis:	It is **wider** and **lower** than the male pelvis. The pubic arch is wide and round, the iliac bone is flatter, and the ischial spines are not prominent. The anterior-posterior and transverse diameters are roughly equal. All of this makes the pelvic basin more spacious.
Describe the shape of an anthropoid pelvis:	It is **heart-shaped** with a wider anterior-posterior diameter than a transverse diameter.
Describe the shape of an android pelvis:	It is **narrower** and **taller** than the gynecoid pelvis.
Describe the shape of a platypelloid pelvis:	It has a wider transverse diameter than an anterior-posterior diameter.
What is the pelvic inlet?	The superior circumference of the lesser pelvis. Its boundaries include the sacral promontory, the pubic ramus and symphysis pubis, and the linea terminalis.
Describe the following:	
Obstetric conjugate:	The shortest pelvic diameter through which the fetal head passes; it can only be measured radiographically; the distance from the sacral promontory to the symphysis pubis; the normal diameter is more than 10 cm
True conjugate:	The AP diameter that lies between the sacral promontory and the superior symphysis pubis
Diagonal conjugate:	Only one measured clinically; the distance between the sacral promontory and the inferior margin of the symphysis pubis

PELVIC ORGANS

What is the major blood supply to the pelvic organs?	Internal iliac artery (aka hypogastric artery)
Describe the branches of the internal iliac artery:	Coming off the common iliac artery, the internal iliac typically but not always divides into anterior and posterior trunks (see Fig. 3.2)

Anterior trunk:	Inferior vesical Middle rectal Obturator Umbilical Internal pudendal Inferior gluteal Uterine Vaginal (can also arise from the uterine arter)	Posterior truck:	Iliolumbar Lateral sacral Superior gluteal

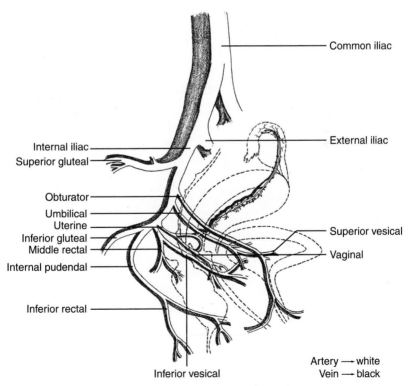

Figure 3.2 Arteries and veins of the female reproductive system.

What is the major blood supply to the vagina?

The vaginal artery, descending branches of the uterine artery, ascending branches of the pudendal artery, and small contributions from the middle and inferior hemorrhoidal vessels (see Fig. 3.3)

What is the innervation to the vagina?

Parasympathetics via S2-S4 for the upper two-thirds and general somatic efferent to the lower one-third via the pudendal nerve

What is the lymphatic drainage of the vagina?

The upper two-thirds drain into the internal and external iliac nodes. The lower one-third drains into the inguinal nodes.

What ligaments support the uterine position in the pelvis?

Uterosacral, cardinal, round, and broad ligaments

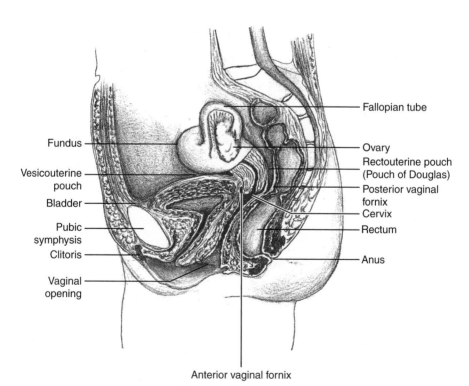

Figure 3.3   Midsagittal view of pelvic viscera.

What are the anatomic portions of the uterus?

Fundus (most superior portion of the uterus, above the entrance of the fallopian tubes)

Corpus (the uterine body)

Isthmus (area where the uterus begins to constrict)

Cervix (inferior portion of the uterus that extends into the vagina)

What is meant by flexion of the uterus?

The angle between the long axis of the uterine body and the cervix; can be anteflexed or retroflexed

What is meant by the terms anteversion and retroversion?

The angle between the cervix and the vagina

What are the histological layers of the uterine wall (from interior to exterior)?

Endometrium (ciliated columnar epithelium, glands, and spiral arteries)

Myometrium (smooth muscle and connective tissue)

Serosa

What are the major blood supplies to the uterus?

Uterine and ovarian arteries (there are extensive anastomoses which allow for ligation of the uterine or internal iliac during hemorrhage to control bleeding without compromising blood supply to the uterus)

Describe the course of the uterine artery in the pelvis:

Arises from the internal iliac → divides into cervicovaginal and uterine branches → uterine branch divides into the fundal, ovarian, and tubal arteries and provides radial arteries that perforate into the uterus

What is the relationship of the uterine artery with the ureter?

The ureter crosses under the artery ("water under the bridge") 2 cm lateral to the cervix in the cardinal ligament

What is the lymphatic drainage of the uterus?

Internal and external iliac nodes (although the fundus can drain into the para-aortic lymph nodes)

Describe the following portions of the cervix:

Portio: The portion of the cervix that is visible from the vagina

Cervical canal: Area in between the internal and external os

External os: Inferior opening of the cervix into the vagina

Internal os: Superior opening of the cervix into the uterine cavity

What is the major blood supply to the cervix?   Cervical branch of the uterine artery

What is the innervation to the cervix?   Autonomics, sympathetics (T12-L3), and parasympathetics (S2-S4)

What is the lymphatic drainage of the cervix?   Internal and external iliacs to the common iliacs

What are the fallopian tubes?   These are 8 to 10 cm tubes that extend laterally from the body of the uterus

What are the histological layers of the fallopian tubes (from interior to exterior)?   Mucosal layer (ciliated columnar epithelium covered in cilia)

Muscular layer (external longitudinal layer and internal circular layer)

Serosa

What are the segments of the fallopian tubes (from medial to lateral)?   Interstitial, isthmic, ampullary, infundibular, and fimbrial

What is the major blood supply to the fallopian tubes?   Uterine and ovarian arteries

What is the lymphatic drainage of the fallopian tubes?   Aortic nodes

What are the histological layers of the ovary (from interior to exterior)?   Medulla (connective tissue and blood supply); cortex (ova and tunica albuginea); germinal epithelium

What is the major blood supply to the ovaries?

Ovarian arteries (arising from aorta just below the level of the renal arteries) and branches of the uterine artery

Where do the right and left ovarian veins drain?

The right ovarian vein drains through the inferior vena cava (IVC) and the left drains through the left renal vein.

Describe the course of the ureter through the abdomen and pelvis:

In the abdomen, it is retroperitoneal on the anterior surface of the psoas muscle. It then crosses the common iliac artery nears its bifurcation and then follows the pelvic wall laterally to the medial broad ligament. It then crosses under the uterine artery and courses medially to enter the cardinal ligaments. It enters the bladder at the trigone.

How is the ureter distinguished during surgery?

1. Ureteral peristalsis
2. Auerbach plexus (only on the ureteral anterior surface)

What are the most common sites of ureteral injury?

1. Pelvic brim
2. Where the ureter crosses the uterine artery
3. Bladder trigone

How can the rectum be differentiated from the rest of the bowel?

It begins after the sigmoid colon where the mesentery ends and it does not have teniae coli or appendices epiploicae.

Describe each of the ligamentous structures in the pelvis.

    Broad ligaments:

Reflections of peritoneum from the lateral margin of the uterus to the pelvic sidewall; contain the uterine vessels and ureters in their base

    Round ligaments:

Homologue of the male gubernaculums; also contain an artery of the round ligament, connects lateral uterine fundus to the upper labia majora

    Uterosacral ligaments:

Extend from posterior-inferior uterus to the presacral fascia

    Cardinal ligaments:

Support the uterus; at base of broad ligament, contain uterine artery
See Fig. 3.4

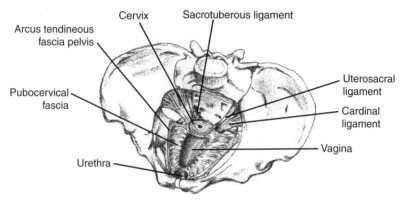

Figure 3.4 Ligaments of the female pelvis.

Describe the clinical manifestations of damage to each of the following nerves:

Femoral nerve:
Problems with hip flexion

Obturator nerve:
Problems with adduction of thigh/hip; loss of sensation in medial thigh

Genitofemoral nerve:
Loss of sensation in perineum

Peroneal nerve:
Foot drop; loss of sensation in lateral lower leg and dorsum of the foot

During which types of surgeries can each of the following nerves be injured?

Femoral nerve:
Abdominal surgery or inguinal node dissection

Obturator nerve:
Radical hysterectomy or node dissection

Genitofemoral nerve:
Radical hysterectomy or node dissection

Peroneal nerve:
Improper placement of legs in stirrups

PERINEUM

What is the perineum?

Area between the mons pubis and the buttocks (see Fig. 3.5)

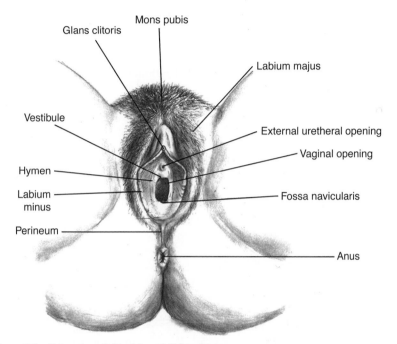

Glans clitoris

Mons pubis

Labium majus

Vestibule

External uretheral opening

Vaginal opening

Hymen

Labium minus

Fossa navicularis

Perineum

Anus

Figure 3.5   External genitalia of the adult female.

What is the major blood supply to the perineum?

Internal pudendal artery

What is the major innervation to the perineum?

Pudendal nerve

What is the lymphatic drainage of the perineum?

Inguinal nodes

Name the muscles of the perineum:	Superficial and deep transverse perineal
	Bulbocavernosus
	Ischiocavernosus
	External anal sphincter
	Urethral sphincter
What is the urogenital diaphragm?	Muscles between the pubis symphysis and the ischial tuberosities that support the perineum
Name the muscles of the urogenital diaphragm:	Urethral sphincter and deep transverse perineal
What is the pelvic diaphragm?	Muscles from the upper pubis and ischium to the rectum that support the perineum
What muscles comprise the pelvic diaphragm?	Levator ani, coccygeal; see Fig. 3.6.

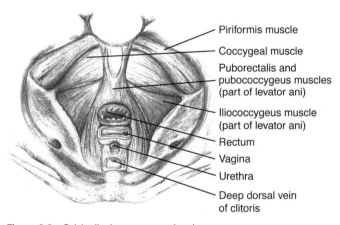

Piriformis muscle

Coccygeal muscle

Puborectalis and pubococcygeus muscles (part of levator ani)

Iliococcygeus muscle (part of levator ani)

Rectum

Vagina

Urethra

Deep dorsal vein of clitoris

Figure 3.6   Pelvic diaphragm—superior view.

What are the superficial muscles of the vulva?	Superior transverse perineal
	Bulbocavernosus
	Ischiocavernosus
	(All lie superficial to the urogenital fascia [perineal membrane])
What are Bartholin glands?	Glands found deep to the vestibule, lateral to the vagina that open into the vestibule

What are Skene glands?	Also called paraurethral glands; they are homologues of the prostate that surround the urethral opening and empty into the vestibule

ABDOMINAL WALL

What are the layers of the abdominal wall?	Skin → subcutaneous fat → outer fatty layer (Camper) of superficial fascia → inner membranous layer (Scarpa) of superficial fascia → anterior rectus sheath → rectus abdominus muscle → posterior rectus sheath → preperitoneal fat subserous or extraperitoneal fascia → parietal peritoneum
Describe the blood supply to the lower abdomen:	Deep circumflex iliac (off of the external iliac) and external pudendal artery
What is the arcuate line?	Above the arcurate line, the posterior aponeurosis of the internal oblique splits. The posterior leaflet and the aponeurosis of the transversus abdominus comprise the posterior portion of the rectus sheath. The anterior leaflet of the external oblique forms the anterior portion.
	Below the arcuate line, the aponeuroses of both leaflets of the internal oblique and the external oblique contribute to the anterior leaflet of the rectus sheath. Only the aponeurosis of the transversus abdominus comprises the posterior portion.
What is the linea alba?	The medial aspect of the rectus abdominus; formed by the fusion of the aponeuroses of the anterior abdominal muscles
What are the linea semilunara?	The lateral borders of the rectum abdominus muscles
What structures pass through the inguinal canal in the female?	Round ligament
	An artery and vein passing to the uterus
	Extraperitoneal fat

Topics in Gynecology

CHAPTER 4

General Gynecology

Menstrual Cycle Physiology

What is the average duration of the menstrual cycle, duration of menses, and amount of blood loss during menses?

The average duration of the menstrual cycle is **28 days (± 7 days)**. The cycle begins with the first day of menstrual flow, which typically last **4 days**. On an average, women lose less than **60 mL of blood** during each menses.

What are the two phases of the menstrual cycle and how long does each last?

1. **Follicular** (or **proliferative**) phase
2. **Luteal** (or **secretory**) phase

These are separated by **ovulation**.

Follicular/luteal describe the ovarian changes, proliferative/secretory describe the endometrial changes.

What causes the variability in the length of the menstrual cycle?

The duration of the follicular phase. The luteal phase is constant and last 14 days.

Describe the hormone pathway involved in the menstrual cycle and name which structures produce each hormone:

The cycle begins in the arcuate nucleus of the **hypothalamus** where **gonadotrophin-releasing hormone (GnRH)** is released in a pulsatile fashion. GnRH stilmulates the **anterior pituitary** to release **follicle-stimulating hormone (FSH)** and **luteinizing hormone (LH)**. In response the ovaries release **estradiol, progesterone and inhibin**. Inhibin down regulates production of FSH. (See Fig. 4.1)

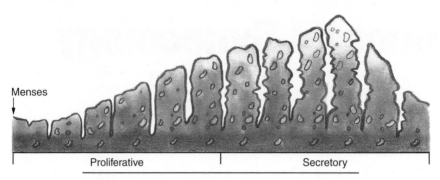

Menses

| Proliferative | Secretory |

Endometrial histology

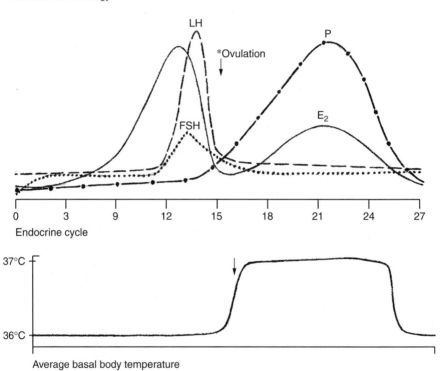

Figure 4.1   The menstrual cycle.

What is happening in the ovary during the menstrual cycle?

Each follicle contains an oocyte arrested in **prophase of meiosis 1**. It is surrounded by pre-granulosa cells and then pre-theca cells. LH stimulates **theca cells** and secrete **androgens (testosterone and androstenedione),** which are aromatized by the granulosa cells into estradiol and estrone. FSH stimulates the granulose cells.

The follicle with the most granulosa cells, FSH receptors, and estradiol production becomes the **dominant follicle** and is released during ovulation. The remaining granulose and thecal cell becomes the **corpus luteum, which** secretes progesterone. If fertilization does not occur, and no HCG is produced, it degenerates into the **corpus albicans.**

What is the function of the corpus luteum?

Secretion of **progesterone** and **estradiol** to sustain the proliferative endometrium for possible implantation. It can maintain a pregnancy until sufficient progesterone is produced by the placenta at 12 weeks estimated gestational age (EGA).

What is happening to hormone levels in the follicular phase?

On day 1 of menses, **estradiol, progesterone**, and **LH** are at their nadir. **FSH and LH levels begin to rise**.

Ovarian Estradiol levels rise by day 4. 72 hours prior to ovulation (day 14 of a 28 day cycle), estradiol peaks and causes an LH surge. Ovulation occurs 30 to 38 hours after the surge.

What is happening to hormone levels in the luteal phase?

The LH surge causes granulosa and theca cells to secrete **progesterone (which increases the basal body temperature)** and **peaks** 3 to 4 days after ovulation.

Estrogen levels decrease immediately after ovulation but slowly rise with the growth of the corpus luteum. Progesterone and estrogen (at low to moderate levels) both act via negative feedback to **suppress LH** and **FSH**. If fertilization and implantation do not occur, progesterone and estradiol levels diminish after 11 days. FSH increases as the corpus luteum regresses.

What is happening to the endometrium in the proliferative phase?

At menses, the **endometrium sloughs off** and only the basalis remains. Increasing estradiol stimulates proliferation of the uterine endometrial glands and elongation of **spiral arteries**. Prior to ovulation it appears as a **"triple stripe"** pattern on ultrasound.

What is happening to the endometrium in the secretory phase?

Progesterone reorganizates the glands (resulting in a more **edematous stroma**), and causes **coiling of the spiral arteries**.

On ultrasound it appears as a **uniformly bright** endometrium. If pregnancy does not occur, the endometrium degenerates.

What are the primary cervical and systemic manifestations of estradiol and progesterone during the menstrual cycle?

Estradiol.

Endocervix: stimulates secretion of thin, **watery mucus**. Produces **"ferning"** pattern when spread on a glass slide; Vagina: promotes **vaginal thickening.**

Progesterone.

Endocervix: **thickens** endocervical **mucus, causing it to become stringy (spinnbarkeit)**; Breast: stimulates acinar glands, causing breasts to round and become tender.

Raises basal body temperature by 0.6°F to 1°F. Causes some women to have the emotional, physical, and behavioral changes of premenstrual syndrome (PMS).

What layer of the endometrium sloughs off during menses?

The **functionalis layer (inner layer)** sloughs off after glandular and stromal degeneration.

What hormone mediates menstrual cramps and how is it synthesized?

Prostaglandins, especially $PGF_{2\alpha}$. It is released by the secretory endometrium in response to progesterone and causes uterine contractions.

Family Planning

CONTRACEPTION OVERVIEW

How many American women use contraception and what are the rates of unintended or mistimed pregnancy in the United States?

Between **89% and 93%**; yet **53%** of births are either unintended or mistimed

What are some of the reasons for contraception failure?

Failure of the method, incorrect use, nonadherence

What are the two measures for effectiveness of a contraceptive method?

1. **Theoretical effectiveness (perfect use)**—the pregnancy rate among women who use the method correctly every time
2. **Actual effectiveness (typical use)**—includes the chances of inconsistent or incorrect use

What factors about each method must be considered when counseling about contraception?

Coital dependence, convenience, cost, duration of action, protection against sexually transmitted infections (STIs), effect on menses, religion, reversibility, acceptability, and side effects

What are the five main classes of contraception?

1. Sterilization
2. Hormonal contraceptivesBarrier methods
3. Rhythm method & coitus interruptus
4. Barrier methods
5. Intrauterine devices (IUD)

What is the failure rate or actual effectiveness of various methods?	IUDs (1%)
	Sterilization (1%-4%)
	Injectable hormonal contraception (< 1%)
	Oral contraceptives (10%)
	Lactation amenorrhea (8%)
	Male condom (20%)
	Diaphragm or cervical cap (16%)
	Female condom (21%)
	Periodic abstinence (25%)
	Withdrawal (30%)
	Spermicide (26%)
	Vasectomy (< 1%)
When is a woman most fertile?	From 1 week prior to ovulation until 3 days following ovulation.
Why are fertility awareness methods unreliable?	Because of irregular cycle lengths and errors in timing or calculation
Is lactation an effective means of birth control?	**Prolactin inhibits GnRH** however, it must be maintained and released approximately every 3 hours. It is associated with an 8% failure rate at 6 months if 80% of the child's nourishment is from breast milk.

STERILIZATION METHODS

What methods are available for surgical sterilization?	**Male:**
	1. **vasectomy**—ligation of vas deferens preventing passage of sperm into seminal fluid
	Female:
	1. **Ligation/removal** of a section of the fallopian tube—involves laparotomy or laparoscopy
	2. **Mechanical blockage**—using rings, coils, clips, or plugs—hysteroscopic or laparoscopy
	3. **Coagulation-induced blockage**—usually through cauterization methods—laparoscopy

What are the overall risks and benefits of female sterilization?	Risks: 1. Anesthesia/surgical complications 2. Ectopic pregnancy—failed procedures can result in risk for ectopic pregnancy 3. Regret of the procedure (especially in younger people) 4. Does not protect against STIs 5. Typically irreversible Benefits: 1. Not coitally dependent 2. Decreased risk of ovarian cancer

Hormonal Contraceptives

What types of hormonal contraceptives are available?	Oral, injectable, implants, rings and patches
What is the general mechanism of action of hormonal methods of contraception?	Progesterone thickens cervical mucus. Low levels of progesterone and estrogen **inhibit ovulation, alter the endometrium**, and **decrease tubal motility.**
Do hormonal contraceptives protect against STIs?	No. Condoms must be used to prevent transmission of STIs.

Oral Contraceptive Pills

What are the types of oral contraceptive pills (OCPs) available?	**Combined estrogen-progesterone** and **progestin-only pills.** Combined may be monophasic or multiphasic.
What is in OCPs?	Progestin pills contain a form of progestin, such as norethindrone. Combined pills contain ethinyl estradiol (EE or E2) at a variety of doses: 20 to 35 µg. Older medications had higher doses of estrogen, 50 µg. There are a variety of progesterones to alter side effect profiles.

When should OCPs be started?

ASAP. However, if menstruation began more than 5 days ago, complete a pregnancy test on day of initiation and use condoms for the first week. If patient does not have a withdrawal bleed in 3 weeks or is on an extended cycle regiment complete a repeat pregnancy test. This quick start method has been proven to improve usage.

In addition to contraception, what other advantages are conferred by taking combined OCPs?

Decreases risk for ovarian cancer, endometrial cancer, pelvic inflammatory disease (PID), colorectal cancer, ectopic pregnancy; decreases acne, anemia, menorrhagia, dysmenorrhea; eliminates ovulation pain (mittelschmerz); regulates menses; protects against benign breast disease, osteoporosis, hirsutism

What are the risks of taking combined OCPs?

Increased risk of **thromboembolic disease/stroke (from 50/100,000-100/100,000 in OCP users) however, risk in pregnancy is double (200/100,000),** adenocarcinoma of the cervix, subarachnoid hemorrhage, and hypertension (which is reverseable on discontinuation). **Older formulations with higher estrogen were associated with myocardial infarction and benign hepatocellular adenoma.**

Is there a risk of developing breast cancer when using combined OCPs?

Experts agree there is **no** association between birth control pills and breast cancer among premenopausal low risk populations.

What are absolute contraindications to the use of combined OCPs?

Personal or family history of thromboembolic disease (Factor V Leiden, Protein S or C abnormalities)

Uncontrolled hypertension

Smokers more than 35-years-old

Cerebrovascular disease/coronary artery disease

Congenital hyperlipidemia

History of an estrogen-dependent tumor

Symptomatic liver disease

Pregnancy

What are relative contraindications to the use of combined OCPs?

Diabetes mellitus for more than 20 years (indicator of peripheral vascular disease)

Smoking

Gallbladder disease (benign disease is not a contraindication)

Hypertension (requires close monitoring and intervention)

Use of some antibiotics, antiepileptics and antivirals will alter OCP and medication metabolism in the liver

The immediate postpartum period (start 4-6 weeks postpartum due to the need to establish milk production)

Migraines/vascular headaches with aura

What are possible side effects of OCPs?

Breakthrough bleeding (especially first 3 months)

Amenorrhea

Depression, mood changes, decreased libido

Nausea

Bloating

Breast tenderness

Headaches

Acne (with some progestin-only pills)

Do OCPs cause weight gain?

No

How do OCPs affect acne?

Progestins worsen acne by increasing sebum production. The estrogen in combined OCPs increases liver production of sex binding hormone globulin, which in turn decreases unbound circulating androgens and decreases acne.

What mediates the increased risk of thromboembolic disease with OCPs?

Estrogen stimulates production of **clotting factors VII and X** and decreases levels of **antithrombin III.**

What is breakthrough bleeding?	**Intermenstrual bleeding** that occurs in up to 30% of women after the initiation of OCPs, it is due to atrophic endometrium (lower systemic estrogen).
	If it persists for more than 4 months, complete examination and possible sonogram for other etiology (STI, polyp, fibroid). Then consider changing to a higher dose of **estrogen** or **lower dose progesterone**.
What is post-pill amenorrhea?	The **failure to menstruate by 3 to 6 months after cessation of OCPs.** It should be worked up please refer to section regarding diagnosis and management of secondary amenorrhea.
What drugs interfere with OCPs effectiveness?	OCPs are metabolized by the **cytochrome P$_{450}$.** Drugs including **anticonvulsants** (phenytoin), **antibiotics** (isoniazid, rifampin, penicillin, tetracycline), and some **antiretrovirals** all induce liver enzymes and result in faster metabolism of systemic medications.
What should be done if the patient must take these drugs?	**Counsel the patient to consider nonhormonal methods such as the copper IUD.**
What should a patient do if she forgot to take pills in following cases?	**One or two pills:** take the missed dose as soon as possible and take the following dose at her regular time.
	Three or more pills: restart a fresh pack of pills. Use a back up method for 1 week and take a pregnancy test if no withdrawal bleed in 3 weeks.

Injectable Contraceptives

What injectable contraceptive is available in the United States?	**Depot medroxyprogesterone acetate** (DMPA or Depo-Provera), a progestin-only injectable
What is its typical use failure rate in the first year?	3%
How is DMPA administered?	**Intramuscular injection** of 150 mg **every 3 months**

When should DMPA be started?

If more than **5 days after the onset of menses, complete a pregnancy test, administer depot, use another method for 1 week, and repeat a pregnancy test in 3 weeks.**

What are the contraindications to the use of DMPA?

Undiagnosed abnormal uterine bleeding, cerebrovascular disease, coronary artery disease, liver disease, breast cancer, active liver disease, pregnancy

In addition to contraception, what other advantages are conferred by DMPA?

Decreased risk of **endometrial cancer, pelvic inflammatory disease (PID), menorrhagia, dysmenorrhea and improvement of endometriosis. Fewer seizures in epileptic patients and fewer crisis in patients with sickle cell disease.** It can be used while breast-feeding.

What are the potential side effects of taking DMPA?

Amenorrhea (50% in 1 year, 80% in 5 years), intermenstrual spotting, decreased bone density **(reverses upon cessation), weight gain** (1 lb per year), acne, headache, mood disorders

How long does it take to restore fertility after DMPA is stopped?

Most women begin to ovulate 10 months after their last injection.

Hormonal Implants, Patches, and Rings

What are contraceptive implants?

Subdermal plastic rod releases progesterone (etonorgestrel). It is placed in the office with local anesthesia and is changed every 3 years.

What is the typical use failure rate in the first year?

0.05%

What are the absolute contraindications to hormonal implants?

Pregnancy, undiagnosed vaginal bleeding, liver disease, breast cancer

What are the main side effects of contraceptive implants?

Intermenstrual spotting, amenorrhea, headache, acne

What is the contraceptive patch?	A **transdermal patch** that delivers **Ethinyl estradiol 20 μg/d and norelgestromin 150 μg/d.** Note: If detached for more than 24 hours, it must be replaced and backup contraception should be used for 7 days.
What is the overall failure rate for the contraceptive patch?	1% however, it is less effective in women weigh greater than 200 lb.
Is there an increased risk of blood clots with the contraceptive patch?	Theoretically, yes. The patch delivers a higher dose of estrogen (area under the curve) than combined OCPs. However, no data demonstrate this to date.
What is the contraceptive vaginal ring?	An **intravaginal plastic ring that releases** ethinyl estradiol 15 μg/d and etonogestrel 120 μg/d.
How is the vaginal ring administered?	If it is inserted more than 5 days after the onset of menses, a backup contraception should be used for 1 week. The ring is taken out after **3 weeks** for a withdrawal bleed. Complete a pregnancy test if no bleeding occurs. Note: If the ring is displaced for more than 3 hours, an additional contraceptive method must be used for 7 days.
What are the potential side effects of the vaginal ring?	Device-related discomfort and other side effects similar to combined OCPs

Emergency Contraception ("Morning-After Pill")

What is emergency contraception (EC)?	A postcoital method of contraception, it is most effective within 72 hours (failure rate 3%). It can be used up to 5 days after unprotected intercourse or failure of implemented method.
How does EC work?	It prevents ovulation and fertilization. **EC will not impact or terminate a pregnancy** that has implanted. There is no evidence that emergency contraceptive pills (ECPs) increase the risk of fetal anomalies or miscarriages.

Which methods are utilized in the United States?	Plan B, Plan B One Step, Next Choice (Levonorgestrel 75 µg × 2 tabs). Note: this is associated with fewer side effects than the **Yuzpe method** (involves taking multiple OCPs to get a high dose of estrogen and progesterone). Copper IUD insertion.
How effective are the Yuzpe method and Plan B at preventing pregnancy?	The Yuzpe method **reduces the risk of pregnancy by 75%,** Plan B **reduces the risk by 89%.**
Who should be prescribed EC?	**Every sexually active woman** at risk of pregnancy should be prescribed EC as a backup in the event of primary contraceptive failure. It is available to persons over 17 years of age with government-issued ID over the counter without a prescription.
What are the major side effects of EC?	**Nausea** and **vomiting. Both are seen more commonly with the Yuzpe method.** Antiemetics may be used prophylactically prior to EC use.

BARRIER METHODS OF CONTRACEPTION

What are the types of barrier methods available?	Male and female condom, diaphragm, cervical cap, contraceptive sponge (no longer manufactured in the US), spermicide
What are the advantages of barrier contraception over other methods?	Many **prevent STI transmission** and they have **no hormonal side effects.**
What are the disadvantages of barrier contraception over other methods?	Coital dependence (less reliable); risk of breakage
Which barrier method is the most effective at preventing STI transmission?	**Male latex condoms,** they have a 20% failure rate.
Do spermicidal condoms offer more protection compared to non-spermicidal condoms?	No

What is the female condom and how it is used?	A **lubricated polyurethane sheath** with two flexible rings, one covers the cervix and the other is external. It can be left in place for 8 hours and should be removed **after intercourse.** The failure rate is approximately 20%.
How are diaphragms and cervical caps used?	They are rubber barriers that are initially sized and fitted by a practitioner. They are filled with spermicide and can be left in place up to 24 to 48 hours and should remain in place for at least 6 hours after intercourse. The failure rate is 16%.
What are the side effects of the diaphragm and cervical cap?	Increased risk of urinary tract infection, epithelial irritation and spotting. Theoretical risk of toxic shock syndrome that has never been observed.
What type of spermicide is available over the counter in the United States?	Nonoxynol-9. It is available as a vaginal cream, film, foam, or gel.
How is spermicide used?	It is placed intravaginally at least 15 minutes prior to intercourse and remains effective for up to 1 hour.
What are the disadvantages of spermicide?	**Failure rate** of 29% No protection against STIs

INTRAUTERINE DEVICES

What are IUDs and how are they administered?	**T-shaped devices** placed in **the uterus (see Fig. 4.2).** Failure rates are less than 1%.
What are the two types of IUDs available and how do they work?	1. **Copper IUD** (*Paragard*) Is spermicidal and alters the composition of the endometrium. It should be changed every 10 years. 2. **Levonorgestrel-releasing IUDs** (*Mirena*) It thickens cervical mucus, alters the endometrium and tubal motility, cause anovulation in 15% of women, and leads to amenorrhea is 20%. It is FDA approved for 5 years.

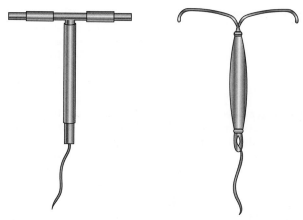

Figure 4.2   Examples of commonly used intrauterine devices.

What are the benefits of IUDs?

Very effective, possible protective effect against endometrial and cervical cancer, cost-effective, quick return of fertility after removal.

Mirena may help reduces menorrhagia, dysmenorrhea, and the risk of pelvic inflammatory disease.

Note: **Copper IUD has the highest level of user satisfaction of any other contraception.**

What are disadvantages or concerns with IUD use?

Menorrhagia and dysmenorrhea with Paraguard.

No protection from STIs.

Risk of postinsertion PID (1/1000), expulsion (3%-11%), perforation at the time of placement (1/1000).

Some persons become colonized with actinomycosis. If no signs of infection are present the IUD can be left in place.

What are contraindications to IUD placement?

Pregnancy, undiagnosed uterine bleeding, PID or endometritis less than 90 days ago, copper allergy or Wilson disease (for Paraguard only), pelvic malignancy, AIDS not well-controlled or on therapy.

Relative contraindications?	Multiple sexual partners, high risk of HIV infection, cervicitis, uterus less than 6 cm or more than 9 cm, fibroids or endometrial cavity distortion. Anemia, dysmenorrhea, or menorrhagia for Paraguard
Should the IUD be removed if a woman is found to have a positive gonorrheal or chlamydial culture?	No. She should first get antibiotics. If she does not improve, the IUD should be removed.

ELECTIVE ABORTION

How common is elective abortion?	47% of US women have one or more elective abortions. 50% of US pregnancies are unplanned and half of these are terminated.
Is there an impact of elective abortion on future pregnancies?	There may be an increased risk of Asherman syndrome (intrauterine synechiae) or abnormal placentation if an infection is present or if multiple procedures are done.
What examinations/tests need to be done before an elective termination of pregnancy?	**Pelvic examination** (to assess uterine size and position); β-**hCG** (to confirm pregnancy); **ultrasound** (to assess dates and confirm intrauterine pregnancy); **hematocrit** and **Rh(D)** status.
	Some providers screen and treat for STIs prior to the procedure
What are the surgical procedure options for evacuation of products of conception (POC)?	Manual vacuum aspiration (**MVA**); suction dilation and curettage (suction **D&C**); dilation and evacuation (**D&E**); dilation and extraction (**D&X**)
What are the risks of these procedures?	Risks of anesthesia, infection, hemorrhage, cervical laceration, uterine perforation and possible organ damage, embolus. The risk of complications from a first trimester abortion is less than 1%.
Does an abortion increase the risk of breast cancer?	No

What should be done if uterine perforation is suspected?

If patient is hemodynamically stable and no suspicion for organ damage is present, patient can be observed with serial hematocrits and examinations. If there is suspected bleeding, extrauterine organs damage, or the vitals are unstable **laparoscopy** is performed with possible **laparotomy.**

How and when is an MVA performed?

Typically before 14 weeks. The cervix is dilated and uterine contents are evacuated using a cannula attached to a handheld vacuum source.

How is a suction D&C performed?

Typically before 14 weeks the cervix is dilated and the uterus is evacuated with an electrical vacuum device.

How is a D&E performed?

From approximately 14 to 24 weeks the cervix is medically or manually prepared at an interval before the procedure, with misoprostol or osmotic dilators (dilopan or laminaria). Mechanical dilation is further performed and uterine contents are evacuated using specialized forceps (Sophers and Bierers). Curettage and/or vacuum are performed to assess for uterine "cri" (gritty texture consistent with complete evacuation).

Are prophylactic antibiotics utilized?

Yes, antibiotics peri-abortion reduces the risk of postoperative infection.

What types of antibiotics can be used prophylactically?

Doxycycline, ofloxacin, or ceftriaxone

What are the various modalities for medical abortion?

They are used up to a gestational age of 49 days.

Intravaginal **misoprostol** (70% effective with one dose).

Oral or IM **methotrexate** followed by intravaginal, oral, or buccal misoprostol 3 to 7 days later (70%-80% effective).

Oral **mifepristone (RU-486)** followed by intravaginal, oral, or buccal **misoprostol** 6 to 72 hours later (92%-98% effective).

How do abortifacient medications work?

Misoprostol: a prostaglandin analogue; increases contractility by directly stimulating the myometrium.

Methotrexate: blocks dihydrofolate reductase, an enzyme necessary for the production of thymidine during DNA synthesis, thus, affecting the rapidly growing cytotrophoblast.

Mifepristone: binds to the progesterone receptor with a greater affinity than progesterone itself, and, therefore, blocks the "pro-gestation" action of progesterone.

What are the side effects of a medical abortion?

Cramping, bleeding (often heavier than a menstrual period)

Gastrointestinal distress: nausea, vomiting, diarrhea

What are the contraindications to a medical abortion?

Allergies to any of the medications, an in situ IUD, anemia (hemoglobin < 10), coagulopathy or usage of anticoagulant, acute liver, adrenal or cardiovascular disease

What is a septic abortion?

Localized or systemic infection after spontaneous or elective abortion

How is a septic abortion managed?

Stabilize and pan-culture the patient, administer broad-specturm parenternal antibiotics, evacuate the uterus, and administer anti-D immunoglobulin if Rh negative.

What antibiotic combinations can be used to treat septic abortion?

Clindamycin and gentamicin with or without ampicillin

Ampicillin and gentamicin and metronidazole

Ticarcillin-clavulanate or piperacillin-tazobactam or imipenem alone

What are the indications for laparotomy or hysterectomy in the management of a septic abortion?

Failure to respond to antibiotics and evacuation, suspicion for abscess, fulminate disease (Clostridium sordelii) or gas gangrene

Who should be given Rh(D)-immune globulin postabortion?

All Rh(D)-negative women who are unsensitized, fetal antigens are present in maternal serum from 6 weeks gestational age.

When does ovulation resume postabortion?

Within 2 weeks, contraception should be started immediately

When do menses resume postabortion?

Usually within 6 weeks (average 4 weeks)

What conditions need to be considered if menses do not resume within 6 weeks?

Pregnancy, gestational trophoblastic disease, Asherman syndrome, other systemic causes of secondary amenorrhea

What instructions should be given postabortion?

Women should be advised to have **nothing per vagina** for 2 weeks after the procedure/passage of POC. Some recommend deferment of pregnancy (if desired) for 2 to 3 months, although there is no data to support this recommendation.

When should a woman return to clinic postabortion?

If she experiences heavy bleeding, fever, or abdominal pain

ECTOPIC PREGNANCY

What is an ectopic pregnancy?

Implantation of the pregnancy into a site outside of the endometrial lining of the uterine cavity (see Fig. 4.3)

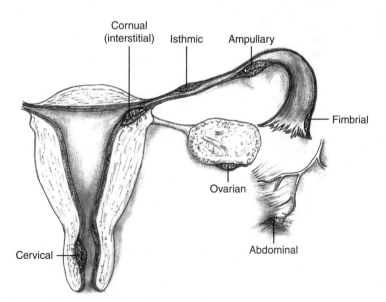

Figure 4.3   Locations of ectopic pregnancies.

What is the most common cause of pregnancy-related death in the first trimester?	Rupture of an ectopic pregnancy
What is the incidence of ectopic pregnancy?	Approximately 2% of pregnancies in the United States are ectopic
What are the major risk factors for ectopic pregnancy?	**History of pelvic inflammatory disease** History of ectopic pregnancy History of tubal surgery or pathology Diethylstilbestrol (DES) exposure in utero Current intrauterine device (IUD) use Current oral contraceptive pill (OCP) use Infertility History of cervicitis Multiple sexual partners Cigarette smoking
Describe the relationship between IUD use and ectopic pregnancy:	Women using an IUD are much less likely to conceive compared to women not using any form of birth control. However, in the unlikely event that they do conceive, there is a greater probability that it will be ectopic.
What are the major symptoms of ectopic pregnancy?	Classic symptoms: **amenorrhea, abdominal/pelvic pain, vaginal bleeding.** Other symptoms: dizziness, nausea, vomiting, diarrhea. Many women are asymptomatic until rupture.
What are the signs on physical examination of ectopic pregnancy?	Many women have a normal physical examination; however, the common signs are Adenexal mass and/or tenderness Mild uterine enlargement Cervical motion tenderness Abdominal tenderness Orthostatic hypotension, tachycardia, and rebound tenderness are all signs of rupture

What is the differential diagnosis of these symptoms?

Threatened abortion

Torsion

Ruptured corpus luteum cyst

Abnormal uterine bleeding

Tubo-ovarian abscess (TOA)

Molar pregnancy

PID

UTI or stones

Pyelonephritis

Diverticulitis

Appendicitis

Pancreatitis

What diagnostic tests can be used to distinguish between these conditions?

β-hCG

Transvaginal ultrasound

What is the difference in β-hCG levels between an intrauterine and ectopic pregnancy?

The rate of β-hCG rise is lower in most cases of ectopic pregnancy.

Where are ectopic pregnancies located and what are the relative frequencies of each (see Fig. 4.3)?

Fallopian tube (95%; ampulla > isthmus > fimbria)

Ovarian (3.2%)

Interstitial or cornual (2.4%)

Abdominal (1.3%)

Cervix (rare)

Hysterotomy scar

What are the causes of tubal implantation?

Conditions that **delay transport** of the egg through the tube

Conditions in the embryo that lead to **premature implantation**

What types of conditions cause a delay in transport of the egg through the tube?

Chronic salpingitis

Salpingitis isthmica nodosa (SIN)

What happens to the endometrium during an ectopic pregnancy?

It still responds to pregnancy hormones and so often exhibits signs of decidual reaction or endometrial thickening.

What is a heterotopic pregnancy?

A **concurrent intrauterine and extrauterine pregnancy**

More common in women pregnant through in vitro fertilization (IVF)

What is the natural course of an ectopic pregnancy?

Rupture, spontaneous regression, or tubal abortion

What is a tubal abortion?

The expulsion of the POC through the fimbria into the abdominal cavity.

The POC can then either regress or reimplant in the abdominal cavity or in the ovary.

At what gestational age do the clinical manifestations of an ectopic pregnancy begin?

At least **6 to 8 weeks** after the LMP

Describe the algorithm for management of a suspected ecoptic pregnancy:

See Fig. 4.4.

What are the treatment options for an ectopic pregnancy?

Methotrexate (for early, unruptured ectopic pregnancies)

Surgery (salpingostomy or salpingectomy)

What are the contraindications of methotrexate used to treat an ectopic pregnancy?

Active hemorrhage

Pregnancy larger than 4 cm

Breastfeeding

Alcoholism

Peptic ulcer disease

Liver or renal disease

Blood dyscrasias

Immunodeficiency

Active pulmonary disease

Heterotopic pregnancy

What is methotrexate's failure rate?

5% to 10%, but higher in more advanced pregnancies

What are the two methods of methotrexate administration for the treatment of an ectopic pregnancy?

1. Give a single intramuscular (IM) dose of methotrexate and then follow β-hCG levels at days 4 and 7. hCG levels should decline by 15% between days 4 and 7.
2. Alternate day IM administration of methotrexate until β-hCG level decreases by 15% in 48 hours.

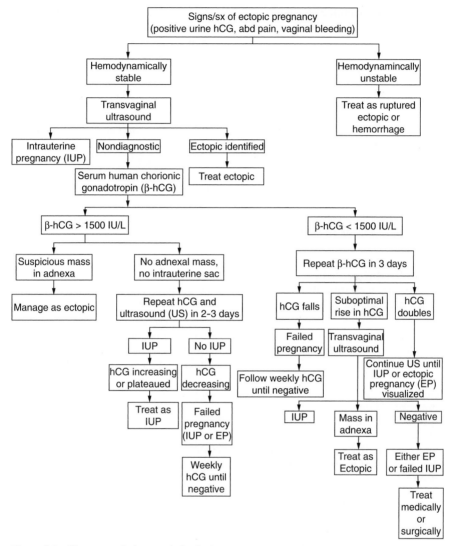

Figure 4.4 Management of suspected ectopic pregnancy.

What are the differences between a salpingostomy and a salpingectomy?

Salpingostomy: an incision is made on the antimesenteric part of the fallopian tube and the POCs are evacuated. The incision is closed by secondary intention.

Salpingectomy: a tubal resection.

What is the discriminatory zone?

A **range of β-hCG levels** (1500-2000 IU/L) in which **a gestational sac should be seen** if there is an intrauterine pregnancy.

If no sac is seen at β-hCG levels above the discriminatory zone, it is a presumed ectopic pregnancy.

How should a patient with a low β-hCG without a visible intrauterine pregnancy be managed?

Both the ultrasound and the β-hCG should be repeated in 48 hours.

If the pregnancy is intrauterine and viable, the **β-hCG should double in 2 days.**

Does a negative pelvic ultrasound rule out the diagnosis of an ectopic pregnancy?

No, an extrauterine pregnancy is visualized in only 50% of ectopic pregnancies.

What is the difference in progesterone levels between an intrauterine and an ectopic pregnancy?

Serum progesterone levels are lower in ectopic pregnancies compared with viable intrauterine pregnancies.

However, the sensitivity and specificity of progesterone levels are too low to make it a screening or diagnostic test for ectopic pregnancy.

What percentage of patients with an ectopic pregnancy experience tubal rupture?

Approximately 18%

In a patient with an ectopic pregnancy, what are the risk factors for tubal rupture?

History of tubal damage/infertility

Induction of ovulation

Never having used contraception

High β-hCG

How does the presence of an ectopic pregnancy affect subsequent pregnancies?

It reduces the chance for a successful pregnancy. A repeat tubal pregnancy occurs in 12% of patients.

GESTATIONAL TROPHOBLASTIC DISEASE

Introduction

What is gestational trophoblastic disease (GTD)?

A group of tumors that **arise from placental tissue** and **secrete β-hCG**

What are the types of GTD?

Hydatidiform mole

Persistent/invasive gestational trophoblastic neoplasia (GTN)

Choriocarcinoma

Placental site trophoblastic tumor (PSTT)

Which of the types of GTD are benign and which are malignant?

Hydatidiform moles are usually benign, whereas invasive GTN, choriocarcinoma, and PSTT are all malignant.

What are the major risk factors for GTD?

Extremes of maternal age

History of prior GTD

When should GTD be suspected clinically?

If there is unusual bleeding after a pregnancy or abortion

What are the signs and symptoms of GTD?

First trimester bleeding

Uterine size/date discrepancy

Pelvic pressure or pain

First trimester preeclampsia

Higher β-hCG than expected

Hyperemesis gravidarum

Hyperthyroidism

Passage of hydropic (grape-like) vesicles

What is the major sign that GTD disease is metastatic?

hCG levels that do not decrease or that increase

Describe the following stages of GTD:

Stage I:

Disease that is limited to uterus

Stage II:

Disease that extends outside the uterus but stays within pelvis or vagina

Stage III:

Disease with pulmonary metastases

Stage IV:

Disease spreads to other sites

Where does metastatic GTD spread?

In order from most likely to least likely:

Lung (80%)

Vagina (30%)

Brain (10%)

Liver (10%)

Other (bowel, kidney, spleen)

What are the good prognostic indicators for GTD?	Short duration between last pregnancy and disease (< 4 months) Low hCG level (< 40,000 IU/L) No metastatic disease to brain or liver No prior chemotherapy
What are the poor prognostic indicators for GTD?	Long duration between last pregnancy and disease (> 4 months) High hCG level (> 40,000 IU/L) Brain or liver metastases Prior chemotherapy Development of disease after a term pregnancy
What is the overall cure rate for GTD?	Over 90%
How does the diagnosis of GTD affect the prognosis for future pregnancies?	It increases the risk of subsequent molar pregnancies; however, this risk is still low (1%).

Hydatidiform Mole

What is a hydatidiform mole?	A localized, usually noninvasive **tumor of the placenta** that results from **aberrant fertilization** leading to proliferation of the trophoblastic tissue.
What is the incidence of a molar pregnancy?	In the United States the incidence is 1 in 1500 pregnancies; however, it is much more common in the developing world.
What is the difference between a complete and a partial hydatidiform mole?	See Table 4.1.
Describe the pathogenesis of a complete mole:	An **"empty" egg** (caused by inactivated or absent maternal chromosomes) is **fertilized by a haploid sperm that then duplicates,** or occasionally by two sperm. This leads to a "normal" diploid karyotype with all chromosomes of paternal origin.

Table 4.1 Difference Between Complete and Partial Mole

	Complete Mole	Partial Mole
Synonyms	Classic or true mole	Incomplete mole
Karyotype	Diploid (46XX or 46XY)	Triploid (XXY or XYY)
Fetal/embryonic tissue	Absent	Present
Uterine size	Often large for dates	Often small for dates
Appearance of trophoblast	Diffuse hyperplasia, often atypia	Focal hyperplasia
Appearance of villi	Diffusely swollen	Focal swelling
Theca lutein cysts	Sometimes present	Never present
hCG levels	> 50,000 IU/L	< 50,000 IU/L
Placental alkaline phosphate levels	Normal	High
Malignant potential	15%-25%	5%-10%

Describe the pathogenesis of a partial mole:

A haploid ovum is fertilized by two haploid sperm, leading to a triploid karyotype.

What is the typical sonographic appearance of a complete mole and a partial mole?

Complete mole: a central heterogeneous mass without an embryo/fetus or any amniotic fluid but with theca lutein cysts; classically described as a **snowstorm pattern.**

Partial mole: a growth-restricted fetus, reduced amniotic fluid, and a Swiss cheese pattern of chorionic villi; no theca lutein cysts.

What are the complications associated with a high hCG?

Ovarian enlargement (with theca lutein cysts)

Hyperemesis gravidarum

Early preeclampsia

Hyperthyroidism (because hCG may stimulate TSH receptors)

How is a molar pregnancy definitively diagnosed?

It is suspected based on ultrasound and hCG levels; however, it must be confirmed with histologic studies of the tissue with analysis of the DNA content.

What is the treatment for a molar pregnancy?

Dilation and curettage (**D&C**; suction curettage is preferred)

Serum hCG levels must be followed weekly until there are three consecutive normal values and then monthly for a total of 6 months of negative levels. During this time, effective contraception *must* be used to avoid misinterpretation of a rising hCG level.

What should be done before surgical evacuation of a complete molar pregnancy?

A **CXR** to assess for metastatic disease.

When can another pregnancy be attempted after the diagnosis of GTN?

The patient should wait for at least a year.

In what percentage of molar pregnancies will trophoblastic tissue persist after evacuation?

19% to 28% of complete moles
2% to 4% of partial moles

When is malignant disease suspected?

After a molar pregnancy when hCG levels rise. This usually represents an invasive mole (75%), but can also represent choriocarcinoma (25%) or a placental site trophoblast tumor (rare).

Or after a nonmolar pregnancy when hCG levels rise. This usually represents choriocarcinoma, but can (rarely) represent a PSTT.

What are the risk factors for development of malignant disease?

Theca-lutein cysts more than 6 cm

Larger uterine size for dates

Advanced maternal age (> 40 years)

History of GTD

Initial hCG more than 100,000 IU/L

Histologic findings of atypia or hyperplasia

When does malignant disease develop?

50% of cases follow a hydatidiform mole, 25% follow a normal pregnancy, and 25% follow an abortion.

What is the major complication associated with malignant GTD?

Hemorrhage—these lesions are highly vascular and often have AVMs, which readily bleed.

Invasive Gestational Trophoblastic Neoplasia

What is an invasive mole?	A molar pregnancy whose chorionic villi invade into the myometrium.
Is an invasive mole more common after a complete mole or a partial mole?	A complete mole
What is the treatment of an invasive mole?	**Methotrexate** and hCG follow-up as with a molar pregnancy (actinomycin-D or etoposide are alternative therapies)
Can an invasive mole regress spontaneously?	Yes

Choriocarcinoma

What is choriocarcinoma?	A malignant carcinoma of the chorionic epithelium, usually after a molar pregnancy.
What is the incidence of choriocarcinoma after a normal gestation, an abortion, and a complete mole?	1 in 16,000; 1 in 15,000; 1 in 40
What are the common signs/symptoms of choriocarcinoma?	**Irregular vaginal bleeding** (typically late postpartum bleeding, but it can present later) Enlarged uterus with bilateral ovarian cysts
What is the ultrasonographic appearance of choriocarcinoma?	An enlarging, heterogeneous, hypervascular uterine mass with areas of hemorrhage and necrosis.
What is the histologic appearance of choriocarcinoma?	Proliferation of cytotrophoblasts and syncytiotrophoblasts that penetrate the musculature and vasculature; no villi present
What percentage of patients with choriocarcinoma develop metastases?	Approximately 50%

What is the treatment for choriocarcinoma?

Chemotherapy (typically **methotrexate** or **actinomycin-D** for low-risk disease and a combination of **methotrexate, actinomycin-D, cyclophosphamide, etoposide,** and **vincristine** for high-risk disease).

Adjuvant hysterectomy decreases the dose of chemotherapy required for remission.

What is the recommended follow-up after treatment of an invasive mole?

Serial hCG follow-up (weekly for 3 months, then monthly) is recommended for **at least a year**. If there are metastases outside of the lung, follow-up is recommended for 2 years.

In both cases, the patient *must* use effective contraception in order to ensure appropriate interpretation of a rise in hCG.

Placental Site Trophoblastic Tumor

What is a PSTT?

A rare malignant tumor that arises from placental intermediate cytotrophoblastic cells.

What are the signs/symptoms of PSTT?

Irregular vaginal bleeding (can be massive hemorrhage)

An enlarging uterus

Amenorrhea

Virilization

Nephrotic syndrome

Metastatic lesions

Is PSTT always associated with high hCG levels?

No, because there is no syncytiotrophoblast proliferation.

What is the ultrasonographic appearance of PSTT?

A hyperechoic intrauterine mass that is invading the myometrial wall and has both cystic and solid areas.

What is the histological appearance of PSTT?

Many mononuclear cells that invade the myometrium; proliferation of intermediate trophoblast cells (no cytotrophoblasts or syncytiotrophoblasts)

What is the treatment for PSTT?	**Hysterectomy** is the first-line therapy because chemotherapy is fairly ineffective and the tumor is usually confined to the uterus.

Sexually Transmitted Diseases and Pelvic Infections

SEXUALLY TRANSMITTED INFECTIONS OF THE LOWER GENITAL TRACT

Condyloma Accuminata

What is condyloma accuminata?	**Benign genital warts**. It is the most common sexually transmitted infection.
How is condyloma accuminata transmitted?	Through skin-to-skin contact; it is primarily transmitted through sexual activity
What is the pathogen and which subtypes are associated more commonly with genital warts?	A DNA virus called human papillomavirus (**HPV**); subtypes **6 and 11**
What are the clinical manifestations of condyloma accuminata?	**Warts** located on the external genitalia, perineum, anus, cervix, mouth, inside the vagina, and urethra. These are generally painless raised, pedunculated/**cauliflower-shaped** lesions but they can vary in number, size, and color (flesh-colored, pinkish-white, grayish-white).
What other disease should be excluded?	**Condyloma lata** of secondary syphilis
How is condyloma accuminata diagnosed?	Visualization by colposcopic examination and cytologic smear. Biopsy can be performed if the diagnosis is uncertain.

What would a biopsy of the specimen reveal?	**Koilocytosis** (vacuolated keratinocyte with peri-nuclear halo). It is often also associated with atypia and dysplasia.
What is the treatment?	For small, less than 2 cm lesions: TCA (trichloroacetic acid) and podophyllum. For larger, more than 2 cm lesions: Cryotherapy and laser excision. If left untreated, visible lesions may resolve on their own, remain unchanged, or increase in size or number.
Can genital warts be cured?	The virus cannot be eradicated once present in the genital tract; therefore, warts can recur.
Should you treat the sexual partner of a patient with genital warts?	Yes. Partners require examination and treatment only if condyloma are present.
What are Buschke-Lowenstein tumors?	**Giant condylomas** caused by HPV that are found in **immunocompromised patients.**
What else can HPV cause?	**Preinvasive and invasive cervical cancer.** Dysplasia is more commonly caused by **subtypes 16, 18, 33, and 35.**
How can HPV infection be prevented?	A quadrivalent recombinant vaccine against HPV serotypes 6, 11, 16, 18 (Gardasil) can be given to females and males between the ages of 9 and 26 Condoms do not offer complete protection for the transmission of HPV

Molluscum Contagiosum

What is genital molluscum contagiosum?	A benign, usually asymptomatic, infection of the vulva caused by poxvirus (a DNA virus)
How is genital molluscum transmitted?	Through sexual contact, casual skin-skin contact, fomites (substances that absorb and transport infectious disease particles), or auto-inoculation from other body sites

What is the typical clinical presentation?	Single or multiple (< 30) small, white, pink, or flesh-colored **dome-shaped** papules with central umbilication in the genital/inguinal area. It is usually asymptomatic but eczema and pruritus may occur.
How does genital molluscum contagiosum present in an immunocompromised person?	Large lesions (> 1 cm) or a clustering of numerous small lesions; intra-oral or peri-oral lesions can arise
What are the differential diagnoses?	Multiple small lesions: condyloma accuminata Large, solitary lesions: basal or squamous cell carcinoma
How is the diagnosis made?	Usually based on clinical manifestations. Excisional biopsy can be performed for definitive diagnosis and will reveal **intracytoplasmic inclusions**
What are the treatment options?	It is usually self-limiting; cosmetic options include curettage or cryotherapy of lesions with liquid nitrogen; topical imiquimod is also used **Sexual partners do not need to be treated**

Pediculosis Pubis (Crabs) and Scabies

What are pediculosis pubis and scabies?	Parasitic infections of the pubic area
What causes pediculosis pubis?	The crab louse *Phthirus pubis*—a blood-sucking parasite that lives on hair shafts and lays eggs (nits)
What causes scabies?	The itch mite *Sarcoptes scabiei*—a parasite that burrows underneath the skin and lays eggs
How are pediculosis pubis and scabies transmitted?	Primarily through sexual contact. Can also be through fomites (clothing, sheets).
What is the typical presentation of these infestations?	Intense pruritus over the genital area, especially at night. Polymorphic papules may be seen in scabies. In adults pruritus often present on abdomen and hands.

How are pediculosis pubis and scabies diagnosed?	Visualization of the parasites or eggs (nits) under a microscope (skin scrapings) or magnifying glass.
What is the treatment?	**Permethrin** 1% cream (first line) Lindane 1% shampoo (second line which is contraindicated in pregnant/ lactating women).
	All clothing and sheets should be washed in hot water and isolated for at least 3 days after treatment. All contacts must be treated.
What other tests should be ordered?	Screening tests for other sexually transmitted diseases (HIV, syphilis, gonorrhea, *chlamydia*)

SEXUALLY TRANSMITTED INFECTIONS CAUSING GENITAL ULCERATIONS

What are the most common infectious causes of genital ulcers in the United States?	Herpes simplex virus (HSV) > syphilis > chancroid > lymphogranuloma venereum (LGV) and granuloma inguinale
Is coinfection with multiple organisms common?	Yes. Making a diagnosis based on the history and physical can be very difficult and requires a thorough workup and knowledge of the most likely causal organism in the specific patient population.
What are some of the most common noninfectious causes of genital ulcers?	Behcet disease, drug reactions, trauma, neoplasm
What are the tests used to diagnose a genital ulcer?	**Darkfield microscopy** (syphilis)
	Serologic tests (syphilis and LGV)
	Gram stain and **viral culture** on selective media (*Haemophilus ducreyi*)
	Tzanck preparation, direct fluorescence antibody (DFA), viral culture, or polymerase chain reaction (PCR) for HSV
	Tissue biopsy (syphilis, granuloma inguinale)

With what other disease are these genital ulcer diseases associated?

HIV

Which of these diseases must be reported to the Department of Health?

Syphilis and HIV

Genital Herpes

What is genital HSV?

A DNA virus **transmitted through infectious secretions** that has a host of clinical manifestations from asymptomatic, or single infection or recurrent, **lifelong disease.**

What is the difference between HSV-1 and HSV-2?

HSV-2 more commonly infects the **genitalia** whereas **HSV-1** more commonly affects the **oral mucosa.**

What is the natural history of the HSV infection?

Primary episode: mucocutaneous infection occurs via direct sexual contact with an infected person. After a 4-day incubation period, ulcerating pustular lesions erupt, often associated with local pain, lymphadenopathy, and systemic symptoms.

Viral latency: after primary infection, there is a period of **viral latency** as the virus ascends along the sensory nerve roots and becomes latent in the dorsal root ganglion.

Reactivation: can occur at any interval when the virus travels back down the sensory nerve. This can either cause a mucocutaneous outbreak (**recurrence**) or sometimes no symptoms may be detected.

What is the strongest risk factor for genital HSV infection?

Multiple lifetime sex partners

What clinical presentation is suggestive of primary genital herpes?

A **prodrome** of 2 to 24 hours characterized by **localized/regional burning and pain**

Systemic symptoms including **fever, malaise, and bilateral inguinal lymphadenopathy**

Grouped vesicles, uniform in size, mixed with multiple, shallow, severely tender ulcers around the vulva, perineum, and perianal area are pathognomonic

Cervical lesions are also common and cause intermittent bleeding and vaginal discharge

Dysuria and urinary retention syndromes may occur because of contact with urethral and vulvar ulcers

Are all primary outbreaks clinically symptomatic?

No. 70% to 80% of infected persons have unrecognized symptoms or completely asymptomatic infections; therefore, transmission can go unrecognized.

Which laboratory tests help make a diagnosis of HSV?

Gold standard: type-specific viral cultures (highest sensitivity and specificity; highest yield if done early when you can attain more vesicle fluid)

Polymerase chain reaction (PCR) (very sensitive, more expensive)

Type-specific serologic testing (best for those with a questionable hx, subclinical infection, or suspicion of a false-negative viral culture)

Tzanck smears

Direct Fluorescence antibody test

What is the presentation of a secondary outbreak?

They vary widely in their frequency, are **milder** and **shorter in duration**, and may not have prodromal symptoms of pain, burning, and itching. Viral shedding can occur for weeks after the appearance of lesions.

What are some precipitating factors of a recurrent outbreak?	Immunodeficiency, trauma, fever, nerve damage, concurrent infection, and sexual intercourse
What are the treatment options for genital herpes?	**Oral acyclovir or valacylovir** for primary and recurrent episodes. It reduces viral shedding and shortens the clinical course. Can also be used prophylactically for patients with frequently recurring episodes, decreasing the recurrence rates by 70% to 80%.
	Intravenous (IV) acyclovir should be considered for severe/disseminated disease or in immunocompromised patients.
	Other therapies include keeping the affected area clean and dry, wearing loose clothing and undergarments, washing hands after contact with affected areas, and using an ice pack or sitz bath for soothing sores.
	All sexual partners should be evaluated for infection.
Screening tests should be considered for what other diseases?	**Syphilis and HIV**

Syphilis

What organism causes syphilis?	*Treponema pallidum (a spirochete)*
How is it transmitted?	Usually via sexual transmission. It enters the body by penetrating intact mucous membranes or by invading epithelial abrasions.
Is it *always* sexually transmitted?	No. Skin contact between any skin abrasions and an ulcer infected with *T. pallidum* can result in infection.
Which population is highest at risk?	African-American heterosexual women and homosexual men in urban areas
What are the clinical manifestations for the three stages of syphilis?	Primary, secondary, and tertiary syphilis

Describe primary syphilis:

Symptoms occur approximately 3 weeks after infection and include:

1. **Painless chancre** (a single, clean-based ulcer usually on labia/vaginal wall/cervix)
2. **Painless lymphadenopathy**

Describe secondary syphilis:

Systemic disease results from hematogenous dissemination that occurs 6 to 8 weeks after infection. Symptoms include a **maculopapular rash on the palms and soles, condyloma latum** (moist, grayish papules-like warts), malaise, fever, arthralgias, pharyngitis, and generalized lymphadenopathy.

Describe tertiary syphilis:

Occurs 3 to 10 years after initial infection. Symptoms include **gummas** (noninfectious granulomatous lesions found in skin and bones), cardiovascular syphilis (**aortitis** or an **aortic aneurysm**), and neurosyphilis **(general paresis, tabes dorsalis, or an Argyll-Robertson pupil).**

What is the latent period?

A period of anywhere from 2 to 20 years that occurs **between the second and third stages** of syphilis. Most patients are asymptomatic (some have recurrences) and are considered noninfectious, although their serologic tests remain positive.

What is the gold standard for diagnosis of syphilis and when can it be used?

Dark field microscopy of a specimen from the primary chancre, condyloma latum, or the maculopapular rash reveals **spirochetes**. It is only useful during the active stages of primary and secondary syphilis.

What other tests are available to help with diagnosis?

Nonspecific and specific serological screening tests:

Nonspecific: venereal Disease Research Laboratory **(VDRL)** and rapid plasma reagin **(RPR). A positive result must be confirmed with a specific treponemal antibody test given high rate of false positives!**

Specific: Fluorescent treponemal antibody absorption **(FTA-ABS),** microhemagglutination assay **(MHA-TP),** and treponemal hemagglutination tests for syphillis **(HATTS).**

How would you interpret the following laboratory results?

Positive VDRL and positive FTA-ABS:

Active treponemal infection

Positive RPR and negative MHA-TP:

False positive

Negative VDRL and positive HATTS:

Successfully treated syphilis

Negative RPR and negative FTA-ABS:

Syphilis unlikely

What other common conditions may cause a false positive nonspecific test result?

Systemic lupus erythematosus (SLE), antiphospholipid antibody syndrome, rheumatic heart disease, pregnancy, infectious mononucleosis, intravenous drug use, viral hepatitis, recent immunization

What is the treatment for syphilis?

Penicillin G or tetracycline (for nonpregnant penicillin allergic patients) for primary, secondary, and early latent syphilis are first-line drugs. PCN desensitization is also preferred. Erythromycin is second-line but is contraindicated in pregnant patients.

What is Jarisch-Herxheimer phenomenon?

A self-limiting, acute worsening of symptoms after antibiotics are started. Symptoms include headache, fever, chills, muscle aches, and other flu-like symptoms.

What diagnosis should be considered for unexplained rashes, arthralgias, neurologic or systemic complaints?

Syphilis

Chancroid

What is chancroid?

An **acute, curable, sexually** transmitted disease caused by *H. ducreyi.* It is uncommon in the United States but is a predominant cause of genital ulcer disease in sub-Saharan Africa.

What clinical presentation highly suggests chancroid?

One to three extremely painful ulcers around the perilabial area that are deep, purulent, and have ragged edges. These are associated with **unilateral, suppurative, painful** swollen inguinal lymph nodes that, in 25% of cases, will rupture, releasing a heavy, foul discharge that is contagious **(suppurative adenopathy = bubo)**. Systemic symptoms (fevers, myalgias) are typically **not** present.

What other infections must be ruled out before a diagnosis of chancroid can be made?

Syphilis, HSV, lymphogranuloma venereum (LGV), and granuloma inguinale

What laboratory tests help make a diagnosis of chancroid?

Culture on selective media isolates *H. ducreyi*

Gram stain of a specimen from the ulcer base or bubo aspirate: reveals gram-negative rods in a chain; referred to as a "school of fish" pattern

PCR

What is the treatment for chancroid?

Azithromycin (oral) or **ceftriaxone** (IM). It is important to treat sexual partners.

Lymphogranuloma Venereum

What is LGV?

A **sexually transmitted ulcerative** disease that occurs in three stages and involves **infection of the lymphatic tissue** in the genital region.

What is the causal agent?

Chlamydia trachomatis; serotypes L1, L2, and L3 are most common

What are key risk factors one should be aware of in the history and physical (H&P)?

Travel and unprotected sex in tropical regions or regions where LGV is endemic (Africa, Southeast Asia, India); anal sex

What are the key physical findings at each stage of this disease?	Stage 1: **small, painless papules/ shallow ulcerations** typically on the vaginal wall.
	Stage 2: **painful unilateral inguinal lymphadenopathy** (groove sign). In women: **bubo** (matted nodes adherent to overlying skin) and lower back/ abdominal/pain due to deep pelvic node involvement.
	Stage 3: **rupture of the bubo** leads to **genitoanorectal syndrome** (strictures and fistulas in the anogenital tract); constitutional symptoms; **proctocolitis**; abscesses.
At what stage do most women present?	Stage 3
Which finding is pathognomic for LGV?	**Groove sign** (inguinal buboes with nonsignificant ulcers)
What other diseases may present with similar cutaneous lesions?	Granuloma inguinale, tuberculosis (TB), early syphilis, and chancroid
What are the most common laboratory tests used to diagnose LGV?	**Complement fixation tests** (used most often)
	Serologic tests for IgG antibodies
	Immunofluorescence on aspirates from bubo for the presence of inclusion bodies
	PCR for *C. trachomatis* or DNA swab from lesion
	Genital or lymph node specimen tested by culture
How is LGV treated?	Oral **doxycycline** or erythromycin for 3 weeks
	Lymph node aspiration if needed
What are some complications of LGV?	Fistulas, strictures, tissue ischemia and necrosis; elephantiasis of the female genitalia (esthiomene)

Granuloma Inguinale (Donovanosis)

What is granuloma inguinale?	A slow, progressive genital ulcerative disease that is primarily sexually transmitted. It is most common in the developing world; it is rare in the United States.
What is the cause?	*Klebsiella granulomatis (previously known as Calymmatobacterium granulomatis)*, a gram-negative pleomorphic bacillus
What are the typical manifestations of granuloma inguinale?	Large, **painless**, and **spreading ulcers** typically in the vulva area; the lesions are clean but have **friable bases with raised, rolled margins that bleed easily**. They are typically **beefy red** in appearance and exude a malodorous discharge. **Inguinal lymphadenopathy is rare.**
What is the classic finding for establishing a diagnosis of granuloma inguinale?	**Donovan bodies** (intracytoplasmic safety pin shaped organisms seen after Giemsa or Wright staining of tissue specimens)
What is the treatment?	**Doxycycline or trimethoprim-sulfamethoxazole** (Tetracycline is no longer recommended because of bacterial resistance)

CERVICITIS

Chlamydia, Gonorrhea, and Other Causes of Cervicitis

What cell types make up the cervix and where are they located?	Columnar epithelium—endocervix Non-keratinizing squamous epithelium—ectocervix
What is mucopurulent cervicitis (MPC)?	Inflammation of the **endocervix** most commonly caused by sexually transmitted organisms. It is characterized by a **yellow-greenish** mucopurulent discharge on visual inspection or on an endocervical swab specimen.

What are the two most common infectious etiologies of MPC and what kind of organisms are they?

1. *C. trachomatis*: gram-negative, obligate intracellular bacterium
2. *Neisseria gonorrhoeae*: gram-negative diplococci

What is ectocervicitis?

Inflammation of the ectocervical epithelium. This squamous epithelium is an extension of the vaginal epithelium and can be infected by the same organisms that cause vaginal infections.

What are some infectious causes of ectocervicitis and what are some key clues, if any, that lead you to that etiology?

Trichomonas: strawberry cervix (small petechiae to large punctuate hemorrhages on the ectocervix)

HSV: ulcerative and hemorrhagic lesions/vesicles during the primary infection

HPV: genital warts, cervical dysplasia on Pap smear

What age group is most frequently affected with cervicitis?

15 to 25 year olds

What are the typical symptoms of MPC?

Vaginal discharge, dysuria, urinary frequency, dyspareunia, postcoital bleeding

What findings are found on clinical examination?

A tender, friable cervix that may also be erythematous and/or edematous.

Patients infected with *C. trachomatis* or *N. gonorrhoeae* are frequently asymptomatic!

What laboratory test supports a diagnosis of MPC?

More than 30 polymorphonuclear (PMN) leukocytes on a Gram-stained specimen from the endocervix

How is the diagnosis of each of the following organisms made?

C. trachomatis: **cell culture** (gold standard, but difficult), nucleic acid amplification tests (NAAT) from urine (good for screening high risk populations), DNA probe, enzyme immunosassay

N. gonorrhoea: **Thayer-Martin agar** culture (gold-standard), DNA probe, enzyme immunoassay

T. vaginalis: visualization of motile trichomonads on **wet mount**

HSV: Tzanck smear test, serologic testing, viral culture

HPV: clinical appearance, cytology

What is the treatment for each of these causes of cervicitis?	*C. trachomatis:* doxycycline for 7 days or azithromycin (single dose)
	N. gonorrhoeae: ceftriaxone (IM) or ciprofloxacin plus doxycycline
	T. vaginalis: metronidazole (PO)
	HSV: acyclovir (PO)
	For all of the above infections, sexual partners also must be treated
What is the treatment for *C. trachomatis* in a pregnant patient or a noncompliant patient?	Azithromycin (single dose PO)
What other organism should be treated in a patient diagnosed with *N. gonorrhoeae?*	*C. trachomatis*
What are some serious complications of cervicitis?	**Pelvic inflammatory disease** (PID), pregnancy and neonatal complications, increased risk of HIV transmission
What are the guidelines for STI screening?	Annual screening of *C. trachomatis* and *N. gonorrhoeae* for all sexually active women less than 25 years of age, or those at high risk more than 25 years of age (new sex partner or multiple sex partners). The CDC also recommends screening of all pregnant women.
What other necessary steps should be taken with a patient diagnosed with an STD-induced cervicitis?	Treat all partners and test for HIV, syphilis, hepatitis B and C

INFECTIONS OF THE UPPER GENITAL TRACT

Pelvic Inflammatory Disease

What is PID?	An acute infection that may involve parts or all of the female genital tract. It is typically initiated by sexually transmitted diseases.

What are the usual presentation/ symptoms/signs of this disease?

The patient is typically a **sexually active female** who presents with two of the three:

lower abdominal pain

adnexal tenderness (usually bilateral)

cervical motion tenderness

While not required to establish the diagnosis of PID, **the presence of one or more of the following enhances the specificity of the minimum criteria: fever (> 101°F); purulent cervical discharge; elevated erythrocyte sedimentation rate (ESR)/C-reactive protein level; leukocytosis**

What are other immediate differential diagnoses of a patient who presents with lower abdominal pain?

Appendicitis, endometriosis, (ruptured) ectopic pregnancy, irritable bowel syndrome, inflammatory bowel disease, ruptured ovarian cyst, miscarriage, gastroenteritis, ovarian torsion, renal colic fibroids, UTI, mesenteric adenitis

For each of the following differential diagnosis related to Ob-Gyn, list the main symptoms/signs that would differentiate between that diagnosis and PID:

Endometriosis:

History of chronic pelvic pain, dysmenorrhea, deep dyspareunia, low sacral back pain, dyschezia, cystic ovarian enlargement, uterosacral tenderness and nodularity, retroflexed uterus

(Ruptured) ectopic pregnancy:

Positive serum hCG, history of amenorrhea, crampy abdominal pain, nausea/vomiting (N/V), dizziness/ light-headedness, palpable tender adnexal mass; other signs depend on extent of rupture and hemorrhage (peritoneal signs, tachycardia, tachypnea, and orthostatic changes)

Ruptured ovarian cyst:

Sudden-onset bi/unilateral lower abdominal pain, rebound tenderness, guarding, N/V

Ovarian torsion:

Intense, progressive unilateral pain combined with tense, tender, and enlarged ovarian mass. History of repetitive, transitory pain. "Wave-like" episodes of N/V may also be experienced

Miscarriage:

Positive serum hCG, amenorrhea, vaginal spotting, crampy abdominal pain

What are the risk factors for PID and what pathogens (if any) are associated with these risk factors?

1. Less than 35 years old; multiple sexual partners; sexual partners with *Chlamydia,* gonorrhea, or other urethritis, nonbarrier protection

    • Common pathogens: *C. trachomatis and N. gonorrhoeae*

2. Instrumentation of the cervix or IUD

    • Common pathogen: *Actinomyces israelii*

3. Bacterial vaginosis (BV)

    • Common pathogens: *Bacteroides, Peptostreptococcus, Escherichia coli*

What is Fitz-Hugh–Curtis (FHC) syndrome?

Focal perihepatitis, causing right upper quadrant tenderness in 15% to 30% of patients with PID. **Right upper quadrant pain does *not* rule out PID!**

Name the diagnostic tests and the expected results that help you make a diagnosis of PID:

β-hCG pregnancy test (rule out ectopic pregnancy or complications of an intrauterine pregnancy)

Microscopic examination of vaginal discharge (wet mount)

Tests for Chlamydia and gonococcus

Urinary analysis (UA) (rule out UTI)

Complete blood count (leukocytosis)

What other methods of evaluation could you consider?

Pelvic ultrasound for evaluation of TOAs

What is the gold standard for diagnosis of PID?

Laparoscopy (usually used in severe cases, patients who require tubo-ovarian drainage, or when the diagnosis is in question)

What are important points to remember regarding treatment?

Always **rule out pregnancy!**

Always use multiple antimicrobial agents to provide coverage for *N. gonorrheae, C. trachomatis*, gram-negative facultative bacteria, streptococci, and anaerobes.

Better to "over diagnose" to prevent sequelae such as scarring, infertility.

Reassess in 48 to 72 hours after initiating treatment! If no improvement, change treatment or diagnosis.

Always treat sexual partners (asymptomatic or symptomatic).

When should you consider inpatient management?	Pregnancy
	Inability to exclude surgical emergency (ie, appendicitis) or uncertain diagnosis
	Failure to respond to outpatient oral therapy within 72 hours
	Inability to tolerate oral therapy
	Severe illness (high fever, peritonitis)
	Presence of a TOA
	Noncompliance, +IUD, +peritoneal signs, +pelvic mass
What are the first-line regimens for inpatient therapy of PID?	**Cefotetan** or **cefoxitin** and **doxycycline**
	Clindamycin and **gentamicin**
What are the first-line regimens for outpatient therapy of PID?	**Ceftriaxone** (or cefoxitin with probenecid) plus doxycycline ± metronidazole
What are complications of PID?	**Tubal factor infertility** (tubes are scarred), ectopic pregnancy, chronic pelvic pain, TOA, perihepatitis (FHC syndrome), adhesions
What is the most likely cause of infertility in a normally menstruating woman of less than 30 years old?	Pelvic inflammatory disease
How can PID be prevented?	**Education** of young women and teenagers-at-risk (primary prevention)
	Annual screening for *Chlamydia* in all sexually active women less than 25 years and women more than 25 years if they have new or multiple partners (secondary prevention)
	Consistent use of barrier contraception
	Oral contraception
	Treatment of sexual partners

Fitz-Hugh–Curtis Syndrome

What is FHC syndrome?	Inflammation of the liver capsule and diaphragm most often associated as an extrapelvic manifestation of PID
What organisms are typically cultured from the infection?	*C. trachomatis* more than *N. gonorrhoeae*

How is the diagnosis of FHC syndrome made?	**Clinical presentation**
	Elevated WBC count and ESR
	Positive cervical and/or abdominal cultures of *C. trachomatis* and/or *N. gonorrhoeae*
What is the gold standard for diagnosis and what are the expected findings?	Diagnostic laparoscopy
	Acute phase: inflammation of the peritoneum and liver capsule
	Chronic phase: **"violin-string" adhesions** of the anterior liver capsule to the anterior abdominal wall or diaphragm
What is the treatment for FHC syndrome?	Medical (same as for PID: doxycycline plus ceftriaxone or ofloxacin plus metronidazole) or surgical (lysis of adhesions)

Tubo-Ovarian Abscess

What is a TOA?	An abscess of the ovary and fallopian tube
In what settings does a TOA develop?	A history of **chronically damaged adnexal tissue with a superimposed recurrent infection.**
	Secondary TOA results from intraperitoneal spread of infection by bowel perforation (appendicitis or diverticulitis) or in association with a pelvic malignancy.
What are the most common pathogens associated with TOA?	Mixed polymicrobial infection with a high prevalence of **anaerobes** *(Bacteroides* and *Peptostreptococcus)* and **gram-negative organisms** *(E. coli* and streptococcal species)
What is the typical presentation of a patient with TOA?	The patient is usually young with a **history of PID**. Typical symptoms and signs include **severe abdominal** and/or **pelvic pain, fever,** leukocytosis, **N/V, rebound tenderness** in lower quadrants.
How does a ruptured TOA present?	As **septic shock**

What tests are used to diagnose TOA?	Pelvic ultrasound (first choice)
	CT (used if ultrasound is uninformative)
	Exploratory laparoscopy
	Culdocentesis
What are the appropriate steps in management of TOA?	Begin IV fluids followed by IV antibiotics. If there is no response, drain the abscess (either IR or surgically).

Pelvic Actinomycosis

What is pelvic actinomycosis?	A very rare infection of the upper genital tract caused by *Actinomyces israelii*, **a gram-positive anaerobic organism**. It is usually part of a polymicrobial infection.
Is it normally part of the female genital tract?	Yes, the presence of *Actinomyces* in the vagina or cervix is neither diagnostic nor predictive of disease.
With which gynecologic diseases has *Actinomyces* been associated?	PID, TOA, chronic endometritis, retroperitoneal fibrosis
With what gynecologic procedure has *Actinomyces* been associated?	IUD placement—*Actinomyces* has been identified in 8% to 20% of women with an IUD
How is the diagnosis of actinomycosis infection made in a symptomatic patient?	Microscopically. An H&E stain reveals sulfur granules and a Gram stain reveals gram-positive filaments
If a Pap smear returns positive for *Actinomyces* on an asymptomatic patient with an IUD, what are the next steps in management?	Antibiotic treatment. Repeat the Pap in 1 year.
When are both removal of the IUD and treatment with antibiotics necessary?	In a patient showing symptoms/signs of a pelvic infection

Pelvic Tuberculosis

| Which bacteria commonly cause pelvic TB? | *Mycobacterium tuberculosis* or *Mycobacterium bovis* |
| How does TB reach the pelvic organs? | Via hematogenous dissemination from either the lung or the GI tract |

What parts of the upper genital tract does TB usually affect?	Fallopian tubes and endometrium
Which population is most affected?	Immigrants from Asia (India), the Middle East, and Latin America
What are the most common presenting complaints of patients with a chronic infection of pelvic TB?	**Infertility**, abnormal uterine bleeding, pelvic pain, and abdominal distension (ascites)
What are some findings on the PE?	Pelvic examination is normal 50% of the time; however, patients may have mild adnexal tenderness and/or bilateral adnexal masses
How is the diagnosis of pelvic TB made?	Positive chest x-ray and lung scan, positive purified protein derivative (PPD), and positive sputum smears/cultures are suggestive. A **positive acid-fast stain and culture from menstrual discharge or biopsy** of the endometrium is diagnostic. Note: **Suspect TB if a patient is not** responding to conventional **antibiotics for bacterial PID.**
What are the histologic findings of the endometrial biopsy?	Classic giant cells, granulomas, and caseous necrosis
What are the next steps in management?	Chest x-ray, intravenous pyelogram, serial gastric washings, and urine cultures (for urinary tract TB)
What is the treatment?	A multidrug regimen consisting INH, rifampicin, pyrazinamide, and ethambutol
What are some complications of pelvic TB?	Infertility and chronic endometritis

VAGINITIS

Introduction

What are the characteristics of normal vaginal discharge?	White or transparent in color, thick, and odorless

What is the normal vaginal pH?	Less than 4.5
What is the microbiology of normal vaginal flora?	There is an average of six different species of bacteria, which are predominantly aerobic. The most common is the **hydrogen peroxide-producing lactobacilli.**
What does microscopy of normal vaginal secretions reveal?	Predominantly squamous epithelial cells, few white blood cells (< 1 per epithelial cells), and possibly a few clue cells
What are the typical symptoms of vaginitis?	Increased vaginal discharge, pruritus, irritation, soreness, odor, dyspareunia, bleeding, dysuria, and mucosal erythema
What are some of the most important etiologies to consider in your differential diagnoses?	Most common infectious causes: bacterial vaginosis > vulvovaginal candidiasis > trichomoniasis
	Less common "infectious" causes: desquamative inflammatory vaginitis, foreign body with secondary infection
	Noninfectious causes: atrophic vaginitis, contact dermatitis, allergens, irritants, hypersensitivity
What laboratory tests are typically ordered to diagnose the etiology of vaginitis?	pH, amine test (whiff test), saline microscopy

Bacterial Vaginosis (Nonspecific Vaginitis)

What is BV?	The most common cause of vaginitis and results from an **alteration of the normal vaginal bacteria flora**. Loss of the normal hydrogen peroxide-producing lactobacilli results in an **overgrowth of anaerobes** such as *Gardnerella vaginalis* and *Mycoplasma hominis*.
What are the key distinguishing symptoms?	"**Musty**" or "**fishy**" vaginal odor; **thin, homogenous, gray-white discharge**

What are risk factors for BV?	Multiple sex partners
	A new sex partner
	Douching
	Lack of vaginal lactobacilli
What are the three major diagnostic findings in BV?	1. **Vaginal pH more than 4.5**
	2. **Positive amine/whiff test** (release of fishy, amine-like odor when vaginal fluid is alkalinized with KOH)
	3. **Saline microscopy reveals more than 20% of clue cells** (vaginal epithelial cells with adherent bacterial clusters)
What are some important complications of BV?	Cervicitis, increased risk of PID, increased risk of HIV infection, preterm delivery, intrapartum and postpartum infections
What is the treatment for BV?	Metronidazole or clindamycin
Do sexual partners need to be treated?	No. BV is not a sexually transmitted disease.

Vulvovaginal Candidiasis

What is vulvovaginal candidiasis (VVC)?	It is a **yeast infection** of the vagina primarily caused by *Candida albicans* because of a change in the vaginal flora.
What are the major risk factors for VVC?	Immunosuppression (**corticosteroids**, AIDS)
	Changes in normal vaginal flora (antibiotics)
	Hormonal changes (**pregnancy**, menstruation, higher dose estrogen OCP)
	Intrauterine devices and vaginal sponges
	Diabetes mellitus
What key symptoms and signs distinguish candidiasis from other causes of *infectious* vaginitis?	Intense vulvovaginal pruritis, soreness, vulvar mucosal erythema and edema, and vaginal discharge that resembles **white "cottage cheese"**

What are other conditions that must be considered in the differential diagnosis?	Hypersensitivity, allergic or chemical reactions, and contact dermatitis or vaginal atrophy
What is the pH of the vagina in patients with VVC?	Normal pH (4-4.5)
How would you definitively diagnose vaginal candidiasis?	Microscopic evaluation of a wet saline or KOH prep of vaginal fluid reveals **hyphae, pseudohyphae, or budding yeast ("spaghetti and meatballs")**
What is the treatment?	Either **oral fluconazole** (single dose in nonpregnant women) or **topical or intravaginal antifungal drugs** (3-7 days). 1% hydrocortisone may be used to relieve external irritative symptoms.
Does the patient's sexual partner need to be treated as well?	No. Candidiasis is not a sexually transmitted disease.

Trichomonas Vaginalis

What is trichomoniasis?	A sexually transmitted vaginal infection caused by the flagellated protozoan, *T. vaginalis*
What are the key presenting characteristics of trichomoniasis?	**Malodorous, purulent, greenish, frothy, profuse watery discharge**; vulvovaginal erythema and irritation, dyspareunia, dysuria; punctate hemorrhages on the cervix (**"strawberry cervix"**)
How is the diagnosis usually made?	**pH of vaginal secretions greater than 5.0** Microscopic examination of a wet saline prep of vaginal fluid reveals **motile trichomonads**
What are some complications of trichomoniasis?	Increased HIV transmission; increased risk of PID; preterm delivery; premature rupture of membranes; low birth weight infants

| What is the treatment? | Oral metronidazole |
| | Sexually partners must be treated |

| What other tests should be considered? | Tests for *N. gonorrhoeae*, *C. trachomatis*, syphilis, HIV, Hepatitis B |

Desquamative Inflammatory Vaginitis

What are the three characteristics of desquamative inflammatory vaginitis?	1. Diffuse, exudative vaginitis
	2. Vaginal-epithelial cell exfoliation
	3. Profuse and purulent vaginal discharge

| What causes inflammatory vaginitis? | Replacement of normal lactobacilli with gram-positive cocci (usually streptococci) |

| What type of patients present with desquamative inflammatory vaginitis? | Premenopausal women with normal estrogen levels |

| How do these patients typically present? | With a purulent vaginal discharge, vulvovaginal burning, dyspareunia, vaginal erythema, and a vulvovaginal-cervical spotted rash |

What are some laboratory findings?	Vaginal secretion pH greater than 4.5
	Increased number of parabasal cells
	Gram-positive cocci (usually streptococci) on Gram-staining

| What is the treatment? | Clindamycin cream intravaginally for 7 days |

Atrophic Vaginitis

| Which women are more likely to be affected by atrophic vaginitis? | Postmenopausal women |

| What causes atrophic vaginitis? | Thinning of the vaginal epithelium because of a reduction of endogenous estrogen. Reduction of lactobacilli and lactic acid increases the vaginal pH and leads to an overgrowth of non-acidophilic organisms |

What are some common symptoms?	Mild vaginal atrophy is usually asymptomatic. Advanced vaginal atrophy can present with vaginal soreness, purulent vaginal discharge, dyspareunia, and postcoital irritation and bleeding
What does a physical examination reveal?	Atrophy of external genitalia, loss of vaginal folds, pale, thin and diffusely erythematous, easily friable vulvovaginal mucosa, and watery or serosanguineous discharge
What do laboratory tests of the vaginal secretions reveal?	pH greater than 5.0 to 7.0 Increased number of leukocytes and parabasal epithelial cells Increased gram-negative rods
What is the treatment?	Topical estrogen vaginal cream

OTHER GYNECOLOGIC INFECTIONS

Postoperative Pelvic Infection

What are some gynecologic postoperative infections?	Cuff and pelvic cellulitis Salpingitis Suppurative pelvic thrombophlebitis TOA with and without rupture
What are the five major causes of fever in the postoperative gynecology patient?	The five "W"s: 1. Wind = pulmonary atelectasis or pneumonia 2. Water = urinary tract infection 3. Walk = deep vein thrombosis (DVT) or superficial phlebitis 4. Wound = infection from the abdominal incision or from a pelvic source 5. Weird drugs = drug-causing fevers (ie, vancomycin)
On what postoperative day does fever because of pelvic infection commonly occur?	Between postoperative day (POD) 2 to 4

What should one think of if fevers continue and there is no clinical response to antibiotics?	Pelvic abscess

Toxic Shock Syndrome

What is toxic shock syndrome (TSS)?	An **acute** illness characterized by **high fevers** which may quickly lead to **hypotensive shock** and **multisystem failure**
What is the cause of toxic shock syndrome?	Preformed exotoxins produced by *Staphylococcus aureus*
In which patients has this syndrome been associated?	**Menstruating women** between age of 12 to 24 years old who use **superabsorbent tampons** Postpartum women Women who use a diaphragm Following surgical procedures
What are the major clinical findings in TSS?	Abrupt onset of **high fevers, vomiting, and diarrhea** Within 48 hours, **signs of shock** occur (temperature $\geq 102.2°F$, dehydration, tachycardia, hypotension) and a **diffuse "sunburn-like" rash** appears over the face, trunk, and proximal extremities **Desquamation (particularly affecting the palms and soles)** may occur 1 to 2 weeks after the onset of illness **Involvement of three or more organ systems (GI, CNS, renal, mucous membrane, skin, cardiac, hepatic) is essential for diagnosis**
What information should be sought during the H&P that is pertinent to this diagnosis?	Ask the patient if she is **menstruating or using tampons!!!** You must perform a vaginal examination and remove the tampon immediately if one is present.
What will the vaginal culture yield in TSS?	Penicillinase-producing *S. aureus*

What is the management and treatment for a patient with TSS?	Assess hemodynamics, treat shock
	IV antibiotics: β-lactamase-resistant antibiotic (nafcillin or oxacillin)
	Vancomycin (for penicillin-allergic patients)

What are the three most common causes of death from TSS?

1. Acute respiratory distress syndrome
2. Intractable hypotension
3. Hemorrhage secondary to DIC

HIV/AIDS

What is HIV?

A single-stranded **RNA retrovirus** that infects **CD4 receptor lymphocytes** and other target cells and causes a progressive **decrease in cellular immunity** leading to AIDS

What are the three means of HIV transmission?

1. Sexual contact
2. Parenteral exposure to blood or bodily fluids (IV drugs, occupational exposure)
3. Vertical transmission (from an infected mother to her fetus)

How do HIV-infected patients initially present?

With mononucleosis-like symptoms such as **fever, weight loss, night sweats**, pharyngitis, lymphadenopathy, erythematous maculopapular rash. This is followed by a long asymptomatic period lasting from months to years.

What are some symptoms of HIV infection in females?

Difficult-to-treat vaginal infections (**candidiasis**, BV, and common STDs)

Increase in frequency, severity, and recurrence of HSV ulcers, HPV infections, and cervical dysplasia

Presence of idiopathic genital ulcers

How is it diagnosed?

Screening test: **ELISA** (detects antibodies to HIV)

Confirmation test: **Western Blot**

When should you use the rapid detection HIV testing?

In urgent care settings, labor and delivery, or emergency room departments only. Specificity is high but false positives and false negatives can occur.

Any positive result should be confirmed with Western Blot.

When can the ELISA test give a false-negative result?

In early infection (< **12 weeks**). All patients with recent exposure need to be tested again after this window period.

What vaccinations should be offered to HIV-infected patients?

Hepatitis B, hepatitis C, influenza, and pneumococcus, TdAP.

Avoid live vaccines (such as MMR).

What is the current treatment regimen for HIV infection?

Two nucleoside reverse transcriptase inhibitors (NRTIs) and one protease inhibitor

Pelvic Pain

CHRONIC PELVIC PAIN

Etiologies

How is chronic pelvic pain (CPP) defined?

It is **noncyclic pain** of nonmenstrual origin that **lasts** more than or equal to **6 month duration** and is located **below the umbilicus.**

The pain is severe enough to **cause functional disability or require medical treatment.**

What is the prevalence of chronic pelvic pain?

Approximately 15% to 20% of women aged 18 to 50 years have chronic pelvic pain of greater than 1-year duration.

What are the most common gynecologic conditions that cause chronic pelvic pain?

Pelvic inflammatory disease (18%-35%); endometriosis; adenomyosis; gynecologic malignancies (late stages); tuberculous salpingitis

How often is endometriosis diagnosed by laparoscopy in women with chronic pelvic pain?

Diagnosis of endometriosis by laparoscopy is made in 33% of women with chronic pelvic pain.

What are the most significant non-gynecological causes of chronic pelvic pain?

Interstitial cystitis, irritable bowel syndrome, chronic coccygeal or back pain, and depression may cause or exacerbate chronic pelvic pain.

What is the association between physical or sexual abuse, and chronic pelvic pain?

About 40% to 50% of women with chronic pelvic pain have a history of some form of abuse

What other mental disorders should be considered in a patient with chronic pelvic pain?

Somatization, opiate abuse, depression

Workup

What information should be gathered when taking the history of the patient's pain?

A thorough review of systems should be performed with emphasis on urinary tract disease, bowel disease, reproductive tract disease, musculoskeletal disorders, and psychoneurologic disorders.

How do the nature and the quality of pain give a clue to the source of the pain?

Somatic pain is usually localized and sharp, indicating a musculoskeletal origin.

Visceral pain is usually vague, aching, and difficult to localize; this may indicate an intraperitoneal or upper reproductive tract etiology.

What are the physical findings that suggest the following etiologies of chronic pelvic pain?

Endometriosis:

Uterosacral ligament nodularity or thickness, cervical stenosis, lateral displacement of the cervix because of shortening of one of the ligaments

Adenomyosis:

Slightly enlarged, globular, tender uterus on examination

Leiomyomata:

Enlarged, mobile uterus with an irregular contour on bimanual or abdominal examination

Pelvic inflammatory disease (PID):

Uterine tenderness or cervical motion tenderness on examination

Neuropathy:

Burning, shock-like, paresthesia, and dysesthesia

Neoplasm:

Adnexal mass, ascites

What is Carnett's sign?

It refers to **increased local tenderness during muscle tensing by raising both legs straight up while lying supine.** This maneuver tightens the rectus abdominis muscles, increasing pain if there is **myofascial pain** (eg, trigger points, entrapped nerve, hernia, myositis).

Visceral sources of pain are associated with less tenderness when abdominal muscles are tensed.

Which laboratory and imaging tests should be ordered in a patient with chronic pelvic pain?

Complete blood count (CBC) with differential and ESR

Pregnancy test

Urinalysis

Fecal occult blood test

Pelvic ultrasound

Chlamydia and gonorrhea cultures

When should MRI or CT scan be used?

Only when abnormalities are found on ultrasound examination

What is the role of laparoscopy in evaluation of women with chronic pelvic pain?

It is indicated in women who have symptoms and signs of endometriosis and/or adhesions. It is also indicated in women with **chronic pelvic pain** who have not had relief of symptoms with nonsteroidal anti-inflammatory drugs (NSAIDs) or estrogen-progestin treatment and have no strong contraindications to laparoscopic surgery.

Treatment

How is endometriosis-associated chronic pelvic pain treated?	Nonsteroidal anti-inflammatory drugs
	Continuous oral contraceptives
	GnRH agonist analogues (nafarelin, goserelin, and leuprolide)
	Progestins (medroxy-progesterone acetate)
In what other sources of chronic pelvic pain are GnRH agonists effective?	Irritable bowel syndrome, pelvic congestion syndrome, and interstitial cystitis also respond to GnRH agonists
When are oral contraceptives indicated for treatment of chronic pelvic pain?	To decrease pain from primary dysmenorrhea
What is the role of antidepressants in treatment of chronic pelvic pain?	Currently, evidence is insufficient to substantiate efficacy of antidepressants for the treatment of chronic pelvic pain. However, adding psychotherapy to medical treatment of chronic pelvic pain appears to improve response over that of medical treatment alone and should be considered.
What is the role of surgery in treatment of chronic pelvic pain?	Excision or destruction of endometriotic tissue or lysis of adhesions have been effective in reducing pelvic pain.
What is presacral neurectomy and is it effective for treatment of chronic pelvic pain?	It is the surgical resection of the superior hypogastric plexus which innervates the cervix, uterus, and proximal fallopian tubes with afferent nociception.
	It may be used to treat centrally located dysmenorrhea but has limited efficacy for chronic pelvic pain or pain that is not central in its location.
What is the main take-home point of treatment for chronic pelvic pain?	Multimodal therapy (medical therapy, surgical therapy, and behavioral/mental health treatment, along with pain consultation) is superior to a single approach.

ACUTE PELVIC PAIN

Etiologies

What are the obstetric and gynecologic differential diagnoses for acute pelvic pain?	Pelvic inflammatory disease
	Adnexal cysts/masses/abscesses with bleeding, torsion, or rupture
	Ectopic pregnancy
	Spontaneous abortion
	Endometritis
	Degeneration, infarction, or torsion of leiomyomas (fibroids)
What are non-gynecologic differential diagnoses for acute pelvic pain?	Appendicitis
	Diverticulitis
	Urinary tract infection or obstruction
	Renal colic
On what additional points should the history taking focus to determine a pelvic etiology?	The regularity and timing of menstrual periods, possibility of pregnancy, presence of vaginal discharge or bleeding, and a recent history of dyspareunia or dysmenorrheal.
How do differences in the clinical and laboratory findings help point out the etiology of acute gynecologic pelvic pain?	See Table 4.2
What is mittelschmerz?	Recurrent acute midcycle abdominal pain because of leakage of prostaglandin-containing follicular fluid at the time of ovulation

Table 4.2 Differential Diagnosis of Acute Gynecologic Pelvic Pain

Disease		Clinical and Laboratory Findings				
	CBC	UA	Pregnancy Test	Culdocentesis	Fever	Nausea and Vomiting
Ruptured ectopic pregnancy	Low Hct	Nml	Positive, beta-hCG low for gestational age	High hematocrit Defibrinated, nonclotting sample with no platelets Crenated red blood cells	No	Unusual
Salpingitis/ PID	High WBC	Occasional WBCs	Generally negative	Yellow, turbid fluid with many white blood cells and some bacteria	Progressively worsening; spiking	Gradual onset with ileus
Hemorrhagic ovarian cyst	Low Hct	Normal	Usually negative	Hematocrit generally < 10%	No	Rare
Torsion of adnexa	Normal	Normal	Generally negative	Minimal clear fluid if obtained early	No	Rare
Degenerating leiomyoma	Normal or elevated white blood cell count	Normal	Generally negative	Normal clear fluid	Possibly	Rare

Reprinted, with permission, from Pearlman MD, Tintinalli JE, eds. *Emergency Care of the Woman.* New York, NY: McGraw-Hill; 1998: 508.

Endometriosis

What is endometriosis?

A benign yet very debilitating gynecologic disease where **endometrial glands and stroma** are present in an **extrauterine location**

To which hormone does ectopic endometrial tissue respond? What is the significance of this?

Estrogen

It **changes in a cyclic manner** according to menstrual changes in estrogen levels. The ectopic tissue can release a small amount of blood into the surrounding tissues leading to repeated **tissue inflammation, pelvic pain, scarring, and eventually adhesions in the reproductive organs, pelvis, and other intestines.**

Who develops endometriosis?

Reproductive-age women and postmenopausal women on estrogen-replacement therapy

What is the prevalence of endometriosis in the United States?

7% of reproductive-age women are diagnosed with endometriosis

What are the two most common symptoms associated with endometriosis and what percentage of women with these complaints are found to have endometriosis?

Chronic pelvic pain (71%-87%)
Infertility (38%)

How does endometriosis lead to infertility?

It causes the **formation of adhesions** that distort the normal uterine/tubal/ovary anatomy, inhibit tubo-ovarian motility, and block ovum release.

The release of other substances (such as **cytokines**) may be "toxic" to normal ovarian function/fertilization/implantation.

What other common complication can endometrial adhesions cause?

Small bowel obstruction

For what other disease is endometriosis a risk factor?

Epithelial ovarian cancer (EOC).

Since both are estrogen-dependent diseases, the presence of endometriosis may indicate a risk for developing EOC.

Do genetic factors increase the risk for endometriosis?

Yes. There is a seven to tenfold increased risk of developing endometriosis if a first-degree relative has been affected by endometriosis. The mode of inheritance is polygenic and multifactorial.

What three leading theories explain the etiology of endometriosis?

1. **Retrograde menstruation:** a reverse flow of endometrial tissue through the fallopian tubes during menses leads to the seeding of endometrial cells in the peritoneal cavity.
2. **Lymphatic and vascular spread:** spread of endometrial cells through lymphatic and vascular channels.
3. **Coelomic metaplasia:** transformation of coelomic epithelium or undifferentiated peritoneal cells into endometrial tissue by an endogenous undefined biochemical factor.

In what sites are endometrial implants found?

Most common: **ovaries**, anterior and posterior cul-de-sac, uterosacral ligaments, posterior uterus, posterior broad ligaments, sigmoid colon, appendix, round ligaments

What symptom is pathognomonic for endometriosis?

Cyclical rectal bleeding

What are endometriomas?

Invasive endometriotic lesions found inside the ovary. Often described as a **"chocolate cyst"** because it contains old blood that has undergone hemolysis.

What are the complications of endometriomas?

Rupture of endometriomas can cause periteonal inflammation, scarring, and pelvic adhesions

What findings are typically found on physical examination?

Tenderness upon pelvic examination during menses (most common finding).

Uterosacral or cul-de-sac nodularity.

Retroverted uterus and limited motion of ovaries and fallopian tubes.

Tender, enlarged adnexal mass (unilateral).

There are often no abnormal findings on physical examination.

What value does CA125 have in the clinical management of endometriosis?

CA125 is not a sensitive diagnostic test for endometriosis (especially in minimal to mild disease). However, it may be used as a **marker to follow medical treatment response** for endometriosis....

Are imaging tests a sensitive modality for diagnosing endometriosis?

No. However, ultrasound, CT, and MRI are useful for detecting pelvic or adnexal masses (ie, endometriomas) or ruling out other causes of pelvic pain. Deeply infiltrating endometriosis that involve the uterosacral ligaments and the cul-de-sac may be detected by MRI.

How is the diagnosis of endometriosis made?

Direct visualization by laparoscopy/ laparotomy with histologic confirmation

What are the characteristic findings of endometriosis found during laparoscopy/laparotomy?.

Classic lesions: brown/black/blue **"powder burn," "gun shot"** lesions, nodules or small cysts containing old hemorrhage surrounded by fibrosis on the serosal surfaces of the peritoneum..

Atypical/subtle lesions: clear vesicles, white opacifications, red, white, yellow/brown plaques, excrescences, scars or lesions of varying sizes.

Note: **Normal appearing peritoneum may have microscopic evidence of endometriosis.**

What histologic findings confirm the diagnosis of endometriosis?

The **presence of two** or more of the following histologic features: endometrial epithelium, endometrial glands, endometrial stroma, hemosiderin-laden macrophages

What is the current classification system for endometriosis staging?

One created by the American Society for Reproductive Medicine. It uses point scores for disease staging and is used primarily for the uniform recording of operative findings.

What are the limitations of this system?

It is not good for correlating disease stage with pain and/or dyspareunia. It also does not predict the chance of pregnancy following treatment.

What is the typical clinical outcome of endometriosis and what is the goal of treatment?

Endometriosis is a progressively deteriorating disease that rarely improves. Elimination of endometriotic implants by medical or surgical intervention provides only temporary relief. However, **the goal of treatment should be to eradicate the lesions, treat endometriosis-related pelvic pain and infertility, and prevent bowel and extra-pelvic complications.**

What factors must be considered when choosing the appropriate treatment regimen?

Patient's desire for future fertility, side effects of medication, cost, and patient's tolerance

What type of medical therapy is most effective for endometriosis?

Hormonal therapy that **suppresses estrogen synthesis** (induces atrophy of ectopic lesions) and/or **disrupts the menstrual cycle** (abrogates or diminishes retrograde bleeding)

What are the most commonly used hormonal medications for the treatment of endometriosis?

Oral contraceptive pills (OCPs): best for minimal to mild pain, reduces menstrual flow

Progestins: good for moderate to severe disease, excellent pain relief, induces atrophy of endometrial implants, few side effects, inexpensive

Danazol: effective for mild to moderate disease, relieves dysmenorrhea, inhibits midcycle LH/FSH surge, induces endometrial atrophy within uterus and ectopically ultimately leads to amenorrhea

GnRH agonists: inhibit pituitary gonadotropin secretion which suppresses ovarian estrogen production, induces amenorrhea, relieves pain

What other nonhormonal medication treats endometriosis-related pain?

Nonsteroidal anti-inflammatory drugs

When is surgery indicated for the treatment of endometriosis?

1. When symptoms have not improved or worsened with medical management
2. When symptoms of endometriosis are severe and incapacitating
3. For advanced disease
4. To treat endometriomas, bowel or urogenital tract obstruction, or anatomically distorted pelvic structures because of adhesions/invasive endometriotic lesions

What are the indications for definitive surgery (hysterectomy with or without removal of the fallopian tubes and ovaries)?

For patients with advanced disease and for those who no longer want/need fertility conservation

What is the impact of medical management versus surgical management on recurrence and infertility?

Similar or higher rates of recurrence have been reported with medical management versus surgical management. Surgery has been reported to improve rates of fertility compared to expectant management.

What is the management of endometriosis-related infertility?

Assisted reproduction technologies (ART) such as IVF

What is adenomyosis?

The presence of **ectopic endometrial glands and stroma within the uterine musculature.**

What is the prevalence of adenomyosis?

It is thought to affect 20% of all women.

What is the classic presentation of a patient with adenomyosis?

A **parous, middle-aged** woman with **menorrhagia** and **dysmenorrhea** with a **symmetrically enlarged, tender, and "boggy"** uterus.

How is the diagnosis of adenomyosis made?

A presumptive diagnosis is based on the clinical presentation in the absence of endometriosis or leiomyomas. A definitive diagnosis requires histologic assessment of the uterine tissue.

What is the differential diagnosis for adenomyosis?	Leiomyoma Intra-abdominal neoplasia Endometriosis PID
Is adenomyosis related to endometriosis?	Although they are both disorders of the ectopic endometrium, they are unrelated.
What is the definitive treatment for adenomyosis?	Hysterectomy
What is the prognosis for adenomyosis?	Good—it is a self-limited process that often becomes asymptomatic after menopause

Benign Pelvic Masses

BENIGN CERVICAL MASSES

Cervical Cysts

What four types of cervical cysts are there?	1. Nabothian 2. Mesonephric 3. Endometrial 4. Adenosis
What are the symptoms of a cervical cyst?	Usually **asymptomatic** but can cause dyspareunia
What is a nabothian cyst and how does it develop?	A discrete mucus-filled cyst that appears grossly as a small translucent or yellow elevation on the cervix. They occur via metaplasia. Sometimes a cleft of **columnar endocervical** epithelium becomes covered by **squamous** epithelium, trapping the mucus secretions and forming cysts.

How are nabothian cysts treated?	Most are asymptomatic and therapy is not needed.
	If symptomatic, treatment can be via excision, electrocautery or cryotherapy.
Which other cervical cyst may be confused with a nabothian cyst?	The mesonephric (Wolffian) cysts are found deep in the stroma of the **ectocervix** and are lined by **Wolffian-type cells**
What conditions are most associated with cervical cysts?	Pregnancy, menopause, and cervicitis

Cervical Polyps

What are cervical polyps?	Small, pedunculated, benign neoplasms of the cervix composed of a vascular connective tissue stroma covered by epithelium. They commonly arise via focal hyperplasia of the endocervix and protrude from the cervical canal out of the external os.
How common are they and in whom do they develop?	Relatively common. They are rare before menarche but may develop after menopause.
How are cervical polyps diagnosed and managed?	Asymptomatic polyps often are discovered on routine pelvic examination. Otherwise they usually present with **intermenstrual** or **postcoital bleeding** or discharge.
	Although carcinoma developing in a polyp is rare, polyps should be **removed** close to their attachment and **pathologically reviewed.**

BENIGN UTERINE MASSES

Leiomyomas

What are uterine leiomyomas?	**Benign** tumors of the **smooth muscle** cells (myometrium) of the uterus; also known as fibroids, fibromyomas, or **myomas**

What are the three types of leiomyomas (see Fig. 4.5)?

1. **Intramural**—located **within the wall of the myometrium** and may distort the shape of the uterine cavity and surface
2. **Submucosal**—originate in the myometrium and **grow toward the endometrial cavity**, protruding into the uterine lumen
3. **Subserosal**—originate in the myometrium and grow out toward **the serosal surface** of the uterus; extend from the uterine surface into the peritoneum and abdominal cavity

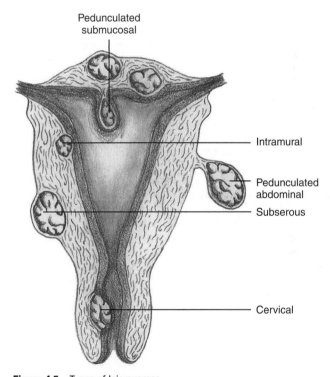

Pedunculated submucosal

Intramural

Pedunculated abdominal

Subserous

Cervical

Figure 4.5   Types of leiomyomas.

What is the prevalence of leiomyomas and in whom do they occur?

Leiomyomas are **hormonally responsive** and are found in **20% to 30% of reproductive-age women**.

What are the risk factors for leiomyomas?

African-American race.

Nulliparity.

Oral contraceptives (OCPs) are mostly protective.

Diet—a diet high in red meat and low in green vegetables has been suggested to increase the risk for fibroids.

Genetics.

Alcohol.

What are the usual presentation/symptoms/signs of fibroids?

Most are **asymptomatic** and so are diagnosed based on the finding of an **irregularly enlarged, mobile uterus** on gynecologic examination

If symptoms do occur, the most common are

Abnormal uterine bleeding (menorrhagia or metrorrhagia)

Pelvic pressure/pain (dysmenorrhea, urinary frequency, constipation, or dyspareunia)

Infertility

Aside from leiomyomas, what are other differential diagnoses of a patient who presents with menorrhagia and pelvic pressure/pain?

Adenomyosis; primary dysmenorrhea; endometriosis; tubo-ovarian abscess; malignancy (cervical, endometrial, or ovarian)

How is the diagnosis of fibroids usually made?

Via ultrasonography

Describe the theoretical mechanisms for increased bleeding associated with leiomyomas:

1. An **alteration in myometrial cells contractile ability** leading to lack of control of bleeding from the endometrial arterioles
2. The endometrium is **unable to respond to hormonal changes** in the menstrual cycle, leading to sloughing off of excess tissue
3. Increased pressure causes **necrosis of the endometrium**, which leads to exposure of the vasculature surfaces and increased bleeding

What other methods of evaluation could you consider for the diagnosis of fibroids?

Hysterosalpingography allows for visualization of submucosal fibroids.

MRI

Hysteroscopy

What causes the growth of leiomyomas?

Their growth is responsive to both **estrogen** and **progesterone**. Estrogen may increase the production of extracellular matrix. Progesterone increases the mitotic activity of myomas and inhibits apoptosis.

What is the molecular pathogenesis of leiomyomas?

First, **normal myocytes transform into abnormal myocytes** either via somatic mutation or in response to injury.

Second, the abnormal myocytes **grow via clonal expansion** into clinically significant tumors.

Molecular alterations that lead to **increased or abnormal vasculature** are also involved in fibroid formation.

What is degeneration of a leiomyoma and what types can occur?

Various histologic and gross changes occur in leiomyomas when they outgrow their blood supply. The types are as follows:

Red degeneration—hemorrhagic changes that occur as a result of rapid growth. Can cause acute pain, low-grade fever, and an elevation in white blood cell (WBC) count; most common during pregnancy

Hyaline degeneration—mildest form of degeneration: hyalization of the smooth muscle of the leiomyoma represented by loss of the whorled pattern and an overall homogenous appearance

Calcification—occurs especially in inactive smooth muscle elements after menopause

When do fibroids need to be treated?

Most women **do not need surgical or medical treatment**. Intervention is indicated with worsening symptom or with a rapidly enlarging uterus.

What are the treatment options for symptomatic leiomyomas?

Progestin supplementation

Prostaglandin synthetase inhibitors— reduce bleeding

Other NSAIDs

GnRH analogs $\rightarrow$ inhibit estrogen which reduces the size of the leiomyoma

Myomectomy $\rightarrow$ indicated in symptomatic women desiring future fertility

Hysterectomy $\rightarrow$ indicated in symptomatic women not desiring future fertility

Embolization of the uterine arteries $\rightarrow$ indicated in symptomatic premenopausal women not desiring fertility and who want to preserve their uterus and avoid surgical intervention

What are the risks of myomectomy?

Intraoperative blood loss; postoperative **hemorrhage; postsurgical adhesions; risk of recurrence**. These risks are higher with myomectomy than with hysterectomy.

What types of complications can occur which are secondary to leiomyomas?

Iron-deficiency anemia

Acute blood loss

Hydroureter or hydronephrosis

Can leiomyomas ever metastasize?

Rarely. In those cases, leiomyomas can grow beyond the uterus or even invade intravascularly to spread to the peritoneum or lung.

What types of metastatic disease can develop from a leiomyoma?

Intravenous leiomyomatosis

Benign metastasizing leiomyoma

Leiomyomatosis peritonealis disseminate

Leiomyosarcoma

Who is most likely to develop a malignancy from a leiomyoma?

Postmenopausal women, especially those presenting with rapid tumor growth, vaginal bleeding, and/or pain

What is a leiomyosarcoma?

A **malignant neoplasm of the uterine smooth** muscle. It occurs most commonly in postmenopausal women, is rapidly expanding, and carries a poor prognosis.

Benign Ovarian Masses

What is the differential diagnosis of an ovarian mass?

Functional ovarian cysts; dermoid cyst; PCOS; endometriomas; ectopic pregnancy; tubo-ovarian complex; malignancy

Functional Ovarian Cysts

What are functional ovarian cysts?

Benign anatomic variations resulting from irregularities in normal ovarian function

What are the three types of functional ovarian cysts and how do they form?

1. **Follicular cysts**: ovulation fails to occur and the remaining fluid does not become reabsorbed but gets accumulated into a cystic structure

2. **Corpus luteum cysts**: the corpus luteum formed after ovulation persists and grows larger than 3 cm

3. **Theca-lutein cysts**: most frequently occur iatrogenically following ovulation induction or in young girls with hypothyroidism. Also may be seen with high levels of hCG (eg, in patients with hydatidiform mole or choriocarcinoma)

What are the typical symptoms (if any) of each of the following types of ovarian cysts?

Follicular:

Typically asymptomatic; can cause midcycle pelvic pain, dyspareunia, and abnormal uterine bleeding

Corpus luteum:

Localized tenderness, amenorrhea, and delayed menstruation (often confused with ectopic pregnancy)

Theca lutein:

Pelvic heaviness/aching, hyperemesis, and breast paresthesias

What is the appearance of each of the following types of cyst?

Follicular: Smooth, thin walled, unilocular

Corpus luteum: More complex, usually yellowish-orange lining consisting of luteinized granulose and theca cells

Theca lutein: Usually bilateral, multicystic, filled with clear, straw-colored fluid. All are usually less than 10 cm.

What is the diagnostic workup for a patient with a suspected functional ovarian cyst?

Pelvic examination; ultrasound; repeat examination and sonography at 6 to 8 weeks; laparoscopy if symptomatic, concern for torsion or persistence after 3 to 6 months

What findings raise your suspicion that a cyst may be neoplastic?

Patient is prepubescent or postmenopausal

Patient has history of another malignancy (especially breast or gastric)

Patient has ascites

Ultrasound findings are significant for: large size, loculations, septa, papillae, or increased blood flow

Continued presence of cyst at 3 to 6 months follow-up

How are asymptomatic functional ovarian cysts treated?

Expectant management with analgesics as needed (usually resolve within weeks)

OCPs are often used; they do not promote faster resolution of the cyst, but reduce the risk of future cyst development

When do functional ovarian cysts need to be treated?

When there is severe pain or when there is suspicion of malignancy, rupture, or torsion

Dermoid Cyst

What is another name for dermoid cyst?	Mature cytic teratoma
What types of cells are contained within a dermoid?	Ectodermal, mesodermal, and endodermal cells. Grossly they often contain hair, teeth, and sebaceous material.
What are symptoms associated with dermoid cysts?	They are often asymptomatic; torsion can occur
How often are dermoid cysts bilateral?	10% to 17%
How are dermoid cysts diagnosed	By their characteristic ultrasonographic appearance (heterogeneous, areas of calcification)
How should dermoids be managed?	Ovarian cystectomy (to prevent future torsion) with copious irrigation to avoid chemical peritonitis from the sebaceous material

Benign Fallopian Tube Masses

What are the types of benign fallopian tube neoplasms?	Paraovarian cysts; paratubal cysts
What is another name for paratubal cysts? Describe them:	Hydatid cysts of Morgagni. They are located near the fimbriated end of the tube, filled with clear fluid, and approximately 1 cm in diameter.
How do these masses usually present?	Usually asymptomatic and the diagnosis is usually made as an incidental finding in the OR

Sexual Dysfunction

What are the four phases of sexual response described by Masters and Johnson

1. **Excitement:** internal or external stimuli
2. **Plateau:** marked degree of vasocongestion throughout the body
3. **Orgasm**
4. **Resolution**

What are the possible etiologies of sexual dysfunction?

1. Change in vascularity (atherosclerosis, pudendal artery insufficiency affecting vaginal vasocongestion)
2. Neurogenic causes (spinal cord dysfunction or injuries)
3. Depression or anxiety disorders
4. Medications (selective serotonin reuptake inhibitor [SSRI], tricyclic antidepressants, H_2 blocker, and some antihypertensive medication)
5. Psychosocial factors (prior history of sexual abuse, religious or cultural expectation, fear of rejection or intimacy, and distorted body image)
6. Hormonal changes (premature ovarian failure and menopause)

What is the prevalence of sexual dysfunction?

Studies show a range of 10% to 60%

What are the types of female sexual dysfunction and what is the main symptom of each?

1. **Sexual desire disorders:** decreased sexual fantasy and/or desire, sexual aversion
2. **Sexual arousal disorders: decreased genital vasocongestion** and lubrication
3. **Orgasmic disorders:** anorgasmia
4. **Sexual pain disorders**: vaginismus, dyspareunia, noncoital sexual pain

What hormones influence vaginal blood flow?

Estrogen and **testosterone** increase vaginal blood flow

Progesterone diminishes vaginal blood flow

What types of therapies are available for the treatment of sexual dysfunction?

1. **Nonpharmacologic therapy:** patient education, lifestyle and behavioral changes should be tried first
2. **Pharmacologic therapy:**

   Estrogen: increases genital blood flow and enhanced lubrication

   Testosterone: may improve libido, data nonconclusive

   Herbal therapy: (eg, St. John's wort, ginseng, yohimbine) generally ineffective

   L-Arginine: increases nitric oxide (NO) leading to genital vasocongestion; needs further study

   Tibolone: used for osteoporosis; has androgenic activity that may improve sexual function

   Sildenafil: a vasodilator; data inconclusive on its benefit for women, not FDA approved

What types of medication or substances can lead to sexual dysfunction?

Alcohol; antihypertensives; illicit drugs; SSRIs

Psychotropic

Antihistaminic

What is hypoactive sexual desire disorder (HSDD)?

Recurrent and persistent lack of sexual fantasies or desires or receptivity to sexual activity that causes personal distress

What is sexual aversion disorder?

It is characterized by a phobia with **avoidance of sexual contact** and severe anxiety associated with contemplation of sexual activity.

What are sexual arousal disorders?

When women experience desire and orgasm, but **lack signs of sexual stimulation**

What is orgasmic dysfunction?

A **persistent delay in or absence of orgasm** after sufficient stimulation and arousal resulting in distress or interpersonal difficulty

What types of orgasmic dysfunction exists?

Primary anorgasmia is found in 5% to 10% of women and is lifelong.

Secondary anorgasmia is often related to relationship problems, medications, medical illness, depression, substance abuse, and self-monitoring/anxiety during arousal.

What types of sexual pain disorders exist and what are they?

Vaginismus (recurrent involuntary contraction of the vaginal musculature during vaginal penetration)

Dyspareunia (general pain that occurs before, during, or after intercourse)

What organic disorders must be ruled out when vaginismus is diagnosed?

Endometriosis; PID; partial imperforate hymen; vaginal stenosis

How is vaginismus treated?

Education; relaxation techniques; kegel exercises; progressive vaginal dilatation

What organic disorders must be ruled out when dyspareunia is diagnosed?

Bartholin cysts; vulvitis; vestibulitis; vaginitis; clitoral irritation/ hypersensitivity; rigid hymenal ring/ introital scar tissue; vaginal atrophy and dryness; pelvic adhesion; fibroid; endometriosis

Benign Conditions of the Vulvavagina

DYSTROPHIES

What are vulvar dystrophies?

A group of disorders characterized by lesions that are **white, intensely pruritic** with or without pain, and may occur with **vulvar epithelial changes. Lesions should be biopsied to rule out malignancy.**

What is vulvar lichen sclerosis?

A **benign, progressive, and chronic dermatologic condition** more common in older women and characterized by **intense pruritus and pain.**

What are other sequelae of lichen sclerosis?

Painful defecation, anal pruritus, dyspareunia, and dysuria.

They may also develop into invasive squamous cell cancer of the vulva.

How does lichen sclerosis appear on clinical examination?

Thin, white, wrinkled skin often resembling **"parchment paper"** or **"cigarette paper"** that is localized to the labia minora and/or labia majora. It may extend toward the anus.

What is the treatment for lichen sclerosis?

Potent topical corticosteroids (Clobetasol)

What other additional steps should be considered in management of these patients?

Strong encouragement of vulvar hygiene.

Given the risk of malignant vulvar cancer, the skin should be examined yearly and suspicious lesions should be biopsied.

What is vulvar lichen planus?

An inflammatory dermatologic condition with unknown etiology that mainly affects the skin and mucous membranes of the oral cavity and genital area.

How does lichen planus clinically present on the vulva?

With either **violaceous papules,** hyperkeratosis, or bright erythematous erosions with a white border or white striae along the margins

How does lichen planus clinically present on the skin and oral mucous membranes?

Skin: eruption of multiple, shiny, polygonal, flat-topped, purple papules with white striae

Oral mucous membranes: white plaques

How is lichen planus different from lichen sclerosis?

The vagina is involved 70% of the time in lichen planus.

What is vulvovaginal-gingival syndrome?

A variant of lichen planus that involves lesions on the vulva, vestibule, vagina, gingival epithelium, and/or skin. These affected areas may or may not occur concurrently.

What is the treatment of lichen planus?

Potent topical corticosteroids

What is vulvar dermatitis?

Also known as vulvar eczema, it is the most common inflammatory skin disease characterized by intense pruritus and irritation.

It can have a familial predisposition (atopic dermatitis) or occur with allergens (contact dermatitis).

What is the end result of constant irritation and scratching in vulvar dermatitis?

Lichen simplex chronicus. It appears as a raised, hyperkeratotic white lesion. Biopsy reveals hyperkeratosis and acanthosis.

What is the difference between lichen simplex chronicus, and lichen sclerosis and lichen planus?

Lichen simplex chronicus is a reactive change whereas lichen sclerosis and lichen planus are primary dystrophies.

What is the treatment?

Medium-to-high-potency topical steroids

What other vulvar dystrophy has the same histologic appearance as lichen simplex chronicus?

Squamous cell hyperplasia

In what setting does lichen simplex chronicus arise?

In patients who have chronic vulvovaginal infections or other causes of chronic irritation.

What is the treatment for squamous cell hyperplasia?

The goal is symptomatic relief. Sitz baths and lubricants are recommended to restore moisture to cells. Medium potency topical steroids are used to decrease inflammation and pruritus.

What is the gold standard for diagnosis of any of these dystrophies?

Biopsy of the lesion

How does psoriasis appear on physical examination of the vulva? How is it treated?

Red moist plaques covered by silver scales. Topical corticosteroids are the treatment of choice.

BENIGN CYSTS

What are the most common benign vulvovaginal cysts?

Bartholin ducts cysts, epidermal, sebaceous, and apocrine sweat gland cysts

Where are Bartholin glands and ducts located?

Deep in the labia majora at about four and eight o'clock positions. They are not palpable in healthy women.

How do Bartholin gland cysts develop?

Infection can cause inflammation and obstruction of the main duct of Bartholin glands leading to cystic dilation. They may enlarge up to 1 to 3 cm and are usually asymptomatic.

What may Bartholin gland cysts develop into?

Bartholin gland abscesses

When symptomatic, what are the acute symptoms and signs of Bartholin gland cysts and abscesses?

Pain, dyspareunia, and difficulty ambulating or sitting. Physical examination may reveal swelling, erythema, edema, and a large fluctuant mass in the medial labia majora.

How are Bartholin gland cysts treated?

Asymptomatic cysts need no intervention or antibiotic treatment.

Symptomatic cysts are incised and drained, and **a catheter is placed to form a tract for the drainage of glandular secretions (Word catheter).**

If this procedure fails, then marsupialization can be done (the creation of a new ductal orifice).

The most definitive procedure for a Bartholin cyst after failure of all previous methods is complete excision of the gland.

What microbes are commonly implicated in Bartholin gland abcesses?

E. coli, N. gonorrhoeae, C. trachomatis, and several anaerobes

How are Bartholin gland abscesses managed and treated?

An aspirate and culture of the abscess should be done. Treatment includes antibiotics such as ceftriaxone and clindamycin, and surgical drainage of the pus.

For the following descriptions, list the most appropriate type of cyst or cyst-related condition:

1. Occurring mostly beneath the labia majora, this cyst occurs when the *sebaceous gland duct becomes obstructed*. They are multiple, smooth, and palpable masses that are generally asymptomatic:

   Sebaceous cyst

2. These cysts are lined by *squamous* epithelial cells and contain oily material. They occur in the setting of vulva surgery or arise from obstruction of pilosebaceous ducts. They are usually small, solitary, and asymptomatic:

   Epidermal cyst

3. Apocrine sweat gland cysts are mainly found in the labium majus and become functional after puberty. They are usually small, multiple, and extremely pruritic. This disease occurs when *keratin obstructs the duct*:

   Fox-Fordyce disease

4. This condition occurs with chronic infection of the apocrine glands and is manifested by multiple painful, pruritic, and subcutaneous abscesses. It may be treated with antibiotics or incision:

   Hidradenomas

5. This cystic vulvar tumor is a rare *congenital anomaly* and located near the urethral meatus. It can be treated with partial excision:

   Skene duct cyst

6. Occlusion of a *persistent processus vaginalis* may cause this hydrocele or cystic tumor:

   Cyst of the canal of Nuck

7. These lateral vaginal wall cysts result from dilation of the *mesonephric duct remnants*:

   Gartner duct cyst

8. This is a benign outgrowth of normal skin. More of a solid tumor than a cyst, it must be removed when it causes discomfort:

   Acrochordon (skin tag)

PYODERMAS AND OTHER NONSEXUALLY TRANSMITTED INFECTIONS OF THE VULVA AND VAGINA

What are the specific types of pyodermas?

Cellulitis, impetigo, folliculitis, furuncles, and carbuncles

What is the most common bacterial etiology for all of these pyodermas?

Staphylococcus aureus

How does impetigo manifest?

Vesicles and pustules form in an area that was recently traumatized. They often rupture and form a characteristic golden crusting.

How is it treated?

Erythromycin or dicloxacillin

What is folliculitis? How does it manifest?

An infection of the hair follicles. It can occur with exposure to whirlpools/hot tubs, antibiotic therapy, and shaving of pubic hair. The lesions are multiple, 5 mm, cluster in groups, erythematous, and pruritic.

What is the recommended treatment for folliculitis?

Warm saline compresses and topical antibiotics

What other pyodermas can occur after an episode of folliculitis? Describe them:

Furuncules: a painful nodular lesion that involves the hair follicle and drains pus

Carbuncles: clusters of furuncles or subcutaneous abscesses that drain pus through multiple hair follicle openings

What is the preferred treatment for furuncules and carbuncles?

Warm compresses to promote spontaneous drainage in furunculosis

Patients with systemic symptoms of furuncules and/or carbuncles warrant empiric oral antibiotic therapy followed by guided therapy based on cultures and sensitivity

What is erysipelas?

Rapidly spreading erythematous lesions of the skin caused by **invasion of the superficial lymphatics by β-hemolytic streptococci**. It usually occurs after trauma or a surgical procedure to the vulva. Pustules, vesicles, and bullae may appear.

How is erysipelas treated?

Oral penicillin or tetracycline

What is hidradenitis suppurativa? How is it treated?

A more severe condition of hidradenomas that occurs when the cysts develop into abscesses and rupture. **Draining sinus tracts develop deep within the skin, and scars, fibrosis, hyperpigmentation, and pitting** can be seen over the vulva. It is treated by drainage and antibiotic therapy.

What is the agent that commonly causes nocturnal perineal itching in children? How is it diagnosed and what is the treatment?

Enterobius vermicularis (pinworm). Apply adhesive tape to the perineum and look for ova under the microscope for diagnosis. Mebendazole is the treatment of choice.

OTHER VULVAR DISORDERS

Trauma to the vulva can occur in both children and women. Straddle-type injuries are the most common cause of vulvar hematomas in children whereas trauma incurred during vaginal delivery is the main etiology in women of reproductive age.

What vessels are most commonly involved in vulvar hematomas?

Branches from the pudendal artery

What are the common symptoms?

Severe perineal pain within the first 24 hours is usually the first symptom of a rapidly expanding vulvar hematoma. Rapid appearance of a tense, palpable, fluctuant, and sensitive tumor of varying size covered by discolored skin readily gives a diagnosis of vulvar hematoma.

How are vulvar hematomas managed?

The two primary modalities are

1. Conservative management with analgesia and ice packs
2. Surgical drainage is warranted for large hematomas (> 3 cm)

CLINICAL VIGNETTES

A 26-year-old female presents to the office with complaints of malodorous, grayish discharge for the past 3 days. She denies dysuria, dyspareunia, or pelvic discomfort. She is sexually active with two partners and intermittently uses condoms. She is concerned as one of her partners was recently treated for Chlamydia. A speculum examination is performed and a sample of vaginal fluid is examined underneath the microscope. Many vaginal epithelial cells with adherent clusters of bacteria are seen on the field.

1. What do you expect the pH of the vaginal fluid to be?
   a. pH less than 4.5
   b. pH greater than 4.5

2. What is the diagnosis?
   a. Bacterial Vaginosis
   b. *Chlamydia trachomatis*
   c. *N. Gonorrhea*
   d. Trichomonas

3. Do you need to treat this STI in her partners?
   a. Yes
   b. No

Answers: 1:b; 2: a; 3: b

Bacterial Vaginosis (BV) is the most common cause of infectious vaginitis and manifests as thin, white/gray discharge with a musty or fishy odor. It is caused by an alteration of the normal flora and an overgrowth of anaerobes such as *Gardnerella vaginalis*. Diagnosis is usually based on a positive amine or "whiff" test; the presence of clue cells (vaginal epithelial cells with clusters of bacteria adhering) in a sample of vaginal fluid when examined under microscopy; and a change in pH of the vaginal fluid (pH > 4.5). BV is considered an STI, however, sexual partners do not need to be treated.

What is the most common female sexual disorder?

a. Orgasmic disorder
b. Sexual arousal disorder
c. Vaginismus
d. Hypoactive sexual desire disorder (HSDD)

Answer: d

The most common sexual dysfunction is HSDD. It is important to screen patients in a comfortable, professional manner for sexual function. Treatment for HSDD is multifaceted with counseling and medications.

A 20-year-old woman is evaluated in urgent care because of 3-day history of fever and lower abdominal pain. She denies urinary frequency, dysuria, flank pain, nausea, or vomiting. Her only medication is an oral contraceptive agent. Her vitals are: temperature 38.4°C, blood pressure 116/68 mm Hg, pulse rate 102/min, and respiration rate 16/min. Examination is significant for lower abdominal tenderness on palpation. There is no flank tenderness. Pelvic examination is positive for cervical motion tenderness and bilateral adnexal tenderness on bimanual examination. The leukocyte count and urinalysis are normal. Urine and serum pregnancy tests are negative. How should she be treated?

    a. Ceftriaxone, IM and Doxycycline, po
    b. Azithromycin, po
    c. Metronidazole, po
    d. Ampicillin and Gentamycin IV

Answer: a

The patient has pelvic inflammatory disease (PID). It is an acute infection of the female genital tract caused by polymicrobes and usually occurs in young, sexually active females. Diagnostic features include abdominal discomfort, uterine or adnexal tenderness, or cervical motion tenderness. Although not required for diagnosis, the presence of one or more of the following enhances the specificity for PID: fever greater than 38.3°C (101.0°F), cervical or vaginal mucopurulent discharge, leukocytes in vaginal secretions, and documentation of gonorrheal or chlamydial infection. All women should be tested for infection with chlamydia and gonorrhea, and undergo a pregnancy test. Antibiotics must treat for both organisms: Outpatients are treated with ceftriaxone and doxycycline with or without metronidazole for 14 days. Metronidazole (choice a) is not an effective treatment for either chlamydia or gonorrhea and is usually added to standard PID regimens if there is an increased risk for anaerobes. Azithromycin (choice b) is sufficient treatment for chlamydia but is no longer recommended as initial treatment for gonorrhea given the high prevalence of resistant strains. Ampicillin and gentamycin (choice d) do not effectively treat gonorrhea and chlamydial infection.

A 25-year-old woman presents to you complaining of two days of fever, fatigue, headache, and painful sores in the genital area. The patient has no previous history of genital lesions. Medical history is unremarkable, and her only medication is an oral contraceptive agent. She does not use condoms. Her last sexual intercourse was 5 days ago. She denies photophobia, neck pain, and nausea and vomiting. Her temperature in the office is 38.0°C (100.5°F). Her physical examination is significant for painful, shallow, ulcerative lesions with some yellow crusting that covers labia bilaterally and vaginal introitus. Inguinal lymphadenopathy is not appreciated on examination. Which of the following tests will reveal the correct diagnosis?

    a. Dark field microscopy of a specimen from the ulcer to reveal spirochetes.
    b. Gram stain of a specimen from an ulcer base to reveal a "school of fish" pattern.
    c. Viral culture for HSV-1 and HSV-2.
    d. Giemsa or Wright staining of tissue specimen to reveal Donovan bodies.

Answer: c

The patient's symptoms and physical findings are consistent with a primary episode of genital herpes simplex virus (HSV) infection, which is more commonly caused by HSV-2. In a primary episode, the virus is passed by direct sexual contact with an infected person. After a 4- day incubation period, ulcerative, painful, pustular lesions erupt, and can be accompanied by local lymphadenopathy and systemic symptoms. The diagnosis of genital herpes is often suspected on clinical grounds but may be confirmed by viral culture or serologic testing. Viral culture for HSV-1 and HSV-2 is a rapid test, with results often available by the next day. The specificity of viral culture approaches 100%, but the sensitivity varies with the quality of specimen handling and the age of the lesion (older, crusted lesions have lower yield).

Dark field microscopy test (choice a) will help in the diagnosis of syphilis. This patient's physical examination does not describe a chancre (painless, single, clean-based ulcer). A positive gram stain that shows a "school of fish" pattern (gram-negative rods in a chain) helps diagnose chancroid. Although this patient does have painful ulcers, the ulcers in chancroid are often deep, purulent, and with ragged edges. They are often associated with painful, suppurative, unilateral inguinal lymph nodes that may rupture (bubo). Lastly, Giemsa or Wright staining which reveals Donovan bodies (choice d) is used to diagnose granuloma inguinale (Donovanosis). These ulcers are typically painless with an ulcer base that is clean but with friable margins that easily bleed and are beefy red in appearance.

A 24-year-old female comes to your office concerned that she is having bloody spotting in between her menstrual periods for the past 2 months. She denies abdominal or pelvic pain. She does not believe she is pregnant as she started combined oral contraceptive pills (OCPs) approximately 2 months ago. What is your next step in management?

   a. **Order a vaginal ultrasound now to assess for endometrial hyperplasia.**
   b. **Order a urine β-hCG test now to assess for pregnancy.**
   c. **Reassure patient that intermenstrual bleeding is common in the first 3 months after starting OCPs and does not require further evaluation.**
   d. **Perform a speculum examination now to examine for any cervical or endometrial infections.**

Answer: c

Intermenstrual ("breakthrough") spotting and bleeding occur in approximately 25% of women during the first 3 months of use. Patients should be counseled to anticipate breakthrough bleeding (choice c). When intermenstrual bleeding occurs after 3 months of use, the patient should be evaluated for causes of bleeding unrelated to oral contraceptive use, including cervical or endometrial infection (choice d), neoplasia (choice a) and pregnancy (choice b). If bleeding persists and is known to be due to combined OCPs, a short course of oral estrogen can be used for management.

A 24-year-old woman is evaluated for worsening pelvic pain just prior to and during menses for the past 5 months. Previously, she had no peri-menstrual pain. She also complains of a 2-year history of dyspareunia, which is now becoming more severe. She has only had two sexual partners and consistently used barrier contraception. She has no history of sexually transmitted infections, pelvic inflammatory disease, abnormal Pap smears or pregnancies. Her physical examination reveals tenderness to palpation in the lower quadrants, with no rebound or guarding. Her external genitalia are normal, and the cervix appears healthy. There is no cervical motion tenderness, but pain is felt on uterine motion. Which of the following tests is the most appropriate next step in diagnosis?

a. Colonoscopy
b. Cystoscopy
c. Hysterosalpingography
d. Transvaginal ultrasonography

Answer: d

This patient has endometriosis. It is a common cause of pelvic pain that is estrogen responsive and therefore changes in a cyclical manner according to menstrual changes in estrogen levels. Diagnostic clues include a change in menstrual discomfort after a history of pain-free menses, lower back pain, dyspareunia, and tenderness upon pelvic examination during menses (most common finding). Transvaginal ultrasonography (choice d) is 100% sensitive and specific for endometriosis **in the ovary.** Laparoscopy with biopsy of endometrial tissue has been the gold standard for diagnosis. Colonoscopy (choice a) is used for symptoms and signs involving the lower gastrointestinal tract (ie, bleeding from the rectum, diarrhea). Cystoscopy (choice b) is usually used to evaluate complaints and signs involving the genitourinary tract (ie, hematuria, dysuria). Lastly, hysterosalpingography (choice c) is indicated in the evaluation of infertility and recurrent miscarriage to rule out mechanical obstruction within the fallopian tube.

A 32-year-old woman comes to your office with complaints of severe lower abdominal cramping, dyspareunia, and anorgasmia for the past 2 years. She was in a monogamous relationship until 6 months ago and is now sexually active with a new partner. She reports no vaginal discharge or abnormal bleeding; she has no history of sexually transmitted diseases and bowel movements are normal. She does report feeling anxious and having trouble sleeping for the past 2 years. On examination, she is intermittently tearful. Her abdomen is soft, with tenderness on palpation of the lower quadrants. Her external genitalia and cervix appear healthy; she has no cervical motion tenderness but does have pain on deep palpation of her uterus. Guaiac stool is negative for blood. What is your next best step in management?

a. Screen for conversion disorder.
b. Screen for malingering.
c. Order a transvaginal ultrasonography.
d. Screen for post-traumatic stress disorder.

Answer: d

This patient has symptoms and signs reflecting chronic pelvic pain (CPP). Chronic pelvic pain is noncyclic pain of nonmenstrual origin that lasts more than 6 months. It is a complex syndrome related to neurologic, psychologic, musculoskeletal, and endocrinologic factors. Many women with CPP have a history of sexual abuse or victimization, so screening for post-traumatic stress disorder (choice d) is recommended. Conversion disorder (choice a) is characterized by complaints of the acute onset of a symptom, usually neurological, typically in the setting of extreme stress. Malingering (choice b) is characterized by the intentional feigning or exaggerating of physical or psychological symptoms for personal gain. This patient does not fit this profile. Although endometriosis is a common cause of chronic pelvic pain, this patient's pain is not cyclical with her menses. Therefore, a vaginal ultrasound (choice c) is unlikely to reveal the cause of her pain.

A 22-year-old female with a pregnancy at 8-weeks gestation asks you to perform an elective termination. All of the below mentioned techniques may be used except which of the following?

a. Manual vacuum curettage
b. Sharp curettage
c. Dilation and extraction
d. Intramuscular methotrexate plus oral misoprostol

Answer: c

Suction or manual vacuum curettage (choice a) is the safest and most effective method for terminating pregnancies of 12 weeks duration or less. If suction curettage cannot be performed, then sharp curettage (dilation and curettage) (choice b) can be used to terminate first trimester pregnancies. Medical abortion agents for first trimester pregnancies include methotrexate and misoprostol, or oral mifepristone (choice d). Dilation and extraction (choice c) is the most common surgical technique for second trimester pregnancy abortion.

A 35-year-old African-American woman presents to your office with complaints of increasingly heavy and prolonged menstrual periods over the past year. She also describes a feeling of "fullness" in her pelvic area. In addition, she reports having mild dyspareunia. She is happily married to her husband and they have two children. They are considering having another child in the near future. Presently, she uses oral contraceptive pills for birth control.

In addition to her chief complaint, she reports feeling "more tired." She attributes this to her job, as she is the vice-president for a consulting company and has recently been working longer hours. Her past medical history is unremarkable. Her physical examination is remarkable for pale conjunctiva on eye examination. On bimanual examination, a large mobile uterus with an irregular contour is appreciated. What is the next most appropriate step in management?

a. Perform an exploratory laparoscopy.
b. Obtain a pelvic ultrasound.
c. Obtain an MRI of the pelvis.
d. Perform an endometrial biopsy.

Answer: b

This patient's symptoms and physical findings are consistent with uterine fibroids or leiomyomas. Leiomyomas are hormonally responsive, benign tumors of the smooth muscle cells of the uterus. They are 2 to 3 times more common in African-American women and are found in 20% to 30% of reproductive-age women. This patient presents with classic symptoms of fibroids: menorrhagia or metrorrhagia, pelvic pressure or pain, dyspareunia, and symptomatic anemia. Diagnosis of fibroids can usually be made via pelvic ultrasonography (choice b). Treatment can include either medical therapy with progestion or GnRH analogues, or surgical therapies including myomectomy, uterine artery embolization, or hysterectomy. An exploratory laparoscopy (choice a) would be indicated if endometriosis was suspected; however, this patient's pain is not cyclical with her menses. An MRI of the pelvis (choice c) is helpful if the clinical suspicion for fibroids is high but the ultrasound is unrevealing (submucosal fibroids may not be detected by ultrasound); however initial imaging is pelvic ultrasonography. An endometrial biopsy (choice d) would be indicated if the ultrasound revealed abnormally increased endometrial thickness.

A 22-year-old female complains of a 1-year history of lower abdominal cramping pain, particularly during the first few days of her menses. She denies dysuria, urinary frequency, or constipation. She has never been sexually active. She denies relief of her abdominal pain with defecation. She has tried acetaminophen but without relief. Her physical examination is significant for mild, lower abdominal tenderness on palpation. No masses or hepatosplenomegaly are appreciated. Bowel sounds are normal. Pelvic examination reveal bilateral lower-abdominal tenderness but otherwise normal. An abdominal x-ray and pelvic ultrasound are normal. Which of the following would you use to treat this patient's pain?

a. Naprosyn
b. Percocet
c. Oral contraceptive pills (OCPs)
d. Colace and senna

Answer: a

This patient has primary dysmenorrhea, a common cause of lower abdominal pain in women in their late teens or early twenties. Dysmenorrhea typically occurs at the onset of menses and is thought to be hormonally-related. Physical examination and imaging are usually negative for anatomic or pathologic abnormalities. Naprosyn and other NSAIDs (choice a) are generally safe and are often effective initial treatment for this symptom. Although OCPs (choice c) may be helpful in treating symptoms of primary dysmenorrheal, an empiric trial of NSAIDs should be initially used. An initial trial of NSAIDs is also preferable to starting pain medications containing low-dose opioids (choice b). The patient denies constipation and there is no evidence of constipation on the abdominal plain film. As well, the timing of her abdominal pain in relation to her menses is inconsistent with a diagnosis of constipation; thus, colace and senna (choice d) would not effectively treat this patient's pain.

CHAPTER 5

Gynecologic Oncology

Cervical Cancer

INTRODUCTION

Describe the three histologic regions of the cervix:

1. **Ectocervix:** the inferior portion of the cervix that is continuous with the vagina; covered with squamous epithelium
2. **Squamocolumnar junction (SCJ):** separates two regions of the cervix (often with overlap)
3. **Endocervix:** the superior portion of the cervix that begins at the external os and continues to the endocervical canal; covered with mucin-secreting **columnar epithelium** and continues into the cuboidal epithelium of the endometrium

Describe the location of the SCJ:

Throughout a woman's life, the SCJ **migrates internally** toward the endocervix via the metaplasia.

What is the transformation zone?

The 1 to 3 cm area of **squamous metaplasia** that separates the endocervix from the ectocervix created from the internal migration of the SCJ. It is the area **most susceptible to the development of cervical neoplasia** because of the metaplastic changes. See Fig. 5.1.

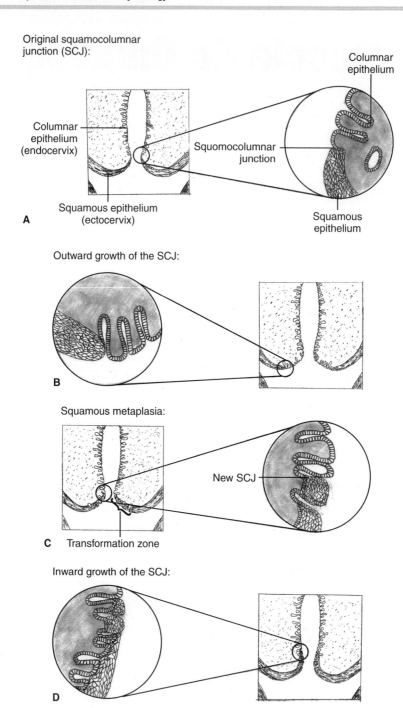

Figure 5.1   The cervical transformation zone.

What is the incidence of cervical cancer?

It is the second leading cause of malignancy in women worldwide but comprises only 1% of all cancer deaths of women in the United States.

Who does cervical cancer affect?

Sexually active women, usually in a bimodal age distribution with peaks in the late 30s and in the early 60s

What are the risk factors for cervical cancer?

HPV infection

Sexual history: early onset of sexual activity; multiple sexual partners; history of sexually transmitted infections (STIs); sex with high-risk partners

Smoking

High parity

Immunosuppression

Low socioeconomic status

Pelvic radiation

Prior history of vulvar or vaginal squamous dysplasia

What is the epidemiologic relationship between HPV infection and cervical cancer?

Human papillomavirus (HPV) is found in nearly all cases of squamous cell cervical cancer and is thought to **contribute to the pathogenesis of** dysplasia. While most HPV infections self-resolve, some progress to genital warts or cervical dysplasia. HPV infection is therefore deemed **necessary but not sufficient** for the development of cervical cancer.

How does HPV infection lead to cervical cancer?

HPV initially infects the basal layer cervical cells, forming **koilocytes** within the cells. HPV can then **integrate into the cells genome,** altering the expression of the cell's regulatory genes. This leads to intraepithelial neoplasia and/or cancer.

What serotypes of HPV most commonly cause cervical cancer?

HPV 16, 18, 31, 33, and 45

In what other types of neoplasia is HPV thought to be a causative agent?

1. **Vaginal intraepithelial neoplasia** (VAIN) and vaginal malignancies
2. **Vulvar intraepithelial neoplasia** (VIN) and vulvar malignancies

What are the types of cervical cancer, how common are each worldwide, and where in relation to the SCJ do they occur?

Squamous cell carcinomas: 80% to 90% of all cervical cancers, occur below the SCJ

Adenocarcinomas: 15% of all cervical cancers (although increasing prevalence), occur above the SCJ

Adenosquamous carcinomas: 3% to 5% of all cervical cancers

Neuroendocrine, small cell carcinomas, clear cell carcinomas, melanomas, lymphomas, and sarcomas can all originate in the cervix but are rare

What are the signs/symptoms of cervical cancer?

Early stages of cervical dysplasia and cancer are asymptomatic. There is no **classic presentation for cervical** cancer but the most common symptom is **abnormal vaginal bleeding** (either postcoital, postmenopausal, or intermenstrual).

Symptoms of late stage disease include: **vaginal discharge,** pain (usually pelvic or lower back pain), weight loss, hematuria (vaginal passage of blood in urine) or hematochezia (passage of blood in stool).

Signs on cervical examination can range from a normal gross appearance with aberrant cytology to a cervix entirely replaced with tumor.

What is the differential diagnosis of these symptoms?

Cervicitis, vaginitis, STI

How is the definitive diagnosis of cervical cancer made?

Cervical biopsy if the lesion is grossly visible. If the lesion is only diagnosable microscopically, a **colposcopic-directed biopsy** or diagnostic **conization** (for microinvasive disease) are modalities for diagnosis.

Upon diagnosis, what other tests need to be done?

A comprehensive physical examination to evaluate metastases, including cervical and vaginal inspection, a rectovaginal examination, and palpation of the liver and lymph nodes (inguinal and supraclavicular)

Laboratory and imaging tests to evaluate for metastases

What do each of the following contribute to the evaluation of cervical cancer?

Chest x-ray:	Identifies lung metastasis.
Intravenous pyelogram:	Identifies bladder involvement, but has been largely replaced by CT, MRI, or cystoscopy.
MRI, CT, or lymphangiography:	Identifies nodal involvement, tumor size, and abdominal/retroperitoneal spread; CT and MRI cannot be used for staging purposes.
Renal function tests:	Identifies urinary tract metastasis.
Liver function tests:	Identifies liver metastasis.
Barium enema:	Identifies colonic metastasis.

How and to where does cervical cancer spread?

Direct extension to contiguous structures

Lymphatic dissemination to any of the pelvic lymph node groups

Hematogenous dissemination most commonly to the **lungs, liver,** and **bone** although it can spread to the large intestine, adrenals, spleen, or brain as well

Intraperitoneal implantation

What are the stages of cervical cancer?

The **FIGO system** is based on the histological assessment, the physical examination, and the laboratory results. See Table 5.1.

What are the overall survival rates for cervical cancer?

The survival rates **depend most significantly on the stage of disease** at diagnosis. The 5-year survival rates for each stage are:

Stage I: over 90%

Stage II: 75%

Stage III: 40%

Stage IV: under 15%

What is the differential diagnosis of a cervical mass?

Nabothian cysts

Glandular hyperplasia

Mesonephric remnants

Reactive glandular changes

Endometriosis

Table 5.1 The Stages of Cervical Cancer

Stage			
I			**Carcinoma confined to the cervix**
	IA		Invasive carcinoma diagnosable only by microscopy
		IA1	Minimal microscopic invasion < 3 mm deep and < 7 mm horizontally
		IA2	Microscopic lesions < 5 mm deep and < 7 mm horizontally
	IB		Clinically visible lesions that are confined to the cervix
II			**Carcinoma extends beyond the cervix, but not to the pelvic wall or lower third of the vagina**
	IIA		No parametrial involvement
	IIB		Parametrial involvement
III			**Carcinoma extends to the pelvic wall and/or lower third of the vagina. Also includes all cases with hydronephrosis**
	IIIA		No extension to pelvic wall, but involvement of lower third of vagina
	IIIB		Extension to pelvic wall or hydronephrosis
IV			**Carcinoma extends beyond the true pelvis or clinically involves the mucosa of the bladder or rectum**
	IVA		Spread to adjacent pelvic organs
	IVB		Spread to distant organs

CERVICAL CANCER SCREENING AND PREVENTION

What is a Pap smear and how is it done?

A cytological examination of the cervix. A small brush scrapes cells from the endocervix and ectocervix. These cells are either spread on a microscopic slide and fixed or placed in a liquid medium for evaluation.

What is the difference between a Pap smear and the thin-layer liquid-based cytology (ThinPrep, SurePath)?

In a **traditional Pap smear,** a spatula or brush is used to collect cells on the ectocervix and then from the endocervix. The specimen is rolled or smeared onto a slide and rapidly fixed. A single slide can be used to examine both ectocervical and endocervical cells.

Liquid-based cytology involves taking cells from the ectocervix and endocervix and placing the specimens in vials containing preservative solutions. The vials are placed in a ThinPrep processor machine and ultimately, the cells are transferred to a slide. This technique results in a monolayer of cells on the slide, which can be read more quickly than conventional cytology slides.

How often should a Pap smear be done?

The general consensus to date is an **annual examination beginning at the age of 21 or by 3 years after the onset of sexual activity.** If a female is over the age of 30 years, low-risk, and has three negative Pap smears, she can then get repeat evaluations every 3 years.

What are some of the limitations of Pap smear screening?

Not all patients have access (the most important limiting factor); it is less successful in diagnosing adenocarcinoma; it has a low sensitivity and therefore a high false-negative rate.

What is the difference between cytology and histology in evaluation of cervical dysplasia?

Cytology is based on the Pap smear. Histology is based on a colposcopic biopsy.

What are the cytological definitions of the Bethesda system?

Low-grade squamous intraepithelial lesion (**LSIL** or LGSIL).

High-grade squamous intraepithelial lesion (**HSIL** or HGSIL).

Atypical squamous cells of undetermined significance (**ASCUS**).

Atypical squamous cells that cannot exclude HSIL (**ASCH**). See Table 5.2.

Table 5.2 The Bethesda System

Bethesda System	Dysplasia/CIN System
Atypical squamous cells of undetermined significance	Squamous atypia
Low-grade squamous intraepithelial lesion	HPV atypia
High-grade squamous intraepithelial lesion	CIN I
	CIN II
	CIN III

Describe the histologic definition of cervical intraepithelial neoplasia (CIN) and of each of the stages:

CIN refers to precancerous pathology that can slowly progress to cervical cancer.

CIN I: formerly known as mild dysplasia, is a **cellular dysplasia confined to the basal one-third of the epithelium.**

CIN II: refers to **lesions confined to the basal two-thirds of the epithelium** that used to be referred to as moderate dysplasia.

CIN III: formerly known as severe dysplasia and carcinoma in situ (CIS), is a **cellular dysplasia that affects more than two-thirds of the epithelium.**

How rapidly does cervical dysplasia progress to cervical cancer?

Cervical cancer in general progresses slowly and mild dysplasia (CIN I) often spontaneously regresses It is estimated that is takes 3 to 10 years for women with CIN III to progress to cervical cancer.

What is colposcopy?

A binocular stereomicroscope that **magnifies the cervix** that is used to visualize changes consistent with dysplasia, allowing for directed biopsy.

What must be seen in order to consider colposcopy satisfactory?

The entirety of the SCJ and the entire lesion in question

What findings on colposcopy are suggestive of cervical cancer?

Abnormal blood vessels; abnormal appearing surface of the cervix; color change

What is endocervical curettage?

A sampling procedure of the endocervix used to retrieve cells further inside the cervical canal that can be visualized with colposcopy.

What should be done if the ECC is positive?

Because there is no tissue orientation, **a positive ECC warrants conization**

What is cervical conization?

A cone-shaped biopsy of the entire SCJ that allows diagnosis via histologic criteria

How is cervical conization done?

Either via **cold knife conization** (scalpel excision in the OR) or **loop electrosurgical excision procedure** (LEEP) (via heated wire)

What are the four common indications for conization in order of their frequency?

1. CIN III
2. Unsatisfactory colposcopy
3. Positive endocervical curettage
4. A discrepancy between Pap smear and biopsy results

What are the risks of cervical conization?

Infection, blood loss, risks from anesthesia, cervical stenosis, and cervical insufficiency

What is the appropriate workup of each of the following abnormal Paps?

LSIL:

Colposcopy.
If ≤ CIN I, the patient can be just followed-up with repeat Pap/colpo.

HSIL:

Warrants a **colposcopy followed by direct ablation or excision.**

ASCUS:

HPV DNA testing. If high-risk HPV+, colposcopy should be done. If high-risk HPV−, then a repeat Pap smear can be done in 12 months.

Alternatively, a repeat Pap smear can be done every 6 months until there are three consecutive negative smears.

Menopausal women may have an atrophic component leading to this cytology, and they can be given **intravaginal estrogen** and followed-up every 6 months.

Women with an infection should be reexamined once their infection is treated.

Immunosuppressed women with ASCUS need colposcopy.

Glandular cell abnormalities:

All glandular cell abnormalities warrant **colposcopy** and **endocervical sampling.**

How often should patients be followed up after treatment of noninvasive abnormalities?	Because of the greater risk of recurrence, patients need to be followed **every 3 to 6 months for 2 years after ablation or excision.**
What types of vaccination is now available to prevent cervical cancer?	**Gardasil,** a quadravalent vaccine protecting against HPV 6, 11, 16, and 18
Who should get this vaccination?	Females (and males) aged between 9 to 26 years
Do vaccinated individuals still need to get Pap smears?	**Yes!** The vaccine only protects against four of the many HPV serotypes that cause cervical cancer.

SQUAMOUS CELL CARCINOMA OF THE CERVIX

Who gets squamous cell carcinoma (SCC) of the cervix?	There is a bimodal age distribution with peaks between 35 and 40 years and between 60 and 65 years.
What are the five prognostic indicators for SCC?	1. **Stage of disease** (most important) 2. Lymph node involvement 3. Tumor size 4. Depth of stromal invasion 5. Invasion of lymphovascular space
What are the treatment options for invasive SCC of the cervix and what are the indications of each?	**Cervical conization:** used for women with Stage Ia1 with no involvement of the lymphovascular space who wish to preserve fertility.
	Radical trachelectomy: involves surgical removal of the cervix and parametria and placement of a cerclage, and can be combined with a laparoscopic or open diagnostic/ therapeutic lymphadenectomy with paraaortic lymph node sampling; used for women with Stage Ia1 with involvement of the lymphovascular space, Stage Ia2 or Stage Ib1 disease who wish to preserve fertility.
	Radical hysterectomy: used for premenopausal women with early stage (up to Stage IIa) cervical cancer who wish to preserve ovarian function.
	Chemoradiotherapy alone: used for women with more advanced disease Chemoradiotherapy versus surgery for Ib2 is controversial.

What is the recommended treatment for each of the following stages of cervical cancer?

Ia1: conization or simple hysterectomy

Ia2–early IIb: radical hysterectomy with a pelvic lymphadenectomy or chemoradiotherapy

Late IIb–IV: chemoradiotherapy or combination chemotherapy

What are the indications for adjuvant chemoradiotherapy?

If a patient has any of the following:

Positive resection margins

Positive lymph nodes

Parametrial involvement

What types of chemotherapy are used for cervical cancer treatment and how do they work?

Cisplatin with or without **5-FU.**

Cisplatin is a cycle-nonspecific alkylating agent that cross-links DNA.

5-FU is a cycle-specific DNA synthesis inhibitor.

What are the main side effects of the following?

   Cisplatin:

Leukopenia, ototoxicity, nephrotoxicity, and peripheral neuropathy

   5-FU:

Fatigue, diarrhea, nausea, vomiting, and myelosuppression

The two main methods of radiation delivery for cervical cancer are external photon beam radiation therapy (RT) and intracavitary brachytherapy. When is each indicated?

Intracavitary brachytherapy alone is adequate treatment for Stage Ia1 disease

External beam RT is generally added to brachytherapy to improve pelvic control with more advanced disease.

What are the side effects of radiation?

Acute side effects: nausea, diarrhea, and skin damage

Long-term complications: **cystitis, proctitis,** vaginal foreshortening, stenosis, and dryness (which leads to **sexual dysfunction**), development of fistulae, small bowel obstruction

What are the complications of surgery?

Postoperative complications: hemorrhage, fever, sepsis, pulmonary embolus, and infection

Long-term complications: bladder dysfunction, strictures of the ureter, lymphocyst formation, and fistula formation

What type of surveillance is indicated in posttreatment for SCC?

Patients need to be evaluated **every 3 months for the first 2 years** after treatment. After these 2 years, they must be seen every 4 months in the third year, every 6 months for 5 years, and annually thereafter. These evaluations must include careful attention to the supraclavicular and inguinal lymph nodes, a rectovaginal examination, and an abdominal examination. A Pap smear must be done at each visit.

What is the treatment for recurrence?

It depends on patient and presentation, however in general, patients who were initially surgically treated may receive radiotherapy. Patients initially treated with radiotherapy may be surgically treated if their recurrence is localized or they may receive chemotherapy.

What are the 5-year survival rates for the following stages of SCC?

Stage I:	85% to 90%
Stage II:	60% to 80%
Stage III:	30%
Stage IV:	10%

ADENOCARCINOMA OF THE CERVIX

What are the types of adenocarcinoma?

Mucinous; endometrioid; clear cell; serous

What is the incidence of cervical adenocarcinoma?

Accounts for 15% of cervical cancers, however this rate has been rising

What are the risk factors for the development of cervical adenocarcinoma?

The same risk factors as for SCC

How is cervical adenocarcinoma classified?

Using the **Bethesda system** which divides it into four subgroups:

1. **Atypical glandular cells** (AGC)—either endocervical, endometrial, or unspecified
2. **AGC favoring neoplasia**—either endocervical, endometrial, or unspecified
3. **Endocervical adenocarcinoma in situ** (AIS)
4. **Adenocarcinoma**

What are some of the theories for the rise in the diagnosis of AIS?

Improved detection

An increase in the prevalence of the pathogenic serotype of HPV (HPV 18)

An increase in oral contraceptive use (more associated with adenocarcinoma than SCC)

What is the epidemiologic relationship between AIS and SCC of the cervix?

About 50% of women found to have adenocarcinoma have concomitant SCC or CIN.

How is AIS diagnosed?

It is usually asymptomatic and is found through the following:

1. **Cervical cytology** with **colposcopy-directed biopsy** (not sensitive)
   a. cold knife conization—best method
   b. electroexcision—may obscure margins
2. **Endocervical curettage** (improves the detection rate if used with the above methods)

What is the microscopic appearance of cervical adenocarcinoma?

Endocervical glands crowded together in a cribiform pattern, lined by atypical columnar epithelial cells. **Multifocal** disease is often found.

What is the gross appearance of cervical adenocarcinomas?

Half are exophytic, some are ulcerative, and some have the lesion within the endocervical canal (and so it is not visible)

What are the treatment options for microinvasive disease/carcinoma in situ?

There is not a consensus; however the following options are acceptable:

1. **Simple hysterectomy** (generally recommended if fertility need not be preserved)
2. Radical hysterectomy
3. Conization (however, margins have poor predictive value for residual disease)
4. Radical trachelectomy

How should a patient be followed after the diagnosis of AIS if she does not have a hysterectomy?

With cervical cytology and endocervical sampling, every 6 months, indefinitely

What are the treatment options for adenocarcinoma?

Similar to that of SCC. However, adenocarcinomas tend to be more bulky and therefore more often warrant radiotherapy, even with earlier stage disease.

What are the prognostic indicators for adenocarcinoma?

Prognosis primarily depends on **stage**. However, in general, adenocarinoma is more aggressive than SCC and so survival rates are slightly lower.

What are the 5-year survival rates for the following stages of adenocarcinoma?

Stage I: 70% to 75%

Stage II: 30% to 40%

Stage III: 20% to 30%

Stage IV: Less than 15%

Vulvar and Vaginal Cancer

VULVAR CANCER OVERVIEW

What are the designations of preinvasive vulvar malignancy?

Vulvar intraepithelial neoplasia, classified into three levels:

VIN-I: mild dysplasia

VIN-II: moderate dysplasia

VIN-III: severe dysplasia or carcinoma in situ

How do each of the preinvasive lesions typically present?

VIN-I and VIN-II present most commonly with **itching, chronic irritation,** and development of a **palpable lesion.**

The lesion typically appears as localized, isolated, raised, whitish areas found most commonly along the posterior vulva and perineal body.

How is VIN treated?

Complete excision. Early cases with limited involvement can be treated with local excision, cryocautery, electrodesiccation, or laser ablation. VIN-III is treated with wide local excision with/without laser ablation.

What is the incidence of vulvar cancer?

Vulvar cancer is the fourth most common gynecologic cancer that affects almost 4000 women in the United States annually.

Whom does vulvar cancer affect?

Typically, postmenopausal women, usually around 65 years of age

What are the risk factors for vulvar cancer?

Infection with certain types of HPV

History of cervical cancer

Immunocompromise

Northern European ancestry

Cigarette smoking

Diabetes

Vulvar dystrophy

Obesity

Vulvar intraepithelial neoplasia

How is the diagnosis of vulvar cancer made?

Biopsy of each lesion leads to a definitive diagnosis as gross appearance is often inconsistent with the underlying cellular morphology.

If there is no obvious lesion, **colposcopy** may be used. The skin can be washed with a dilute **acetic acid solution** to accentuate any lesions or aberrant vascular patterns.

What other test should be ordered after biopsy?

A synchronous secondary malignancy is found in over 20% of patients with vulvar cancer and so screenings for a secondary malignancy as well as for metastasis should be done.

Screenings may include: **CXR; IVP; LFTs; renal function tests; CT scan.**

If the lesion is located near the anus then a **barium enema** is warranted and if the lesion is located near the urethra then cystoscopy is warranted.

What is the differential diagnosis of a suspected vulvar cancer?

Epidermal inclusion cysts; seborrheic keratoses

Lentigo condyloma acuminata

Bartholin gland disorders; lichen sclerosus

Acrochordons; hidradenomas

What are the types of vulvar cancer?

Over 90% of vulvar cancers are primary cancers.

Types of primary vulvar cancers include: **squamous cell carcinomas** (90%); **melanomas** (5%); Bartholin gland carcinomas; basal cell carcinomas; sarcomas; lymphomas; endodermal sinus tumors.

Metastasizing cancers to the vulva include **cervical, endometrial, renal, and urethral cancers.**

SQUAMOUS CELL VULVAR CANCER

What are the signs/symptoms of squamous cell vulvar cancer?

Itching, burning, irritation, and/or the development of a **palpable lesion** (plaque, ulcer, or mass).

Bleeding, ulceration, abnormal discharge, dysuria, or an enlarged groin lymph node are usually associated with more advanced disease.

What are the two subtypes of squamous cell carcinoma of the vulva?

1. **Keratinizing type**—occurs in older women; associated with other vulvar dystrophies such as lichen sclerosis but not with HPV; usually unifocal
2. **Warty or basaloid type**—found in younger women; associated with HPV, VIN, and cigarette smoking; usually multifocal

How does squamous cell vulvar cancer spread?

Direct extension: to the vagina, urethra, or anus

Lymphatic dissemination: occurs via the superficial inguinal nodes into the deep inguinal and femoral nodes and finally into the pelvic lymphatics

Hematogenous dissemination: rare; occurs mostly in patients who also have lymphatic dissemination; spreads to lung, liver, and bone

How common is lymphatic spread and what factors predict whether it occurs?

Lymphatic spread **occurs in 30%** of vulvar cancers and its likelihood increases with the size of the lesion and the depth of invasion.

What are the stages of vulvar cancer?

The FIGO system is used to stage vulvar cancer and is based on both the microscopic evaluation of the removed tumor as well as of the regional lymph nodes (see Table 5.3).

Table 5.3 The Stages of Vulvar Cancer

Stage		
Stage 0		
	Tis	Carcinoma in situ; intraepithelial carcinoma
Stage I		
	T1 N0 M0	Tumor confined to the vulva and/or perineum; < 2 cm in diameter; no palpable nodes
Stage II		
	T2 N0 M0	Tumor confined to the vulva and/or perineum; > 2 cm in diameter; no palpable nodes
Stage III		
	T3 N0 M0	Tumor of any size with: (1) adjacent spread to
	T3 N1 M0	the lower urethra and/or the vagina, or the
	T1 N1 M0	anus; and/or (2) unilateral regional lymph
	T2 N1 M0	node metastasis
Stage IVA		
	T1 N2 M0	Tumor invades any of the following: upper
	T2 N2 M0	urethra, bladder mucosa, rectal mucosa, pelvic
	T3 N2 M0	and/or bilateral regional lymph node
	T4 N-any M0	metastasis
Stage IVB		
	T-any N-any M1	Any distant metastasis including pelvic lymph nodes

How is squamous cell vulvar cancer treated?

In general, treatment needs to be **individualized** using the most conservative treatment that will lead to cure of the disease. The possible modalities are listed below:

1. **Groin node dissection** with either **wide local excision** or **radical vulvectomy** is the mainstay of treatment
2. **Adjuvant radiation therapy** can be added postoperative in patients with either positive inguinal nodes or close/positive surgical margins or preoperatively in patients with advanced disease.
3. **Chemoradiotherapy** can be used for advanced stage disease where surgery is associated with high morbidity and mortality.
4. Adjunctive chemotherapy alone is only of limited value.

When is node dissection warranted and how is it done?

All patients with more than 1 mm of stromal invasion require an inguinal femoral lymphadenectomy.

Unilateral lesions only need node dissection on the ipsilateral side if these nodes are negative.

Midline or bilateral lesions warrant bilateral node dissection.

What is the difference between the following?

Wide local excision:

Surgical excision of the lesion down to the layer of underlying fascia that must include at least 1 cm negative surgical margins

Radical vulvectomy:

Excision of both the labia majora and the mons pubis down to the layer of underlying fascia

What are the complications of radical vulvectomy and groin dissection?

Wound infection and **breakdown** (occurs in 40%-50% of cases)

Chronic leg edema (occurs in 30% of cases)

Depression, poor body image, sexual dysfunction

Less commonly: UTIs, deep vein thrombosis (DVT), PE, MI, seromas, hemorrhage, femoral nerve injury, chronic cellulitis, femoral hernias, and fistula development

What are the most important predictors of recurrence and survival?

Lymph node involvement (most important predictor); lesion size

What is the treatment for recurrent disease?

Further surgical resection or **radiotherapy.** Metastatic recurrences are treated with chemotherapy (usually cisplatin, cyclophosphamide, methotrexate, bleomycin, or mitomycin C).

What type of surveillance is indicated posttreatment for vulvar cancer?

Biannual inspection as well as palpation of the vulva and inguinal lymph nodes

What are the survival rates for squamous cell vulvar cancer?

The average 5-year survival rate for all stages is around 70%. If there is no lymphatic spread, survival rates reach up to 90%, but if spread has extended to the deep pelvic nodes, 5-year survival rate drops below 20%.

What is a verrucous carcinoma and how does it present?

A type of squamous cell cancer that grossly has a cauliflower-like appearance.

Who develops verrucous carcinoma?

Usually postmenopausal women; it is associated with HPV infection

How is verrucous carcinoma treated?

Radical local excision

What is the prognosis for verrucous carcinoma?

Good—it grows slowly, does not metastasize often. However, it can be locally destructive.

VULVAR MELANOMA

How does vulvar melanoma present?

Typically in postmenopausal Caucasian women as a **raised pigmented lesion,** usually on the labia minora or clitoris. It is often asymptomatic, however it can present with **itchiness, irritation,** or **bleeding**.

What is the etiology of a vulvar melanoma?

Melanomas can arise either de novo or from a prior nevus.

How is vulvar melanoma staged?

Using the **Breslow** criteria

Because of the direct association of survival with depth, this system measures the thickness of the lesion from the surface to the deepest point of invasion.

How is vulvar melanoma treated?

Local excision with wide margins.

Groin lymph node dissection is needed for lesions with more than 1 mm invasion.

Sentinal lymph node sampling may also be warranted in women with central primary lesions.

Chemotherapy and radiotherapy do not have good results.

What are survival rates for vulvar melanoma?

Survival is near 100% if the melanoma has not invaded more than 1 mm, but rates decline with increasing dermal depth.

BARTHOLIN GLAND CARCINOMA

What is Bartholin gland carcinoma?

An uncommon type of **adenocarcinoma** that arises mainly from the **epithelium** of the Bartholin ducts/glands.

How does a Bartholin gland carcinoma present?

It typically presents either as an **asymptomatic vulvar mass** or as **perineal pain,** usually in women in their 50s. Because of this, any Bartholin gland enlargement in postmenopausal women must be biopsied.

What are the criteria required to diagnose a vulvar tumor as a Bartholin gland carcinoma?

1. Tumor in the posterior vulva.
2. Tumor is deep in the labia majora.
3. The overlying skin is infracted.
4. There is some recognizable normal gland present.

How is Bartholin gland carcinoma treated?

Because metastasis is common, treatment usually involves a **radical vulvectomy, bilateral lymphadenectomy,** and postoperative **radiation therapy**

What is the survival rate for a Bartholin gland carcinoma?

The 5-year survival is only 50% to 60% as recurrences are common.

BASAL CELL CARCINOMA

What is basal cell carcinoma of the vulva and how does it present?

A rare vulvar cancer that typically presents in postmenopausal Caucasian women as a **vulvar lesion** that has **rolled edges** with **central ulceration** (a "rodent ulcer") usually on the labia majora.

How is basal cell carcinoma treated?

Wide local excision without lymph node dissection.

They are associated with the presence of other malignancies, so treatment also involves a search for concomitant disease.

What are the survival rates for basal cell carcinoma?

Survival rates are overall good; while they are locally aggressive, lymphatic metastasis is rare.

VULVAR SARCOMA

What are the most common types of vulvar sarcoma?

Leiomyosarcoma and **rhabdomyosarcoma**

How does leiomyosarcoma usually present?

As an **enlarging, painful lesion** of the labia majora

How is a leiomyosarcoma treated?

Wide local excision (lymph node involvement is rare)

| In whom is vulvar rhabdomyosarcoma most common? | Children |
| How is vulvar rhabdomyosarcoma treated? | Primary chemotherapy followed by surgery |

PAGET DISEASE OF THE VULVA

What is Paget disease of the vulva and how does it present?	An extensive intraepithelial adenocarcinoma
	It is most commonly found in white women aged 60 to 80 years and it grossly appears as **multifocal, well-demarcated areas of a bright red background with white, hyperkeratotic areas.**
How does Paget disease usually present?	With **pruritis** and **vulvar soreness**
What is the histological appearance of Paget lesions?	Similar to Paget disease of the breast—large pale apocrine cells directly below the epithelium
What is the diagnostic workup for Paget disease?	About 20% to 30% of Paget disease patients will have a noncontiguous carcinoma (especially of the breast, colon, cervix, bladder, or gallbladder) and so evaluation should include an extensive evaluation for these.
What is the treatment for Paget disease?	Either wide local excision or a simple vulvectomy
What is the prognosis of Paget disease?	Local recurrence is common.
	Increased depth of invasion and involvement of the lymph nodes lead to a poorer prognosis.

VAGINAL CANCER OVERVIEW

| Describe preinvasive vaginal malignancy: | Called **vaginal intraepithelial neoplasia (VAIN).** It is squamous atypia without invasion and is classified by depth of involvement. |

What are the designations of preinvasive vaginal malignancy?

VAIN I: involves lower one-third of the epithelium

VAIN II: involves lower two-thirds of the epithelium

VAIN III: involves more than two-thirds of the epithelium; includes carcinoma in situ

How does VAIN typically present?

Usually asymptomatic, but can present as postcoital spotting or **vaginal discharge**

What are the options for VAIN treatment and what are the benefits of each?

Excision: the mainstay of therapy; allows histologic diagnosis

Ablation: well-tolerated but may require repeat administration

Topical chemotherapy: good for multifocal disease or difficult to access lesions

Radiation therapy: a last resort therapy if all else has failed or is contraindicated

Observation: for mild cases

What factors should be considered when deciding on therapeutic modalities for VAIN?

Previous treatment failures; presence of multifocal disease; risks of surgery; desire to preserve sexual function; whether invasive disease has been definitively excluded.

What is the incidence of vaginal cancer and VAIN?

One case per 100,000 women in the United States.

However, the diagnosis of VAIN has been steadily increasing (likely secondary to increased awareness).

What is the most common type of vaginal cancer?

Metastatic cancer from other primary sites, especially cervix

What are the types of primary vaginal cancer?

Squamous cell carcinomas (most common); melanoma; sarcoma; adenocarcinoma

How is the diagnosis of vaginal cancer made?

Digital palpation and **colposcopy** (with acetic acid and Lugol iodine to enhance visualization).

Biopsy of suspicious areas is the definitive diagnostic tool.

| In whom should you aggressively search for VAIN/vaginal cancer? | Postmenopausal women with an abnormal Pap smear; any woman with an abnormal Pap smear without any cervical lesions |

SQUAMOUS CELL VAGINAL CARCINOMA

What are the risk factors for squamous cell vaginal cancer?	HPV infection; HIV infection; increased number of sexual partners; early age at coitarche; smoking; prior lower genital neoplasia
What are the explanations for the association between squamous cell vaginal cancer and other genital neoplasia?	**Extension of disease** → CIN of VIN may spread contiguously to the vagina **Common etiologic factors** → vulvar, cervical, and vaginal cancer share many common etiologies (such as HPV exposure) **Prior radiation** → treatment of prior neoplasia increases susceptibility to later cancers
What are the symptoms of squamous cell vaginal cancer?	Up to one-fifth of all women are **asymptomatic** but are found to have a vaginal mass or atypical Pap smear. Symptoms can include **abnormal vaginal bleeding, vaginal discharge,** vaginal mass, urinary/GI complaints, and pelvic pain.
Where are squamous cell vaginal lesions typically located?	In the **upper one-third of the vagina,** especially the **posterior wall**
How is vaginal cancer staged?	Using the FIGO system which is clinically done using information obtained from the physical examination, cystoscopy, proctoscopy, and x-rays (see Table 5.4).
What are the common primary sites for metastatic vaginal cancer?	Endometrium, breast, cervix, rectum, vulva, kidney, ovary

Table 5.4 The Stages of Vaginal Cancer

Stage		
I		Carcinoma confined to the vaginal mucosa
II		Submucosal infiltration into parametrium, but not extending out to pelvic wall
	IIA	Subvaginal infiltration; no parametrial involvement
	IIB	Parametrial infiltration; not extending to pelvic wall
III		Carcinoma extends to the pelvic wall
IV		Carcinoma extends beyond the true pelvis
	IVA	Infiltration of the mucosa of bladder or rectum or extends outside true pelvis
	IVB	Distant metastatic disease

How do these cancers spread to the vagina?	Either through direct extension or via lymphatic or hematogenous spread
To where and by what routes do primary vaginal cancer spread?	**Direct extension** to bladder, rectum, urethra, parametria, and bony pelvis **Lymphatic spread** to pelvic and paraaortic lymph nodes **Hematogenous dissemination** to lungs, liver, and bone (usually occurs late)
What are the treatment options for vaginal cancer and when is each used?	**Radiation:** the main treatment modality; used with or without surgery for large Stage I or Stages II to IV lesions **Surgery:** used for small, localized Stage I cancer in the upper vagina **Chemotherapy:** sometimes used in combination with radiation with advanced disease, however not shown to be more effective
What are the side effects of treatment?	Fistulas (rectovaginal or vesicovaginal); vaginal or rectal strictures; radiation cystitis or proctitis; vaginal stenosis; radiation-induced menopause

What considerations need to be taken into account when deciding on a treatment modality?	Stage of tumor; proximity of tumor to structures that preclude radiotherapy; anatomical constraints of surgery; future sexual function
What predicts survival rates?	Stage of cancer at presentation
What are the average 5-year survival rates for each stage?	
Stage 0:	95%
Stage 1:	67%
Stage 2:	39%
Stage 3:	33%
Stage 4:	19%

OTHER VAGINAL CANCERS

What is vaginal melanoma and how does it typically present?	A rare but aggressive malignancy of the vaginal mucosa. Occurs in middle-aged Caucasian women and presents as a **dark-colored mass or ulceration,** usually in the distal one-third of the vaginal wall.
What is the 5-year survival rate of vaginal melanoma?	A dismal 10%
When does adenocarcinoma of the vagina typically present?	Usually in women under 20 years
In utero exposure to what leads to vaginal adenocarcinoma?	**DES** (diethylstilbestrol)—it leads to the **clear cell variant** of adenocarcinoma
What is the risk of developing clear cell adenocarcinoma if exposed?	1 in 1000; higher risk is associated with those exposed before 12 weeks of gestation
How does clear cell carcinoma of the vagina present?	As a polypoid vaginal mass in a young woman. DES was discontinued in 1971, so most cases have already been discovered.
What are the major types of vaginal sarcomas?	Rhabdomyosarcomas; leiomyosarcomas; endometrial stromal sarcomas; malignant mixed müllerian tumors
What is the most common form of vaginal sarcoma?	**Embryonal rhabdomyosarcoma or sarcoma botryoides**

What is sarcoma botryoides and how does it present?

A **very aggressive malignant** tumor that presents in early childhood as a vaginal mass that resembles a **bunch of grapes**

How is sarcoma botryoides treated?

Preoperative chemotherapy followed by surgery or radiation

Uterine Cancer

ENDOMETRIAL CANCER

What is endometrial cancer?

An **estrogen-dependent neoplasm** of the endometrium that begins with proliferation of normal endometrial tissue. Over time, hyperplasia of the glandular elements becomes anaplastic and then neoplastic, with invasion of the underlying stroma, myometrium, and vascular spaces.

There are two types of endometrial cancer based on light microscopic appearance, clinical behavior, and epidemiology, Type 1 and Type II. What are these types?

Type 1: these have an endometrioid histology and comprise 70% to 80% of newly diagnosed cases of endometrial cancer in the United States. They are associated with unopposed estrogen exposure and are often preceded by premalignant disease.

Type II: these have nonendometrioid histology (usually papillary serous or clear cell) with an aggressive clinical course. Hormonal risk factors have not been identified, and there is no readily observed premalignant phase.

How common is endometrial cancer and in whom does it occur?

It is the **most common** gynecologic cancer; 75% of these cancers occur in **postmenopausal women**.

What are the major symptoms of endometrial cancer?

Abnormal uterine bleeding (primarily postmenopausal bleeding)

What are the roles of estrogen and progesterone in endometrial cancer?

Estrogen stimulates endometrial growth while **progesterone has antiproliferative** effects. Long-term unopposed estrogen stimulation can eventually lead to atypical endometrial hyperplasia and endometrial cancer.

What are the main etiologies for chronically elevated estrogen levels?

Exogenous unopposed estrogen (ie, estrogen replacement therapy); chronic anovulation (ie, polycystic ovarian syndrome [PCOS]); estrogen-producing tumors (ie, granulosa cell tumors); obesity

What are the risk factors for endometrial cancer?

Obesity; diet; diabetes; hypertension; early menarche/late menopause; nulliparity; PCOS (infertility); tamoxifen treatment for breast cancer; family predisposition (hereditary nonpolyposis colorectal cancer [HNPCC]/Lynch syndrome II)

What are protective factors against endometrial cancer?

Combined oral contraceptives; exercise; multiparity; smoking (through increased hepatic metabolism of estrogen)

What is the relationship between endometrial hyperplasia and endometrial cancer?

Endometrial hyperplasia is a benign condition associated with hyperestrogenic states. Atypical hyperplasia is a precancerous condition.

What characteristics are used to classify endometrial hyperplasia?

Glandular/stromal architecture (simplex or complex)

Nuclear atypia (present or absent)

Which histologic feature of endometrial hyperplasia confers the greatest risk for cancer?

Nuclear atypia

What are the four types of endometrial hyperplasia and what is the risk of cancer for each?

1. Simple hyperplasia without atypia 1%
2. Complex hyperplasia without atypia 3%
3. Simple hyperplasia with atypia 8%
4. Complex hyperplasia with atypia 40%

What are the general guidelines for the treatment of endometrial hyperplasia?

If nuclear atypia is absent, treat with progesterone. If nuclear atypia is present, hysterectomy is recommended.

How should atypical endometrial cells on a Pap smear be worked up?

They warrant an endometrial biopsy for further evaluation.

What is the differential diagnosis for abnormal uterine bleeding in the premenopausal woman?

Complications of early pregnancy; other gynecologic neoplasms; leiomymata; endometrial hyperplasia/polyps; cervical polyps; intrauterine device; hemophilias

What are your differential diagnoses for abnormal uterine bleeding in the postmenopausal woman?

Atrophic vaginitis; exogenous estrogens; other gynecologic neoplasms; endometrial hyperplasia/polyps

What is the gold standard for diagnosing endometrial cancer?

Hysteroscopy with dilation and curettage **(D&C)**

Is CA-125 a useful laboratory test to help with diagnosis?

In advanced disease, CA-125 may be elevated; however, it is not useful in the diagnosis or management.

What are the different subtypes of endometrial cancer?

1. **Endometrioid adenocarcinoma** (80%)
2. Papillary serous carcinoma (5%-10%)
3. Clear cell carcinoma (1%-5%)

How does endometrial cancer spread?

Most commonly through **direct extension,** but it can also spread trans-tubally, lymphatically, or hematogenously.

What lymph nodes are involved in endometrial cancer metastases?

Pelvic and paraaortic lymph nodes

How is tumor grading for endometrial cancer determined?

By tumor histology (architecture and nuclear atypia)

What are the three different tumor grades for endometrial cancer?

1. Grade 1: well-differentiated (~95% glandular tissue, 5% solid pattern)
2. Grade 2: moderately differentiated (~50% to 95% glandular tissue, 5%-50% solid pattern)
3. Grade 3: poorly differentiated (< 50% glandular tissue, > 50% solid pattern)

How is endometrial cancer staged?

Surgically (by the spread of the cancer) based on abdominal exploration, pelvic washings, total abdominal hysterectomy with bilateral salpingo-oophorectomy (TAH/BSO), and pelvic and periaortic lymph node biopsies

What is the staging system for endometrial cancer?

See Table 5.5.

Table 5.5 Stages of Endometrial Cancer

Stage	Description	Endometrial Tumors	5-Year Survival
Stage I: Involvement limited to the uterus	Ia: invasion < half of myometrium Ib: invasion > half of myometrium	75%	80%-95%
Stage II: Extension to and involvement of the cervix	IIa: extension to endocervical glands only IIb: cervical stromal invasion	11%	65%-75%
Stage III: Local spread	IIIa: invasion of serosa and/or adnexa, and/or positive peritoneal cytology IIIb: vaginal metastases IIIc: metastasis to pelvic and/or paraaortic lymph nodes	11%	30%-60%
Stage IV: Distant spread	IVa: invasion of the bladder and bowel IVb: distant metastasis including intraabdominal and/or inguinal lymph nodes	3%	5%-20%

How is endometrial cancer treated?

TAH/BSO with lymph node dissection

What is the role of adjuvant therapy in endometrial cancer?

It is dependent on whether the patient is at low, intermediate, or high risk for disease recurrence. Below are general guidelines for adjuvant postoperative treatment:

Low risk (Stage Ia): no adjuvant treatment warranted (Stage Ia, grade 3) Vaginal brachytherapy

Intermediate-risk (Stage Ic, Stage II): vaginal brachytherapy

High risk (Stage III, IV): pelvic/abdominal radiation therapy ± chemotherapy

Name the chemotherapeutic agents used in endometrial cancer and their major toxicities:

Doxorubicin (cardiotoxicity)

Cisplatin (ototoxicity, neuropathy, nephrotoxicity, nausea)

Paclitaxel (bone marrow suppression, allergic reaction)

What is the recommended treatment for women who have early-stage disease and wish to preserve their fertility?

Trial of progestins after careful counseling

What factors worsen the prognosis for endometrial cancer?

Advanced stage; higher pathologic grade; histologic subtype; increase in myometrial invasion; lymph/vascular space invasion

What is the appropriate follow-up after treatment of endometrial cancer?

Monitor patients every 3 to 4 months for the next 2 to 3 years, then twice yearly with a comprehensive pelvic examination

What is the overall prognosis for endometrial cancer?

Without major adverse risk factors, treatment with a TAH/BSO may result in a 5-year survival greater than 95%.

What is the screening recommendation for the general population?

Screening is not warranted for women who are asymptomatic.

What is the screening recommendation for women with/at risk for HNPCC?

Annual endometrial biopsies by the age of 35 years

UTERINE SARCOMA

What is a uterine sarcoma?

A very aggressive tumor that arises from the myometrium.

How common is it and who does it affect?

It is a very rare cancer (3%-4% of all uterine malignancies) and commonly affects women over 40 years old.

What are risk factors for uterine sarcoma?

History of pelvic radiation

Long-term use of tamoxifen

What are the main types of sarcomas?

Mixed müllerian tumors (carcinosarcoma); leiomyosarcoma; endometrial stromal sarcoma (ESS); undifferentiated sarcoma

How do uterine sarcomas present clinically?	**Abnormal uterine bleeding; rapidly enlarging uterus;** malodorous vaginal discharge; pelvic pressure and pain; part of the tumor may protrude from the cervical os
What is the major differential diagnosis of uterine sarcoma?	Uterine leiomyomas
What preoperative examinations may help with the diagnosis of a uterine sarcoma?	Endometrial biopsy; dilation and fractional curettage
How is the definitive diagnosis of uterine sarcoma made?	Exploratory laparotomy with a pathologic diagnosis
What is the role of imaging studies in uterine sarcomas?	Imaging studies cannot distinguish between a sarcoma or other uterine tumors. A CT scan of the thorax is recommended because uterine sarcoma commonly metastasizes to the lung.
What is the staging system for uterine sarcomas?	Staging is done surgically and is a modification of the system used for endometrial cancer.
What is the treatment for uterine sarcomas?	TAH/BSO, pelvic/paraaortic lymph node dissection, and pelvic washings
What is the role of adjuvant therapy?	Stage I and II pelvic radiation therapy
What is the overall prognosis for sarcomas?	Generally, they have worse prognosis than endometrial cancers of a similar stage.

Ovarian Cancer

INTRODUCTION

How common is ovarian cancer?	It is the second most common gynecologic malignancy, but the **leading cause of mortality** among women who develop a gynecologic malignancy, and the **fifth most common cause of cancer-related female deaths in the United States.** The lifetime risk of developing ovarian cancer is 1.4% (1 in 70).

Why is ovarian cancer the leading cause of mortality among women with gynecologic cancers?	Symptoms of early-stage ovarian cancer are ill-defined and many women will not seek medical attention. Often, the cancer is detected at its advanced stages when it has spread beyond the ovaries.
How are ovarian tumors categorized?	**Epithelial origin; germ cell tumors; sex cord-stromal tumors; cancer metastatic to the ovary** (usually from primary tumors of the breast, GI tract, or genital tract)
Which ovarian tumor is the most common?	Epithelial (~90% of all ovarian tumors)

EPITHELIAL OVARIAN CANCER

What age group does Epithelial Ovarian Cancer (EOC) affect?	Predominantly **postmenopausal** women. Median age is 62 years old.
What are the risk factors for development of EOC?	**Family history of breast cancer or EOC** **Personal history of breast cancer** **Advanced age** Obesity/high fat diet Infertility/nulliparity Talc Endometriosis
What factors are protective against development of EOC?	**OCPs; tubal ligation;** breastfeeding (history of); pregnancy; multiparity
What percent of EOC develops sporadically? What percent are because of genetic predisposition?	90% are sporadic; 10% are genetic predisposition
What is one feature that distinguishes hereditary ovarian cancer from a somatic cause?	The onset of ovarian cancer occurs **10 years earlier** in hereditary syndromes

With what hereditary syndromes has ovarian cancer been associated? Describe them.

Breast and ovarian cancer: associated with BRCA-1 and 2 mutations (autosomal dominant), higher frequencies in Ashkenazi Jews

Lynch II Syndrome (hereditary nonpolyposis colon cancer— HNPCC): colorectal cancer is hallmark, also commonly found are endometrial, urogenital, and other GI primaries

Site-specific ovarian cancer: strong genetic link, autosomal dominant, usually two or more first-degree relatives have the disease

What are current screening recommendations for women at high risk?

Prophylactic genetic screening

CA-125 and transvaginal ultrasound every 6 to 12 months beginning between ages 25 and 35 years

What other preventative surgical procedure is recommended for women with a presumed hereditary ovarian cancer syndrome?

Prophylactic oophorectomy who have completed childbearing or/by 35 years of age

What are the subtypes of EOC and how common is each type?

Serous 75% to 80%

Mucinous 10%

Endometrioid 10%

Clear cell less than 1%

Transitional cell less than 1%

Undifferentiated less than 10%

What are some key features that describe each tumor type?

Serous: often bilateral if malignant, extraovarian spread common, histological finding of **psammoma bodies**

Mucinous: unilateral, **large size,** resembles the endocervix

Endometrioid: resembles the endometrium

Clear cell: "mesonephroid," "clear cells" similar to renal carcinoma, **hypercalcemia**

Transitional cell: "Brenner tumors," **transitional epithelium,** unilateral, benign, or malignant

Undifferentiated: no distinguishable histologic features

At what cancer stage is EOC usually diagnosed?

75% of ovarian cancers are detected at **Stage III or IV**. Five-year survival rate is 5% to 35%

What is the typical presentation of a patient with ovarian cancer?

A **postmenopausal woman** who presents with any or a combination of these:

1. **Abdominal distension** from ascites or pelvic mass
2. **Pelvic pressure**
3. **Nausea, early satiety,** weight loss, bowel obstruction
4. Dyspnea because of a pleural effusion (metastasis to the lungs)

How does ovarian cancer spread?

Ovarian cancer cells are found in peritoneal fluid (ascites) which carries them to distant abdominal sites.

Should the ovaries on a postmenopausal woman be palpable on examination?

Women who are more than 1 year postmenopause should have atrophic, nonpalpable ovaries.

An ovarian enlargement in a postmenopausal woman is cancer until proven otherwise.

What findings on the physical examination would lead you to believe this is an ovarian malignancy?

A **solid, fixed, irregular pelvic mass** associated with an upper abdominal mass (omental caking) and/or ascites

What is meant by omental caking?

Ovarian cancer metastasis to the omentum causing a fixed upper abdominal mass with ascites, very common in advanced disease

What is the initial step to evaluate an ovarian lesion?

Ultrasound

What other radiographic tests should be ordered in a patient suspected of having EOC?

Abdominal-pelvic CT: to determine the extent of metastases

Chest x-ray: to determine the presence of a pleural effusion

What tumor marker is often elevated in advanced stage ovarian cancer? What is its value?

CA-125 is elevated in 80% of cases with advanced ovarian cancer. It is not as useful in premenopausal women or for early stage disease. It is most useful to **evaluate the progression/regression of disease following treatment.**

| What is the "gold standard" to diagnose EOC? | Exploratory laparotomy/laparoscopy and histopathologic diagnosis |

| How is ovarian cancer staged? | Surgically |

| Describe the stages of ovarian cancer and their prognoses: | See Table 5.6. |

Table 5.6 The Stages of Ovarian Cancer

Stage	Description	5-Year survival
Stage I: Tumor limited to the ovaries	1a: one ovary involved and capsule intact 1b: both ovaries involved and capsule intact 1c: 1a or 1b and tumor on the ovary; ruptured capsule; malignant ascites and positive peritoneal washings for malignant cells	> 90%
Stage II: Spread of the tumor to the pelvis	IIa: uterus/oviducts are involved IIb: other pelvic structures are involved IIc: IIa or IIb and tumor on the ovary; ruptured capsule; malignant ascites and positive peritoneal washings for malignant cells	60%-75%
Stage III: Spread to the abdominal cavity	IIIa: microscopic seeding of the abdominal peritoneal surfaces; negative nodes IIIb: < 2 cm implants on the abdominal peritoneal surface IIIc: > 2 cm implants on the abdominal peritoneal surface and/or positive retroperitoneal or inguinal lymph nodes	25%-40%
Stage IV: Distant metastasis	Liver, splenic, or pulmonary parenchymal metastasis Malignant pleural effusion Metastases to the supraclavicular lymph nodes or skin	5%

| Which lymph nodes are typically involved in advanced ovarian cancer? | Pelvic and paraaortic lymph nodes |

| What is the optimal treatment for advanced ovarian cancer disease? | Surgical debulking and chemotherapy. Debulking includes TAH/BSO, omentectomy and lymph node dissection. |

What is the most effective chemotherapeutic regimen?	A combination of **paclitaxel plus cisplatin**
What are the most common side effects of chemotherapy?	Nausea, vomiting, alopecia, diarrhea, nephrotoxicity, myelosuppression
What are poor prognostic factors?	Stage III or IV disease; advanced age; short disease-free interval; residual tumor after primary surgery

Nonepithelial Ovarian Cancer

OVARIAN GERM CELL TUMORS

What percent of all ovarian neoplasms are germ cell tumors (GCTs)?	20% to 25%
From what embryologic origin do ovarian GCTs arise?	From the totipotential germ cells that normally differentiate into the three germ layers.
What are the GCT subtypes?	Dysgerminoma
	Endodermal sinus tumor (yolk sac tumor)
	Immature teratoma
	Embryonal carcinoma
	Choriocarcinoma
	Mixed GCTs
At what age do these malignancies occur?	It is a disease of children and young women (usually between 10 and 30 years).
What are the typical clinical symptoms and signs?	Acute abdominal pain (from rupture or torsion); rapid abdominal enlargement (because of either the mass or ascites); fever; vaginal bleeding
How does the time of diagnosis differ from that of EOC?	Patients usually present at Stage Ia

For each of the following scenarios, identify the correct GCT:

A 20-year-old woman presents with acute onset of lower abdominal pain and pelvic mass. Serum tests reveal an elevated level of alpha-fetoprotein (AFP). Intraoperative examination reveals bilateral ovarian masses and intraperitoneal dissemination. Tumor biopsy reveals Schiller-Duval bodies.

Endodermal sinus tumor (yolk sac tumor)

These tumors are rare, found in young females. They may secrete estrogen, causing precocious puberty and abnormal vaginal bleeding. β-hCG is commonly elevated and serves as a tumor marker.

Embryonal carcinoma and choriocarcinoma

A young female presents with abdominal enlargement. Radiographic films reveal a unilateral mass with calcification. Tumor markers are not present. Histology of the removed specimen reveals the presence of a poorly differentiated tumor consisting of hair, teeth, cartilage, bone, and muscle.

Immature (malignant) teratoma

This tumor is the female counterpart of the male seminoma and commonly occurs in adolescents and young females. It is the most common of the malignant OGCTs and typically presents as a rapidly growing unilateral mass. Lactic dehydrogenase (LDH) may be elevated.

Dysgerminoma

A young female presents with tachycardia, palpitations, anxiety, and tremors. The pituitary and thyroid appear normal on examination and radiographic films. The patient is later found to have a mature teratoma consisting of thyroid tissue.

Mixed GCTs

These neoplasms contain two or more germ cell elements. A dysgerminoma and endodermal sinus tumor occur together most frequently. LDH, AFP, and β-hCG may be elevated.

Struma ovarii

| Which GCTs are benign? | Gonadoblastomas and mature cystic teratomas |

| What laboratory test should be ordered prior to definitive diagnosis and treatment? | Serum ovarian tumor marker panel for β-hCG, AFP, LDH |

| What is the treatment plan for malignant GCTs? | Unilateral adnexectomy (fertility preserving) and complete surgical staging; adjuvant chemotherapy |

| How are GCTs staged? | Similar to EOC staging |

| How effective is chemotherapy in malignant GCTs? | GCTs are very chemosensitive |

| For which tumors is chemotherapy recommended? | For all resected Stage I GCTs except Stage Ia dysgerminoma and Stage Ia, grade 1 unruptured immature teratoma |

| What chemotherapeutic agents are used? | **Bleomycin, etoposide, and cisplatin (BEP)** is the preferred regimen |

List the chemotherapeutic agent that causes the toxicities listed below:

| Nephrotoxicity: | Cisplatin |

| Pulmonary fibrosis: | Bleomycin |

| Blood dyscrasias: | Etoposide |

| How do you monitor the response to chemotherapy? | Based on the physical examination and decrease in the serum tumor marker levels (if initially elevated) |

| What is the prognosis of GCTs? | Much better than EOC. Depending on the GCT, 5-year survival ranges from 60% to 95%. |

OVARIAN SEX CORD-STROMAL TUMORS

| What percent of all ovarian tumors are sex cord-stromal tumors? | 5% to 8% of all primary ovarian neoplasms |

| From what embryologic origin do ovarian sex cord-stromal tumors arise? | They develop from the cells that surround the oocytes, including those that **produce ovarian hormones.** |

What are the ovarian sex cord-stromal tumor subtypes?

Granulosa cell tumors

Ovarian thecoma

Ovarian fibroma

Sertoli-Leydig cell tumors

What are the typical clinical symptoms and signs?

Estrogen-producing tumors may cause **precocious puberty** in young girls, and **endometrial hyperplasia** and **abnormal vaginal bleeding** in postmenopausal women. Androgen producing tumors cause **virilization, acne, and gynecomastia.**

In the following scenarios, identify the correct sex cord-stromal tumor:

Most women present with a unilateral adnexal mass between the second and third decade. Virilization, hirsutism, acne, and menstrual abnormalities commonly occur. Testosterone levels may be elevated.

Sertoli-Leydig cell tumors

A postmenopausal woman presents with a unilateral benign solid mass that is not hormone secreting.

Ovarian fibroma

These tumors are estrogen producing and cause precocious puberty in young females and abnormal vaginal bleeding in postmenopausal women. Inhibin may be elevated.

Granulosa/thecoma

What is Meigs syndrome?

It is the association of an **ovarian fibroma** with **ascites** and/or **pleural effusion.**

With what other syndrome are ovarian fibromas associated?

Gorlin syndome (nevoid basal cell carcinoma syndrome): an autosomal dominant disease characterized by its association with **basal cell cancers, brain tumors, odontogenic keratocysts,** and **mesenteric cysts**

What are Call-Exner bodies and for what tumor are they nearly pathogonomic?

They are small, fluid-filled cavities in between granulosa cells of ovarian follicles that contain eosinophilic fluid. They are associated with **granulosa cell tumors.**

What other cancer is associated with granulosa cell tumors/ovarian thecomas?	With estrogen-producing tumors, **endometrial adenocarcinoma** must be considered. **These women must have an endometrial biopsy.**
How are ovarian sex cord-stromal tumors staged?	Similarly to EOC
What is the surgical treatment?	TAH/BSO or unilateral oophorectomy for women who wish to preserve their fertility and who have low-stage/grade neoplasms A D&C or an endometrial biopsy must be performed for estrogen secreting tumors.
Is adjuvant therapy recommended?	Chemotherapy is not recommended for low-stage/grade neoplasms. Data is inconclusive for more advanced stages.
What is the prognosis for these tumors?	In general, very good. For early-stage cancers, 5-year survival rates range between 70% to 90%.
What follow-up procedures are recommended for the hormone-producing cancers?	Serial pelvic examinations and serum tumor marker levels

TUMORS METASTATIC TO THE OVARY

What percent of ovarian tumors are metastatic?	5%
What are the primary tumors that metastasize to the ovary?	**Breast; gastrointestinal tract;** acute leukemia and lymphoma (rare)
How do metastatic tumors to the ovary clinically present?	Oftentimes they present like primary ovarian (pelvic mass, ascites, early satiety, and change in bowel habits.) Occasionally they may present as an asymptomatic pelvic mass
What are gastric tumors metastatic to the ovaries called?	Krukenberg tumors

What primary ovarian tumor does Krukenberg tumors resemble in histology?	Mucin-secreting adenocarcinoma of the ovary
What histologic feature is pathognomonic for Krukenberg tumors?	Signet ring cells
What can be used to differentiate between a primary mucinous ovarian tumor and metastatic colon cancer?	Immunohistochemistry (cytokeratin expression)
Describe the cytokeratin expression pattern of each of the following:	Primary mucinous ovarian: CK7 positive; CK20 negative
	Metastases from a primary mucinous adenocarcinoma of the colon: CK7 negative; CK20 positive
What is the overall prognosis in patients who have cancers metastatic to the ovary?	Survival following surgery and chemotherapy is very poor, ranging from 4 to 12 months

FALLOPIAN TUBE CANCER

How common is fallopian tube cancer?	Primary carcinoma is **very rare**, accounting for 0.3% of primary gynecologic malignancies.
	Secondary carcinoma from metastases of ovarian, endometrium, gastrointestinal (GI), or breast cancers are more common.
What are risk factors for fallopian tube cancers?	A mutation in the BRCA1 or BRCA2 gene. Women with these mutations who are planning prophylactic oophorectomies should also have their fallopian tubes removed.
What is the most common type of fallopian tube cancer?	Papillary serous adenocarcinoma
What other types of fallopian tube cancers are there?	Adenosquamous carcinoma and sarcoma

How does the cancer spread?	It spreads through the tubal ostia into the peritoneal cavity and also through lymphatics to the paraaortic and pelvic lymph nodes.
Where does fallopian tube cancer commonly metastasize?	Ovaries, uterus, and pelvic and paraaortic nodes
What is the classic clinical presentation?	**Latzko triad: serosanguineous vaginal discharge, pelvic pain, and a pelvic mass**
What is hydrops tubae profluens?	The spontaneous or pressure-induced release of clear or blood-tinged vaginal discharge followed by shrinkage of an adnexal mass and relief of cramping pain. It is pathognomonic for fallopian tube cancer.
What preoperative evidence suggests fallopian tube cancer?	Positive vaginal cytology for abnormal cells with a negative workup for endometrial or cervical cancer suggests fallopian tube carcinoma.
What is the role of CA-125 in fallopian tube cancer?	CA-125 levels are sensitive markers for response to chemotherapy and recurrence.
How is staging for fallopian cell cancers determined?	Surgically; it is staged similarly to epithelial ovarian cancer
What is the treatment?	Total abdominal hysterectomy with bilateral salpingo-oophorectomy (TAH/ BSO), lymph node sampling, infracolic omentectomy, and peritoneal washings
	Chemotherapy consisting of carboplatin and paxlitaxel is recommended after surgery.
What is the prognosis?	Similar to ovarian cancer. The overall 5-year survival rate is 56%.

CLINICAL VIGNETTES

A 19-year-old female comes to you for an initial gynecologic visit. She tells you that she has never engaged in sexual intercourse. She then requests a Pap smear.

1. What do you do next?
   a. Agree to her request and prepare to perform a screening Pap smear now.
   b. Tell her that she never needs a screening Pap smear unless she has engaged in sex.
   c. Inform her that she does not need to have her first screening Pap smear until age 21 years.
   d. Inform her that she does not need her first screening Pap smear until 3 years after her first sexual intercourse.

2. She is concerned about human papilloma virus and asks how she can prevent from getting it. What should you tell her?
   a. Gardasil vaccine can be given in boys and girls ages 9 to 26 years
   b. Limit number of sexual partners
   c. Podophyllin cream
   d. Both a+b
   e. Both b+c

Answers: 1: c; 2: d

In 2010, the American College of Obstetricians and Gynecologists (ACOG) issued new Pap smear guidelines. These recommendations state that women can have their first screening Pap smear at age 21 regardless of prior sexual activity; women in their 20s should have a Pap smear every 2 years; women age 30 or older who have had three normal Pap smears in a row should have a Pap smear every 3 years; Pap smear screening can be stopped in women 65 to 70 years old and above who have had three or more normal Pap smears in a row; women who have had a hysterectomy should no longer have Pap smears if the hysterectomy was for noncancerous reasons and they don't have a history of severely abnormal Pap smears. If a woman had a hysterectomy but still has a cervix, she will need to continue routine Pap smears; these guidelines are to be followed regardless if the vaccine was given or not.

The quadrivalent vaccine Gardasil is now FDA approved for both boys and girls. Prevention with condoms and limiting the number of sexual partners will decrease risk of HPV and cervical cancer. Remember condoms do not prevent against all HPV infection.

A 42-year-old woman presents to your office with complaints of a 6-month history of intense and painful vulvar itching. She also states that she can feel a "small lump." She denies any vaginal bleeding. Examination of the vulva reveals a small fleshy outgrowth on her left labia majora. A biopsy is performed and pathology reveals squamous cell carcinoma in situ. Which of the following statements is the most appropriate next step in the management of this patient?

a. Postoperative radiation is recommended
b. Care observation for the next 6 months to see if the growth enlarges or remains the same is recommended
c. Colposcopy of the vagina and cervix as part of pretreatment evaluation
d. Total vulvectomy is recommended
e. Groin dissection is necessary

Answer: c

Ninety percent of vulvar cancers are squamous cell carcinomas and are associated with HPV 16 and 18 strains in premenopausal women. Moreover, there is evidence that some high grade vulvar and vaginal intraepithelial neoplasia may be monoclonal lesions derived from high grade or malignant cervical disease. Colposcopy of the vagina and cervix (choice c) are recommended as part of the pretreatment evaluation to help guide appropriate medical or surgical therapies.

A 31-year-old female receives results of her Pap smear performed 2 weeks ago. According to her pathology report, her smear is positive for atypical squamous cells of undetermined significance (ASGUS). Her HPV DNA test is positive for a high-risk strain. She then undergoes satisfactory colposcopy with punch biopsy of two abnormal areas on her cervix and endocervical curettage (ECC). Two weeks after, the gynecologist calls the patient to inform her that the pathology of both specimens is consistent with low-grade squamous intraepithelial lesion (LSIL); however, brushings from the ECC are negative for abnormal cells and the HPV DNA test is negative. What is the next best step in management?

a. Tell the patient that she can resume routine screening and no follow-up surveillance is necessary because her HPV DNA test is negative, therefore indicating that the virus has been cleared.
b. Recommend follow-up cervical cytology testing at 6 and 12 months or HPV testing at 12 months.
c. Perform a conization of the entire squamo-columnar junction.
d. Recommend local ablation of the abnormal lesions.

Answer: b

This patient has LSIL (~CIN1). Overall spontaneous regression rates of LSIL are approximately 60% and may reach 90% in young women. Therefore, expectant management with follow-up Pap smears at 6 and 12 months or HPV testing at 12 months is recommended (choice b). Colposcopy should be repeated if repeat cytology shows ASC or greater or if HPV DNA testing is positive for a high risk type. After two negative smears or a negative HPV DNA test, routine screening may be resumed. This patient has biopsy-proven low-grade cervical dysplasia regardless of the negative result of her HPV test. The patient needs close monitoring as 11% of women with CIN1 can progress to CIN2 or CIN3. Telling the patient she can resume routine screening would be negligent (choice a). Local ablation (choice d) is recommended as primary treatment if CIN1 persists greater than 24 month, and if colposcopy is satisfactory and the ECC is negative for glandular or squamous lesions. Excisional modalities (choice c) are recommended if colposcopy is not optimal, the ECC reveals abnormalities, or if there is recurrent disease after am ablation. A conization may help exclude the presence of an underlying high-grade or invasive lesion.

A 59-year-old woman presents to her gynecologist with complaints of abdominal distension and discomfort for three months. She also reports having bloating and feeling "too full to eat." Her physical examination is significant for a distended abdomen. A palpable mass is also appreciated along her anterior abdominal wall. An enlarged right ovary is appreciated on her vaginal examination. A CT scan of the chest, abdomen and pelvis reveals enlarged ovaries, right greater than left. There is also omental thickening, several small implants on the peritoneum, and moderate ascites. The findings are consistent with ovarian malignancy. What is the next best step in management?

   a. Proceed to an exploratory laparotomy for surgical staging and debulking.
   b. Perform a MRI of brain to determine if there are brain metastases.
   c. Start palliative chemotherapy now.
   d. Perform a diagnostic and therapeutic paracentesis.

Answer: a

This patient likely has a diagnosis of advanced epithelial ovarian cancer but needs histologic diagnosis and staging. Surgery (choice a) is the cornerstone of therapy regardless of stage or cell type. Surgical staging involves complete abdominal exploration, biopsies of peritoneal and intraabdominal lesions, biopsies of pelvic and paraaortic lymph nodes, intact removal of the tumor, infracolic omentectomy, hysterectomy, cytoreductive surgery to remove all disease, and samples of ascites or peritoneal washings for cytology. Paracentesis (choice d) is not advocated as a routine procedure for diagnostic purposes as false-negative results may occur in up to 40% of patients with widespread intraabdominal disease. An MRI of brain (choice b) is not necessary at this time as the patient does not have symptoms or signs of neurologic disease. Without proper diagnosis or staging of the cancer, the choice of chemotherapy cannot be made (choice c).

You are the medical student rotating with the gynecologic oncology service for 1 month. A patient is found to have a locally invasive vaginal cancer in the lower one-third portion of her vagina. The attending asks you to name the most likely lymph nodes involved in her disease based on anatomical lymphatic drainage patterns. What is your response?

   a. Inguinal
   b. Hypogastric
   c. Internal iliac
   d. External iliac

Answer: a

The lower one-third of the vagina drains in to the inguinal lymph nodes (choice a) whereas the upper two-thirds drain in to the internal (choice c) and external (choice d) iliac nodes. The hypogastric lymph node system (choice b) is an alternative name to the internal iliac nodes.

CHAPTER 6

Urogynecology

Urinary Infections

ACUTE CYSTITIS

What is the prevalence and incidence of acute cystitis?

50% to 60% of women report having had cystitis at some point in their life. Young, sexually active women have on an average 0.5 episodes per year; postmenopausal women have on an average of 0.1 episodes per year.

Describe the symptoms of acute cystitis:

Abrupt onset of: **dysuria, urinary** frequency and urgency, suprapubic **or low back pain**, possible hematuria (in hemorrhagic cystitis)

What is the differential diagnosis for these symptoms?

Urethritis; vaginitis; pyelonephritis

For each differential diagnosis, list the main symptoms/signs that would differentiate it from acute cystitis:

Urethritis: urethral discharge, more gradual onset, history of new sexual partner

Vaginitis: vaginal discharge/odor, pruritis, dyspareunia, external dysuria, absence of urinary frequency or urgency

Pyelonephritis: elevated temperature, costovertebral angle (CVA) tenderness, nausea/vomiting

How is the diagnosis of acute cystitis definitively made?

Most cases can be diagnosed on **history and physical examination alone.** The examiner should specifically look for signs of vaginitis, cervicitis, urethral discharge, or herpetic ulcerations.

Gonococcus (GC) and *Chlamydia* **cultures** should be done if urethritis is suspected.

Urinalysis should also be done, looking for pyuria or hematuria.

What are the most common pathogens that cause acute cystitis?

Escherichia coli (80%)

Staphylococcus saprophyticus (5%-15%)

Proteus mirabilis, Klebsiella, enterococci, *Pseudomonas, Serratia, Providencia,* staphylococci, and fungi (rare, more common in complicated cases)

What are the risk factors for the development of acute cystitis?

Increased sexual intercourse; newly sexually active; postmenopausal; diabetes, sickle cell anemia, immunosuppressed conditions; abnormalities of the genitourinary tract; use of spermicide, especially with a diaphragm; history of a recent UTI; recent hospitalization

What factors suggest the presence of a complicated urinary infection?

Patient characteristics: elderly patient; pregnancy

Medical history: hospital-acquired infection; indwelling catheter/recurrent instrumentation; functional or anatomic abnormality of the urinary tract; recent antibiotic use; diabetes; immunosuppression

What is the prognostic significance of a complicated urinary infection?

Complicated infections are associated with increased rates of failing therapy

What are the treatment options for uncomplicated acute cystitis?

Trimethoprim-sulfamethoxazole for 3 days

Nitrofurantoin for 3 to 5 days

Fluoroquinolone for 3 days

No follow-up is needed unless symptoms recur

What are the treatment options for complicated acute cystitis?

Treat initially with **broad spectrum antibiotics** (such as fluoroquinolones) and then tailor therapy based on the culture results. These patients should be treated for **7 to 14 days. Pregnant patients can be treated for 3 to 7 days with broad spectrum antibiotics (such as nitrofurantoin).** They need to be followed-up to ensure resolution of symptoms.

How often does cystitis recur?

20%; the vast majority of these are because of exogenous reinfection

What is considered recurrent cystitis?

More than three UTIs per year or more than two UTIs within a 6-month period

What are the risk factors of recurrent cystitis?

Sexual intercourse; use of spermicide, especially with a diaphragm; recent antimicrobial use; genetic predisposition; urinary incontinence, cystocele, elevated post-void residual volume

How is recurrent cystitis treated?

Cultures need to be taken to rule out resistance to prior treatment. For patients with multiple reinfections, treatment consists of one of four options:

1. **Behavioral changes** (change contraceptive methods, early postcoital voiding)
2. **Continuous low-dose antibiotic** prophylaxis
3. **Postcoital low-dose antibiotic prophylaxis**
4. **Self-start therapy** when symptoms begin

In postmenopausal women with frequent infections, **topical estrogen** is often used, with or without concomitant use of prophylactic antibiotics.

Is cranberry juice an effective home remedy for preventing UTIs?

Cranberry juice inhibits pathogens from adhering to uroepithelial cells, which can reduce the incidence of UTI. It is not effective in the treatment of UTI.

What percentage of reproductive-age women have asymptomatic bacteriuria?

3% to 6%

What are the risk factors for the development of asymptomatic bacteriuria?

Diabetes; advanced age; presence of an indwelling bladder catheter

Should asymptomatic bacteriuria be treated?

No, unless the woman is at high risk

Who are the high-risk women that need treatment for their asymptomatic bacteriuria?

Pregnant women; women with indwelling catheters; renal transplant recipients; women with spinal cord injury; prior to invasive procedures

URETHRITIS

Describe the signs and symptoms of urethritis:

Dysuria, but with a more **gradual** onset and **milder** symptoms than with acute cystitis, often associated with abnormal vaginal discharge or bleeding (because of related cervicitis)

A **mucopurulent discharge from the urethral os** is usually found on examination.

What are the risk factors for urethritis?

History of an STD; new sexual partner in past weeks; partner with urethral symptoms

How is the diagnosis definitively made?

Pyuria on urinalysis and mucopurulent cervicitis or herpetic lesions are usually found. A positive GC, *Chlamydia*, or herpes test result can confirm the diagnosis.

What are the most common pathogens that cause urethritis?

Most common: *Chlamydia trachomatis* (5%-20%) *Neisseria gonorrhea* (<10%) **Genital herpes**

Others: *Candida, Trichomonas*

What is irritant urethritis?

Dysuria that occurs as a reaction to an irritant such as a condom, tampon, or any other product inserted into the vagina

ACUTE PYELONEPHRITIS

Describe the symptoms of acute pyelonephritis:

Typical presentation: flank pain, fever (>38°C), CVA tenderness, nausea/vomiting, ± cystitis symptoms

What is the differential diagnosis for acute pyelonephritis?

Gastrointestinal: **cholecystitis, appendicitis, pancreatitis, diverticulitis**

Gynecologic, pelvic inflammatory disease **(PID), ectopic pregnancy**

Pulmonary: **lower lobe pneumonia**

Genitourinary: **urinary calculi**

How is the diagnosis definitively made?

Most patients can be diagnosed based on history and physical examination alone.

Urinalysis: **pyuria** is almost always found; **white cell casts**, if found, indicate renal origin; **gram-negative bacteria** on Gram stain

Urine cultures and possible blood cultures should be taken at time of diagnosis for antimicrobial susceptibility.

What is the most common pathogen that causes acute pyelonephritis?

E. coli (70%-95%); *S. saprophyticus* (5%-20%)

What are the risk factors associated with developing uncomplicated acute pyelonephritis?

Increased sexual intercourse; history of UTI within past year; diabetes; stress incontinence within the past 30 days; a new sexual partner within the past year; spermicide use; family history of UTIs

How is acute pyelonephritis treated?

Outpatient treatment: **trimethoprim-sulfamethoxazole** or a **quinolone** for 10 to 14 days; if enterococcus is suspected, add amoxicillin until cultures return.

Inpatient treatment: indicated if patient is noncompliant, cannot tolerate PO, is severely ill, or is pregnant; initial treatment is **ceftriaxone, ampicillin** and **gentamycin,** or **aztreonam.**

What should be done if flank pain does not resolve after 2-3 days?

An ultrasound or CT to rule out perinephric or intrarenal abcess or ureteral obstruction

Pelvic Organ Prolapse

How significant is pelvic organ prolapse (POP) in women in the United States?

The lifetime risk for undergoing surgery for urinary incontinence or prolapse is 11%. The risk of requiring a repeat procedure may be as high as 29%.

What is meant by POP?

Refers to the relaxation of the normal connective tissue supports of any of the pelvic organs (uterus, vaginal apex, bladder, rectum) and its associated vaginal segment from its normal anatomic location

What are the most common POP abnormalities? Describe each defect:

Cystocele:

An anterior vaginal wall defect/prolapse that includes the bladder. See Fig. 6.1.

Enterocele:

An apical vaginal wall defect/prolapse in which bowel is contained within the prolapsed segment. See Fig. 6.2.

Rectocele:

A posterior vaginal wall defect/prolapse that includes the rectum. See Fig. 6.3.

Uterine prolapse:

An apical vaginal wall defect where the cervix/uterus descends with strain from its normal anatomic site.

Sometimes associated with cervical elongation.

Vault prolapse:

A defect of the apex of the vagina, most commonly found post-hysterectomy.

Defects in which pelvic floor muscles/supporting structures allow POP?

The uterosacral and cardinal ligaments, the levator ani muscles, and the endopelvic connective tissue. See Figs. 6.4 and 6.5.

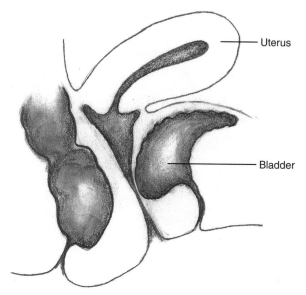

Figure 6.1   Anterior vaginal prolapse—cystocele.

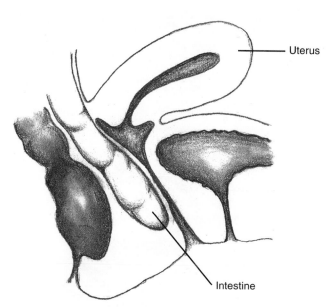

Figure 6.2   Apical prolapse—enterocele.

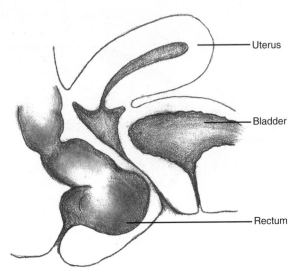

Figure 6.3   Posterior vaginal wall prolapse—rectocele.

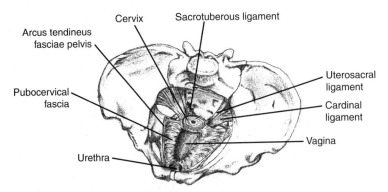

Figure 6.4   Ligaments of the female pelvis.

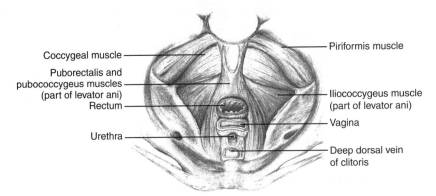

Figure 6.5   Pelvic diaphragm—superior view.

What are the risk factors for POP?

Advancing age; multiparity (vaginal deliveries); obesity; history of pelvic surgery (particularly hysterectomy); increased intra-abdominal pressure (ie, chronic straining during constipation, chronic coughing (COPD), heavy lifting); postpartum muscle weakness (ie, levator ani); loss of innervation; connective tissue disorders; tumor/masses; genetic predisposition

What is the most common symptom of POP?

Many women are asymptomatic. **The most specific complaint for POP is when the woman can see or feel a bulge of tissue that protrudes to or past the vaginal opening. Other symptoms include:** stress incontinence, urinary frequency or hesitancy, feeling of incomplete emptying of the bladder, defecatory symptoms, and coital laxity.

How is POP diagnosed?

It is based upon the findings of physical examination. The patient should be examined in both upright and recumbent (dorsal lithotomy) positions with valsalva maneuver and each area of vaginal anatomy should be described separately.

What are the grading systems used to evaluate and diagnose POP?

While there are several different classifications, currently the two most commonly used are:

1. The Pelvic Organ Prolapse Quantification (POP-Q) system
2. The Baden Walker Halfway system

What does the POPQ system involve?

The POPQ system was created to use objective measurements in centimeters using the hymenal ring as a reference point. It involves quantitative measurements of various points representing anterior, apical, posterior, and basal vaginal prolapse. These points are then used to determine the stage of the prolapse.

Explain the Baden–Walker Halfway System:

It is a less detailed grading system for evaluation of POP displacement compared to the POPQ system, but it is still widely used in clinical practice (see Table 6.1).

Table 6.1 Baden–Walker Halfway System for the Evaluation of POP on Physical Examination

Grade	Displacement of Prolapse
0	No prolapse
1	Halfway to the hymen
2	At the hymen
3	Halfway out of the hymen
4	Total prolapse

What is the management for women with asymptomatic POP?

Observation at regular intervals

Kegel exercises can improve the tone of the muscular floor upon which the pelvic organs rest

What is the management for women with symptomatic POP?

Nonsurgical treatment such as pessaries and symptom-directed therapies (ie, weight loss, pelvic floor muscles rehabilitation, behavior modifications)

Surgical intervention

What is a pessary?

It is a prosthesis usually made out of rubber or silicone-based material with a spring frame that is placed in the vaginal vault to support the prolapsing vaginal walls or uterus. There are several types available which come in varying shapes and sizes. See Fig. 6.6.

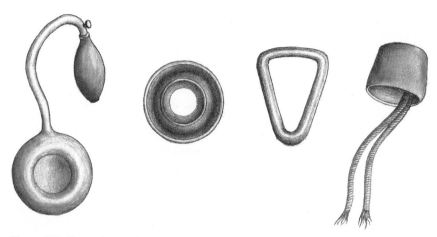

Figure 6.6 Types of pessaries.

When is a pessary contraindicated?

Allergy to the product material
Untreated vaginitis
Pelvic inflammatory disease
A patient who is unable/unlikely to follow-up

When is surgery indicated?

When a patient is symptomatic from her prolapse and has been counseled regarding her treatment options

What is the traditional procedure for an anterior vaginal prolapse (cystocele)? What does it involve?

Anterior vaginal colporrhaphy: dissecting the vaginal epithelium from the underlying fibromuscular connective tissue and bladder, and plicating the vaginal muscularis across the midline

What is the traditional procedure for a posterior vaginal prolapse (rectocele)? What does it involve?

Posterior vaginal colporrhaphy: dissecting the vaginal epithelium from the underlying fibromuscular connective tissue and rectum, and plicating the vaginal muscularis across the midline

What are the different surgical options for treatment of an apical prolapse (enterocele)?

Colpocleisis: usually reserved for severe uterovaginal prolapse. It is an obliterative procedure that closes off the genital hiatus, and therefore should only be considered in patients who do not desire future sexual intercourse. It is minimally invasive, so it is a good consideration for patients in whom major surgery is contraindicated.

Sacrospinous ligament fixation: attachment of the vaginal apex to the sacrospinous ligament, usually unilaterally.

Iliococcygeus suspension: attachment of the vaginal apex to the iliococcygeus muscle, either uni- or bilaterally.

Uterosacral ligament suspension: attachment of the vaginal apex to the uterosacral ligament bilaterally.

Abdominal sacral colpopexy: an abdominal procedure attaching the vaginal apex to the sacral promontory.

Laparoscopic/robotic sacral colpopexy: a laparoscopic or robotic assisted procedure attaching the vaginal apex to the sacral promontory.

Transvaginal apical prolapse repair with mesh: a vaginal procedure using mesh kits to support the vaginal apex as well as the anterior and posterior compartments.

When is a hysterectomy warranted?

For treatment of uterine prolapse or if concomitant uterine pathology is present at the time of prolapse surgery

Urinary Incontinence

INTRODUCTION

Name the factors involved in normal urethral closure:

Extrinsic factors: the levator ani muscles, endopelvic fascia, ligamentous attachments

Intrinsic factors: striated and smooth muscle of the urethral wall, vascular congestion of the submucosal venous plexus, urethral epithelial folds, urethral elasticity, α-adrenergic receptors in the urethra (urethral tone)

Describe the factors involved in normal bladder function:

Bladder filling: increased outlet resistance via muscle fiber recruitment; the detrusor is inactive

Full bladder: a micturition reflex is sent to the brain by tension-stretch receptors, cortical control mechanisms then permit or do not permit this reflex

Bladder emptying: voluntary relaxation of the pelvic floor and urethra, sustained contraction of the detrusor muscle

Describe the action of the detrusor muscle:

It is the **involuntary smooth muscle** wall of the bladder that **reflexively contracts** after voluntary relaxation of the pelvic floor and urethral musculature

Describe the innervation to the lower urinary tract:

1. **Sympathetic** system—controls **bladder storage**
   a. α-receptors: located mainly in the urethra and bladder neck, stimulation increases urethral tone (promotes closure)
   b. β-receptors: located mainly in the bladder body, stimulation decreases bladder tone
2. **Parasympathetic** system—controls **bladder emptying**
   a. stimulation of muscarinic receptors increases bladder contraction
3. **Somatic system**—innervation of the pelvic floor and the external urethral sphincter

What is the differential diagnosis of urinary incontinence?

Infection: cystitis

Anatomic: fistula (vesicovaginal or ureterovaginal), ectopic ureter

Neuro/Psych: dementia, normal pressure hydrocephalus

Medications: diuretics, caffeine, sedatives

Endocrine: diabetes mellitus, diabetes insipidus

What is meant by the following symptoms?

Urgency:

Sudden pressing desire to urinate

Nocturia:

Waking at night more than one time to urinate

Overactive bladder:

A syndrome of urgency, frequency, and nocturia ± urge incontinence

Continuous urinary incontinence:

Constant dribbling of small amounts of urine

Daytime frequency:

Subjective voiding too often by day

Describe the symptoms of the following major types of incontinence:

Stress incontinence:

Involuntary leakage with increased intra-abdominal pressure (eg, with exertion, sneezing, or coughing)

Urge incontinence:

Involuntary leakage immediately preceeded by a feeling of urgency; often precipitated by running water, hand washing, or cold temperatures

Mixed incontinence:

Involuntary leakage associated with urgency and increased intra-abdominal pressure

Overflow incontinence:

Leakage associated with significant urinary retention, which exceeds the storage capacity of the bladder (usually associated with neurogenic conditions)

What type of incontinence do the following symptoms suggest?

Leakage when coughing/sneezing/exercising:

Stress incontinence

Leakage associated with a strong desire to void:

Urge incontinence

Many voids per day:

Urge or overflow incontinence or possible infection

Continual dripping with shifting positions:

Overflow incontinence or sphincter impairment

Nocturia or incontinence associated with intercourse:

Urge incontinence

Painful urination:

Obstruction, infection, or urge incontinence

What are the known risk factors for urinary incontinence?

Childbearing; advanced age; obesity; family history; chronic cough; ascites; pelvic masses

What age-related changes contribute to the development of urinary incontinence?

The prevalence of detrusor overactivity increases with age

Total bladder capacity diminishes

Urinary flow rate decreases

Postvoiding residual increases

The urethral mucosal epithelium becomes atrophic secondary to low estrogen levels

Is incontinence a part of normal aging?

No, however the prevalence and severity of incontinence increases with age

PATIENT EVALUATION

What are the pertinent factors to ask about when taking a history?

Review of symptoms: how often leakage occurs, what provokes urine loss, how much urine is leaked, what makes the problem better/worse, any prior treatment that has been tried

General medical history: systemic illnesses (such as diabetes, vascular insufficiency, chronic pulmonary disease, or any neurologic condition)

Past surgical history

Current medications

What types of medications can sometimes cause urinary incontinence?

Benzodiazepines; α-agonists (OTC cold medications); α-antagonists (antihypertensives); calcium channel blockers; ACE inhibitors (by increasing cough); alcohol

What should be done on physical examination and what tests should be done?

General examination: look for signs of other medical problems as well as for alertness/functional status

Pelvic examination: look for signs of atrophy, infection, fistulae, diverticulum, pelvic organ prolapse

Urinalysis and Culture

Labs: metabolic panel (renal function, glucose, calcium), vitamin B_{12} (in the elderly), glucose

Measurement of **postvoid residual urine** (especially in high-risk patients)

Give out a frequency/volume **bladder diary** for the patient to record her symptoms

What are normal values for the following?

    Daily urine output:

1500 to 2500 mL

    Average void volume:

250 mL

    Functional bladder capacity:

400 to 600 mL

    Voids per day:

7 to 8 times

Is routine urodynamic testing indicated in the evaluation of urinary incontinence?

No.

While it is the gold standard, it is not always necessary to make the diagnosis. It should be considered if empiric therapy has failed or prior to any surgical intervention.

Describe the following urodynamic tests:

Multichannel urodynamic testing:	Produces a biophysical profile of the patient's bladder and urethra. Used for patients with mixed incontinence, prior bladder surgeries, or suspected intrinsic sphincter deficiency.
Cystometry:	Measures the pressure–volume relationship of the bladder. **Filling cystometry** measures bladder pressure during filling; fluid is infused while pressure is continually monitored. The point of urgency, point of leakage, and total capacity are recorded. **Voiding cystometry** (also known as pressure-flow study) measures the urine flow rate and correlates it with the detrusor pressure.
Urethral pressure profile:	Measures urethral closure and sphincteric integrity.

STRESS INCONTINENCE

What is the prevalence of stress incontinence?	20% to 30% of women complain of stress incontinence.
Describe the pathophysiology of stress incontinence:	With weakening of the pelvic muscles and endofascia, **urethral support is impaired.** Rising intra-abdominal pressure (because of sneezing, coughing, or exercise) leads to the intravesicular pressure rising higher than the pressure of the urethral closure mechanism. This leads to urine leakage.
What are the risk factors for the development of stress incontinence?	Advanced age; denervation and/or **connective tissue injuries** from childbirth or surgery; **previous surgery for prolapse and/or incontinence; low estrogen levels; chronically increased intra-abdominal pressure; collagen vascular disorders**
What is intrinsic urethral sphincter deficiency?	A less common cause of stress incontinence wherein there is **complete failure of urethral closure**; usually because of **scarring** from a past operation or occasionally from severe atrophy in postmenopausal women

Does demonstration of urine leakage during coughing always indicate stress incontinence?

No. It could also be detrusor overactivity, detrusor hyperactivity with impaired contractility (DHIC), or overflow incontinence.

What is the Q-tip test?

Insertion of a cotton swab into the urethra at the bladder neck. It is positive (indicates stress incontinence) if the angle of the cotton swab changes by more than 30° with strain.

How does the timing between the increased pressure and incontinence affect the diagnosis?

Immediate leakage with pressure suggests **stress incontinence. A delay** between the maneuver and the leakage suggests **detrusor overactivity**.

What is the treatment for stress incontinence?

Nonsurgical: muscle strengthening, pessaries, medications (usually ineffective)

Surgical: **pubovesical sling** or **collagen injections**

URGE INCONTINENCE

How common is urge incontinence?

It is the second most common form of incontinence and the most common form of incontinence in older women.

Describe the pathophysiology of urge incontinence:

Involuntary **detrusor overactivity** or bladder contractions

What are some of the causes of detrusor overactivity?

Advanced age; disruption of **inhibitory pathways** (stroke, cervical stenosis, diabetes, Alzheimer disease, Parkinson disease); **bladder irritation** (infection, stones, cancer); **idiopathic**

What is interstitial cystitis?

Urgency and **frequent voiding of small amounts** of urine, often associated with dysuria or pain. Most commonly diagnosed in younger women.

What is DHIC?

Detrusor hyperactivity with impaired contractility. It is characterized by both urgency and an elevated postvoid residual.

What is the treatment for urge incontinence?	Behavioral: bladder retraining
	Medication: anticholinergics and/or β-adrenergics; botox injections into the detrusor
	Surgical: neuromodulation implants (interstim); surgical denervation (usually ineffective); correction pelvic organ prolapse if significant

MIXED INCONTINENCE

What are the symptoms of mixed incontinence?	Leakage associated with urgency and with increased intra-abdominal pressure
Describe the pathophysiology of mixed incontinence	Combination of both **detrusor overactivity and stress incontinence, sometimes compounded by impaired urethral sphincter function**
What is the treatment for mixed incontinence?	Individualized care based on the primary complaint and the individual's characteristics

OVERFLOW INCONTINENCE

What are the symptoms of overflow incontinence?	Continual **dribbling** associated with incomplete bladder emptying
Describe the pathophysiology of overflow incontinence:	There is **underactivity of the detrusor muscle** resulting in failure of full bladder emptying. This leaves a **large postvoid residual** which leads to leakage with increased intra-abdominal pressure. It can also be caused by bladder outlet **obstruction**, usually in women with significant pelvic organ prolapse.
What are some of the causes of underactivity of the detrusor muscle?	Neurogenic bladder (eg, from diabetes, vitamin B_{12} deficiency, Parkinson disease, multiple sclerosis); prior bladder surgery; chronic, long-standing overdistention

TREATMENT

What are the three categories of treatment options for urinary incontinence?	Lifestyle/behavioral changes; medications; surgery (should be tried in that order)
What types of lifestyle changes are associated with an improvement in urinary incontinence?	Limiting fluid intake (no more than 2 L/day) Avoidance of caffeine and alcohol Smoking cessation Treatment of cough (for stress incontinence) Treatment of constipation Weight loss and increased physical activity
What types of behavioral changes are associated with an improvement in urinary incontinence?	**Bladder training; pelvic muscle exercises**
Describe bladder training:	**Timed voiding** while awake, with gradually increasing intervals between voids; **relaxation and distractive techniques** to suppress urgency in between voids
What is the theory behind bladder training?	The central nervous system and pelvic musculature can be **trained to inhibit detrusor contractions** by becoming gradually accustomed to accommodating larger bladder volumes.
What is supplemental biofeedback?	Vaginal or anorectal biofeedback mechanisms used to help patients identify and use their pelvic musculature in response to a sense of urgency
For which type of incontinence is bladder training most useful?	Urge incontinence
What are pelvic muscle exercises?	Also known as **Kegel** exercises, they involve isometric repetitions of exercises in order to strengthen the levator ani muscles

For which types of incontinence are pelvic muscle exercises effective?

Urge, stress, or mixed incontinence

In which types of incontinence is pharmacotherapy warranted?

Urge and mixed incontinence

What types of medications are used to treat urinary incontinence?

Antimuscarinics: oxybutynin; tolterodine; trospium; solifenacin; darifenacine

α-adrenergic agonists: duloxetine; tricyclic antidepressants (TCAs) (imipramine); topical estrogens; botulinum toxin

What is a continence pessary?

A device that can be used to treat incontinence because of pelvic floor prolapse

What types of surgical options are effective for urge incontinence?

Sacral nerve modulation; augmentation cystoplasty

What types of surgical options are effective for stress incontinence?

Minimally invasive midurethral anti-incontinence procedures (Tension free vaginal tape [TVT], Tension free vaginal tape-obturator [TVTO])

Retropubic bladder neck suspension (Burch or Marshall–Marchetti–Krantz [MMK] colposuspension)

Sling procedures

Periurethral bulking injections

Should an indwelling urinary catheter be used to alleviate symptoms of incontinence?

As these are associated with high morbidity, they should only be considered in selected cases as a last resort.

Describe the midurethral anti-incontinence procedures:

These are minimally invasive, vaginal surgical procedures using synthetic mesh material placed at the level of the midurethra in a tension-free manner (TVT/ TVTO)

What complications are associated with the midurethral anti-incontinence procedures?

Postoperative voiding dysfunction

Urinary retention

Erosion of mesh material

Describe the retropubic bladder neck suspension procedures:	An abdominal procedure that uses the periurethral vaginal tissue to support the urethrovesical junction via sutures to Cooper's ligament (Burch) or to the pubic symphysis (MMK)
What complications are associated with the retropubic bladder neck suspension procedure?	Enterocele formation; postoperative voiding dysfunction; urinary retention
Describe suburethral sling procedures:	Elevation of the urethrovesical junction and introduction of mechanical compression of the urethra using autologous or synthetic graft material
What are the complications of a sling procedure?	Postoperative voiding dysfunction; urinary retention; erosion of graft material
Describe periurethral bulking agents procedures:	Elevation of the urethrovesical junction and introduction of mechanical compression of the urethra using autologous or synthetic graft material

CLINICAL VIGNETTES

A 34-year-old G1P0 at 24 and 4/7 weeks gestation presents with suprapubic pain, dysuria, and frequency in the last 2 days. She is afebrile. Her urinalysis shows 2+ LE, greater than 10 WBC/ high power field, and nitrite negative. She is allergic to penicillin. What is your first step?

a. Start ciprofloxacin for 3 days.
b. Start ciprofloxacin for 7 days for a complicated UTI.
c. Obtain urine cultures and treat based on results.
d. Start nitrofurantoin for 7 days for suspected complicated UTI.
e. This patient is pregnant and an ultrasound should be ordered to r/o pyelonephritis and treat based on the result.

Answer: d

The patient has a UTI in pregnancy and should be treated for 5 to 7 days. Ciprofloxacin (choices a and b) is contraindicated during pregnancy. Her complaints are suggestive for a UTI and therefore, there is no need to wait for a diagnostic urine culture at this time (choice c). However, it could be sent concomitant to starting treatment. There is no need to obtain sonogram at this time (choice e).

A 72-year-old P3 comes to your office for a well-woman examination. She has no complaints. On examination you note a grade 2 prolapse (Baden Walker) of her uterus. The patient is aware of it but is not bothered by it. What is your first step?

a. Do nothing unless patient becomes symptomatic.
b. Prescribe oxybutynin to prevent urinary obstruction symptoms from developing.
c. Try to convince patient to undergo surgical correction in order to prevent complications in the future.
d. Give the patient a pessary in order to reduce the uterus back to place.
e. Tell the patient to refrain from strenuous activity in order to prevent incarceration of the uterus.

Answer: a

There is no need for surgical or medical treatment of an asymptomatic prolapse. Her prolapse may progress as time passes but there is a low risk of complications.

KO is a 36-year-old G2P2 reports that since her last delivery, 2 years ago, she has leakage of urine when changing position from lying to standing and when she coughs. Occasionally she has to urinate urgently but cannot make it to the bathroom in time and loses urine. She denies dysuria. What is your plan?

a. Treat empirically with antibiotics for a UTI.
b. Schedule the patient for a laparoscopic burch colposuspension.
c. Perform multichannel urodynamic testing to evaluate the bladder performance.
d. Inform the patient that her condition is related to her vaginal delivery and it has no good treatment except waiting for it to resolve on its own.

Answer: c

The patient has mixed symptoms and needs further evaluation. There is no need for surgery until the diagnosis is established (choice b). Although the condition may be related to her vaginal delivery, at this stage it will not recover on its own. There are great treatment options (choice d). The condition has been ongoing for 2 years and is unlikely to be a UTI (choice a).

A 56-year-old G1P1 has urge incontinence for the last 3 years. She has been on every possible medication for this indication without relief. She comes crying to your office because it is ruining her life. She wants surgical treatment. What can you offer her?

a. Place a pubovaginal sling to prevent urine leakage.
b. Insert a suprapubic tube to continuously drain the bladder and prevent leakage.
c. Perform sacral nerve neuromodulation for the treatment of her urge incontinence.
d. Perform periurethral injections of bulking agents to prevent leakage of urine.

Answer: c

A sling does not correct urge incontinence (choice a). A suprapubic tube is much too aggressive for this condition (choice b). Periurethral injections treat stress incontinence (choice d). Neuromodulation has good success rates with urge incontinence.

Timed voiding is most indicated for which condition?
   a. Stress incontinence
   b. Urge incontinence
   c. Mixed incontinence
   d. Overflow incontinence
   e. Global incontinence

Answer: b

Timed voiding while awake, with gradually increasing intervals between voids, suppresses urgency in between voids. It may also partly help mixed incontinence.

CHAPTER 7

Reproductive Endocrinology and Infertility

Adolescent Development

INTRODUCTION

What types of changes occur during puberty?	Development of secondary sexual characteristics Growth Changes in body composition Achievement of fertility
What is meant by the following terms?	
Thelarche:	Breast development
Pubarche:	Development of pubic hair
Menarche:	Beginning of menses
What is the typical sequence of events in puberty for girls?	**Thelarche** (breast development) → **Pubarche** (pubic hair growth) → peak growth spurt → **menarche**
What is the average time duration of puberty and when does it start?	4.5 years is the average duration of puberty. On an average, thelarche begins at 10 years and menarche at 12 years of age.
What are the Tanner stages?	A **staging system** for the sequence of **pubertal development**. Divides the development of secondary sex characteristics into five stages.

Describe the Tanner stages for breast development in females:

Stage 1: prepubertal

Stage 2: elevation of breast and papilla; enlargement of areola; breast bud stage

Stage 3: further enlargement of breast and areola; increased glandular tissue

Stage 4: areola and papilla project above the breast

Stage 5: recession of areola, projection of papilla only, mature stage

Describe the Tanner stages for pubic hair development:

Stage 1: vellus hairs only, prepubertal

Stage 2: sparse growth of slightly pigmented hair

Stage 3: hair growth spreads and becomes darker, coarser, and more curly

Stage 4: adult hair type, but no spread to medial thigh

Stage 5: medial spread with inverse triangle distribution

What happens to the external genitalia during puberty?

Estrogen stimulation leads to thickening of the mons pubis, growth of the labia majora, rounding of the labia minora, thickening of the hymen, elongation of the vagina.

What happens to the uterus during puberty?

The myometrium thickens, altering the uterine shape. The endometrium thickens gradually and then more rapidly before menarche.

Describe the pattern of growth that occurs in puberty:

Growth affects both the trunk and the limbs, with the limbs (especially the distal portions thereof) growing before the rest of the body. Girls have their growth spurt before boys and the peak growth occurs approximately 6 months prior to menarche.

What happens to the long bones during puberty?

Long bones lengthen and their epiphyses close

What are some of the unwelcome physiological changes that occur as a result of puberty?

Acne; psychological changes—boys develop a more positive and girls experience a diminished self-image; scoliosis; myopia

CONGENITAL ANOMALIES

What is suggested by clitoral enlargement?

Exposure to high levels of **androgens**. Proper evaluation to exclude any intersex conditions is warranted.

What is imperforate hymen?

A persistent urogenital membrane

What are the symptoms of an imperforate hymen?

It is rare to make this diagnosis before puberty. Symptoms include **primary amenorrhea, pelvic pain, tender posterior vaginal canal on rectal examination,** and difficulty with urination/defecation.

What are some of the potential complications associated with an untreated imperforate hymen?

Endometriosis and vaginal adenosis

What is a vaginal septum?

An absence of fusion of the müllerian ducts and/or urogenital sinuses leading to an obstructive lesion in the vagina. This leads to obstructive symptoms similar to those of an imperforate hymen.

What is vaginal agenesis?

Usually associated with Mayer-Rokitansky-Küster-Hauser syndrome. It involves normal-appearing external genitalia with agenesis of the vagina superior to the hymen (upper 2/3rd). It is usually associated with uterine and cervical agenesis.

It can associated be associated with testicular feminization. These patients have testes instead of ovaries and need to have them removed.

What are the symptoms of vaginal agenesis?

Primary amenorrhea and **pelvic pain**

How is vaginal agenesis treated?

Creation of a vagina by use of either **serial vaginal dilation** or surgical reconstruction with a **vaginoplasty procedure**

What are the various congenital anomalies of the uterus and how common are each? Describe each:

Arcuate uterus (15%): small septum with minimal cavity indentation

Incomplete septum (13%): partial fusion resulting in a septum that does not completely divide the horns

Complete uterine septum (9%): partial fusion that completely divides the uterine horns

Bicornate uterus (37%): partial fusion leading to a midline septum (can be partial or complete)

Uterine didelphys (11%): failure of fusion resulting in two separate uterine bodies

Unicornuate uterus (4%): agenesis of one Müllerian duct, with an absence of the corresponding fallopian tube and round ligament

What are the symptoms of these uterine anomalies?

Usually asymptomatic

Retention of menstrual flow

Infertility

Recurrent pregnancy loss

Preterm delivery

What does the palpation of an inguinal mass in an adolescent patient suggest?

Possible aberrant gonad (often with testicular elements)

How should an aberrant gonad be managed?

A **karyotype** should be done and a **biopsy** of the gonad should be done. If it is an ovary, it should be returned to the peritoneal cavity. If it is a testis, it should be removed.

ACCELERATED SEXUAL MATURATION

What is premature thelarche and how is it managed?

Isolated development of breasts before 8 years of age. No intervention is required if other signs of precocious puberty do not develop.

What is premature pubarche and how is it managed?

Isolated appearance of public or axillary hair before 6 to 7 years of age. It generally represents premature secretion of androgens from the adrenal gland. Evaluation of the adrenal and gonadal function should be done to exclude precocious puberty.

What is premature menarche and how is it managed?

Isolated cyclic vaginal bleeding without any other signs of sexual development. It is usually related to increased end-organ sensitivity to estrogen and it does not require any intervention.

What is sexual precocity?

Onset of sexual maturation before 2.5 times the standard deviation of the normal age for that population

How is precocious puberty classified?

GnRH dependent and GnRH independent

What is GnRH-dependent precocious puberty?

Also called central precocious puberty (CPP); premature activation of the hypothalamic-pituitary axis with premature gonadotropin secretion

What is GnRH-independent precocious puberty?

Sex steroids are present independent of the release of pituitary gonadotropins. This is a pseudoprecocious puberty.

What are some of the causes of GnRH-independent precocious puberty?

Congenital adrenal hyperplasia

Tumors of the adrenal gland

Tumors of the gonads

hCG-secreting tumors

McCune-Albright syndrome

Exogenous steroids

What is the workup for precocious puberty?

1. History: age of onset, progression, family history
2. Physical examination (PE): growth velocity changes, acne, breast development, genital changes
3. Laboratory: luteinizing hormone (**LH**), follicle-stimulating hormone (**FSH**), estradiol, **GnRH-stimulation test**
4. Imaging: skeletal survey and bone scan to determine bone age, pelvic ultrasound, abdominal CT (of adrenals), brain MRI

What are the results of the laboratory tests in GnRH-dependent precocious puberty?	Normal pubertal range
What is the treatment for GnRH-dependent precocious puberty?	GnRH analogues, which induce down-regulation of the receptor function, creating an inhibition of the hypothalamic-pituitary-ovarian axis
What is McCune-Albright syndrome?	A genetic disorder with a classic triad of precocious puberty, polyostotic fibrous dysplasia, and café-au-lait skin lesions

DELAYED SEXUAL MATURATION

What is delayed sexual maturation?	Absence of pubertal changes after 2.5 times the standard deviation of the mean age for a population (eg, absence of thelarche by age 13 and menarche by age 15)
What is the proper evaluation for a patient with delayed sexual maturation?	1. History: previous growth patterns and pubertal development, other medical disorders 2. PE: height and weight, Tanner staging, pelvic examination (for congenital anomalies and obstruction) 3. Labs/imaging: vaginal smear (for cytohormonal evaluation), karyotype, pelvic ultrasound, FSH
What does breast development signify?	Prior gonadal function (adequate release of estrogen)
What does the absence of pubic hair signify?	Androgen insensitivity
What is the differential diagnosis of a patient with delayed menarche and adequate secondary sexual characteristics?	Pregnancy Anatomic genital abnormalities Inappropriate positive feedback Complete androgen insensitivity syndrome
How are patients with delayed menarche and inadequate secondary sexual characteristics classified?	By their FSH level

What is the differential diagnosis of a patient with delayed menarche and inadequate secondary sexual characteristics?	Low FSH: constitutional delay; weight loss (extreme dieting, drug abuse, extreme exercise); Kallmann syndrome; pituitary destruction
	High FSH: Turner syndrome; ovarian destruction (chemotherapy, radiation, infection, autoimmune); resistant ovary syndrome
What is Kallmann syndrome?	A rare genetic syndrome causing **hypogonadotropic hypogonadism** and **anosmia**
What is the differential diagnosis of a patient with delayed menarche and virilization?	1. Enzyme deficiency (such as 21α-hydroxylase deficiency) 2. Neoplasia 3. Male pseudohermaphroditism

Disorders of the Menstrual Cycle, Uterus, and Endometrium

PMS

What is premenstrual syndrome?	A cyclical pattern of **emotional, physical, and/or behavioral** changes that occur in the **luteal phase** of the menstrual cycle and remit during menses. Symptoms cause **significant disability**, and it is *not* an exacerbation of an underlying psychiatric disorder. A more severe variant is **premenstrual dysphoric disorder**.
What is the incidence of PMS and in whom does it occur?	The incidence ranges from 5% to 90% of women.
	Approximately 70% have some symptoms of PMS and 5% have the more severe PMDD.
	It occurs mostly in women in their mid-20s to 40s.

What are the symptoms of PMS?

At least one of the following which is temporally related to the menstrual cycle with a symptom-free follicular phase:

1. **Affective lability**
2. **Anxiety or tension**
3. **Depressed mood, hopelessness,** or **self-deprecating thoughts**
4. **Persistent anger or irritability**

Other symptoms include decreased interest/avoidance of usual activities, decreased productivity, lethargy, changes in appetite/cravings, reproducible patterns of physical complaints (ie, headaches, weight gain, breast tenderness), difficulty concentrating, sleep disturbances, and a sense of being overwhelmed.

What are the treatment options for PMS?

Education of the patient and her family

Dietary changes/Exercise

NSAIDs

Diuretics

Anxiolytic/antidepressant medications

Vitamin B$_6$

DYSMENORRHEA

What is dysmenorrhea and what are the two types?

Dysmenorrhea is **pain with menses** either due to **pelvic pathology (secondary dysmenorrhea)** or **without pelvic pathology (primary dysmenorrhea)**.

What is the incidence of dysmenorrhea and in whom does it occur?

Dysmenorrhea occurs in approximately **15% to 75% of women. Primary dysmenorrhea** is most common in **younger** women, whereas the incidence of **secondary dysmenorrhea** increases with age.

What is the etiology of primary dysmenorrhea?

An excess of **prostaglandin F$_{2\alpha}$** produced in the endometrium.

It stimulates smooth muscle, leading to uterine contractions and uterine ischemia.

What are the clinical signs and symptoms of primary dysmenorrhea?

Pain typically begins **at menstruation** and subsides after 1 to 3 days. It is characterized as **cramping, labor-like pain**, typically in the **lower abdomen** and **suprapubic** area, radiating to the back. The pain can be associated with **nausea, vomiting**, and **diarrhea.**

What is the treatment of primary dysmenorrhea?

NSAIDs therapy is first-line. Other options include **heat, exercise**, and **oral contraceptives.** In severe, refractory cases, **presacral neurectomy** is a last resort.

Secondary dysmenorrhea should be suspected if symptoms are refractory to NSAIDs or OCPs.

How do NSAIDs and OCPs work to treat dysmenorrhea?

NSAIDs work by **inhibiting prostaglandin production.**

OCPs work by **decreasing prostaglandin production** through suppression of ovulation.

What are the gynecologic causes of secondary dysmenorrhea?

Extrauterine causes:
 Endometriosis
 Neoplasm
 Inflammation (eg, PID)
 Adhesions

Intramural causes:
 Adenomyosis
 Leiomyomata

Intrauterine causes:
 Leiomyomata
 Polyps
 IUDs
 Infection
 Cervical stenosis/lesions

For a patient with dysmenorrhea, what primary diagnosis do each of the following findings suggest?

Uterine asymmetry:

Myomas or other tumors

Symmetrical enlargement of uterus:

Adenomyosis

Painful nodules in posterior cul-de-sac:

Endometriosis

Restricted motion of the uterus:

Endometriosis or pelvic scarring/ adhesions from prior infection

What is the treatment for secondary dysmenorrhea?

Treatment of the underlying condition is the primary modality.

However, when this is not possible, **NSAIDs** and low-dose **oral contraceptives** sometimes offer symptomatic therapy.

What other underlying diseases are exacerbated by menstruation?

Women with **migraines** or tension headaches can have increased frequency of headaches at the time of menstruation. Asthma patients occasionally report worsening of symptoms with menses. These effects are thought to be due to increased prostaglandin production.

DYSFUNCTIONAL UTERINE BLEEDING

Describe what is meant by the following patterns of abnormal bleeding:

Hypomenorrhea:

A **decreased amount** of bleeding at **regular intervals**

Intermenstrual bleeding:

Bleeding of variable amounts occurring **between regular menstrual periods**

Menorrhagia:

Prolonged or excessive uterine bleeding occurring at **regular** intervals Synonymous with **hypermenorrhea**

Metrorrhagia:

Uterine bleeding occurring at **irregular intervals**

Polymenorrhea:

Uterine bleeding occurring at **intervals of less than 21 days**

Oligomenorrhea:

Menstrual bleeding at intervals of longer than 35 days

What is dysfunctional uterine bleeding?

Dysfunctional uterine bleeding (DUB) is a diagnosis of exclusion that consists of **irregular menstruation unrelated to anatomic lesions.**

What is the physiologic cause of DUB?

A **hyperestrogenic** state. Because of **anovulation**, these women have **noncyclic estrogen** levels that **stimulate endometrial growth**. Once the **endometrium outgrows its blood supply**, it sloughs off, leading to irregular, often heavy bleeding.

How can you clinically differentiate between ovulatory cycles and anovulatory cycles?

Ovulatory cycles are **regular** in their length. Anovulatory cycle bleeding is much more **irregular.**

What must be ruled out before the diagnosis of DUB can be made?

Organic causes of abnormal bleeding such as **leiomyomas, inflammation** (cervicitis, endometritis), **carcinomas, cervical/endometrial polyps, vaginal lesions, blood dyscrasia,** and **iatrogenic causes** (IUDs, fertility drugs)

Note: **Abnormal uterine bleeding in a postmenopausal woman is cancer until proven otherwise.**

What conditions are often associated with DUB?

Obesity

Polycystic ovarian disease

Adrenal hyperplasia

Perimenopause

In whom does DUB occur?

Half of all patients with DUB are **peri- or postmenopausal**. Another **20%** are **adolescents.**

What type of bleeding pattern is seen in women with high estrogen levels and with low estrogen levels?

High levels of **estrogen** cause the endometrium to build up beyond its blood supply. This leads to **prolonged amenorrhea followed by profuse bleeding.**

Low levels of **estrogen** cause **intermittent spotting of a prolonged duration, but can cause heavy bleeding from denuded, dyssynchronous endometrium.**

What is the initial workup for abnormal bleeding?

A thorough **menstrual history, bimanual examination,** and **Pap smear.**

A TSH may also be ordered as thyroid disease can affect bleeding patterns.

In each scenario, what additional tests should be done and why?

An ovulatory woman:

Transvaginal ultrasound, sonohysterogram, or **D&C with hysteroscopy** (gold standard)

An anovulatory woman:

β-hCG: pregnancy

CBC: infection

Coagulation profile: blood dyscrasia

Endocrine tests (FSH, LH, TSH, prolactin): premature ovarian failure, polycystic ovarian syndrome (PCOS), prolactinoma, hypothyroidism

Age more than 35 years and all postmenopausal women:

Endometrial biopsy: endometrial carcinoma

What are the risks of unrecognized DUB?

Hemorrhage, endometrial hyperplasia, and/or **cancer**

What is the goal of treatment for DUB?

To convert the proliferative endometrium into secretory endometrium

How is anovulatory DUB treated?

OCPs.

Cyclic progesterone therapy (eg, medroxyprogesterone daily for 10 days of each month).

DUB associated with heavy bleeding is treated with **high-dose estrogen or progestins.**

Endometrial ablation or uterine artery embolization can also be used if patient is refractory to oral and IV estrogen therapy.

A **D&C** can be done if patient is hemodynamically unstable.

How is ovulatory DUB treated?

Ovulatory DUB is treated primarily with OCPs.

AMENORRHEA

What is amenorrhea and what are the two subtypes?

Amenorrhea is the **absence of menstruation.**

1. **Primary amenorrhea: no history of menstruation**
2. **Secondary amenorrhea:** previous menstruation but **failure to menstruate over 6 months** or **for three cycle intervals**

What are the four main etiologies of amenorrhea?	1. **Pregnancy.** 2. **Hypothalamic-pituitary dysfunction:** the pulsatile secretion of GnRH is altered such that the pituitary gland ceases secreting FSH and LH. This results in the absence of regular ovulation and menstruation origin. 3. **Ovarian dysfunction:** the ovarian follicles are resistant to stimulation by FSH and LH. 4. **Anatomic dysfunction:** genital outflow tract obstruction, either congenital (such as imperforate hymen) or from the development of scar tissue. The most common cause of obstruction is Asherman syndrome (scarring of the uterine cavity).
What are the common causes of hypothalamic-pituitary dysfunction?	Functional: weight loss, excessive exercise, obesity Drug induced: marijuana, sedatives Malignancy: prolactinoma, craniopharyngioma, hypothalamic hamartoma Psychogenic: anxiety, anorexia Other: head injury, chronic disease, empty sella syndrome, Sheehan syndrome
How is amenorrhea due to hypothalamic-pituitary dysfunction diagnosed?	**Low serum levels** of **FSH** and **LH** are diagnostic. **Prolactin** is usually normal, except in a prolactinoma.
What are the common causes of ovarian dysfunction that lead to primary amenorrhea?	Gonadal dysgenesis: Turner syndrome Mosaicism 17-hydroxylase deficiency Gonadal agenesis
What are the common causes of ovarian dysfunction that lead to secondary amenorrhea?	Pregnancy Menopause Autoimmune ovarian failure (Blizzard syndrome) Premature ovarian failure Alkylating chemotherapy

How is amenorrhea due to ovarian dysfunction diagnosed?

As the ovaries fail, serum FSH level rises

How can estrogen deficiency due to hypothalamic-pituitary failure be differentiated from that due to ovarian failure?

Estrogen deficiency secondary to **hypothalamic-pituitary failure** usually does **not** cause **hot flashes. Ovarian failure** may **cause hot flashes.**

What genital outflow obstructions lead to primary amenorrhea?

Müllerian anomalies (eg, imperforate hymen)

Müllerian agenesis

What genital outflow obstructions lead to secondary amenorrhea?

Asherman syndrome

What laboratory tests are indicated in the evaluation of a patient with secondary amenorrhea?

β-hCG

TSH

Prolactin

FSH

Progesterone challenge test

What diagnoses are suggested by the following lab results?

↑ β-hCG:

Pregnancy

↑ TSH:

Hypothyroidism

↑ Prolactin:

Hyperprolactinemia from a pituitary tumor, idiopathic, or due to medications (eg, dopamine antagonists)

↑ FSH:

Postmenopausal state or ovarian failure

↓ FSH:

Hypothalamic disorder or pituitary dysfunction

Note: **if the gonadotropins are high, the problem is at the level of the ovary. If the gonadotropins are low, the problem is in the hypothalamus or pituitary.**

What further test must be done if the patient is found to be hypogonadotropic?

Imaging of the sella turcica, either via **CT scan** or **MRI.**

Abnormal imaging suggests a pituitary tumor, whereas normal imaging is assumed to signify a hypothalamic problem.

What further test must be done if the patient is found to be hypergonadotropic?

A **karyotype** to diagnose mosaicism with a Y chromosome

What is the progesterone challenge test and what is the procedure?

The patient is given oral **progesterone**. **Withdrawal bleeding** is observed after a few days.

What does withdrawal bleeding in the progesterone challenge test indicate?

Withdrawal bleeding indicates that the patient is **chronically anovulatory** or **oligo-ovulatory**. Ovulation had not occurred and so no endogenous progesterone was made. Causes of anovulation include hypothalamic dysfunction, polycystic ovarian syndrome, Cushing syndrome, or an ovarian tumor.

What does the absence of withdrawal bleeding in the progesterone challenge test indicate?

The absence of withdrawal bleeding indicates that the patient is either **hypoestrogenic** or has an **anatomic obstruction**.

What is the next step if withdrawal bleeding does not occur?

An **estrogen–progesterone test, imaging**

What is an estrogen–progesterone test and what do the results indicate?

The estradiol and progesterone test entails giving a small dose of **estradiol daily for 28 days** and adding **progesterone for the last 7 days**. This differentiates a hypoestrogenic state from an anatomic obstruction. **Withdrawal bleeding** indicates **inadequate estrogen**. If withdrawal bleeding does **not** occur within a few days, **anatomic obstruction** is the diagnosis.

What is the treatment for amenorrhea due to the following?

Hypothalamic anovulation:

Induction of ovulation with **gonadotropins if pregnancy desired, otherwise OCPs.**

A prolactinoma:

Dopamine agonists. Rarely, surgical excision.

Premature ovarian failure:

Exogenous **estrogen** replacement.

Genital tract obstruction:

Surgery to restore genital tract integrity.

Infertility

EVALUATION OF INFERTILITY

How is infertility defined?

It is defined as the **inability to conceive after 12 months** of frequent intercourse without use of contraception.

What is the definition of fecundability?

It is the probability of achieving pregnancy in one menstrual cycle.

What is the prevalence of infertility?

About 13% (range from 7%-28%) depending on the age of the woman

What is the difference between primary and secondary infertility?

Primary infertility pertains to those who have never conceived, whereas secondary infertility is applied to those who have conceived in the past.

What percent of infertility is because of male factors, female factors, both and unknown etiology?

Male factor (23%)

Female factors (40%-50%)

Both (27%)

Unknown etiology (15%-20%)

What are the most common factors that comprise female factor infertility?

Ovulatory disorders (25%)

Endometriosis (15%)

Pelvic adhesions (12%)

Tubal blockage (11%)

Other tubal abnormalities (11%)

Hyperprolactinemia (7%)

What is the first test to perform for infertility if the history and physical from the infertile couple offer no clues?

Semen analysis

What are the relevant characteristics of normal semen?

Volume: 2 to 5 mL

Concentration: greater than or equal to 20 million per mL

Motility: 50% should be motile, 25% should have rapid progressive motility

Morphology: lower limit of normal is 10% to 15%

What hormone tests should be ordered if the sperm concentration is less than 5 million per mL?

Follicle-stimulating hormone (FSH), luteinizing hormone (LH), and testosterone

What is the next step in evaluation of infertility if the semen analysis is normal?

Ovulatory function

What percent of female factor fertility can be attributed to ovulatory dysfunction?

25%

What are risk factors for premature ovarian failure?

Exposure to cytotoxic drugs, pelvic radiation therapy, autoimmune diseases, previous ovarian surgery, family history of early menopause

What are the methods to evaluate ovulatory function?

Menstrual history, basal-body-temperature (BBT) chart, serum progesterone levels in the mid-luteal phase, sonogram, urinary LH kits, and/or endometrial biopsy

How is anovulation classified and what is the mechanism of that type of anovulation?

1. **Hypogonadotropic hypogonadal anovulation (hypothalamic amenorrhea)**—low GnRH or pituitary unresponsiveness to GnRH, resulting in low serum FSH and estradiol levels. Can be seen in stress- or exercise-related amenorrhea, anorexia nervosa, Kallmann syndrome, or CNS tumors.
2. **Normogonadotropic normo-estrogenic anovulation**—most prevalent subtype. Normal GnRH secretion, estradiol and FSH levels with either normal or elevated LH concentrations. Includes women with polycystic ovary syndrome (PCOS).
3. **Hypergonadotropic hypoestrogenic anovulation**—ovarian failure is the primary cause.
4. **Hyperprolactinemic anovulation**—hyperprolactinemia inhibits gonadotropin and, therefore, estrogen secretion.

What other endocrine abnormalities may result in infertility?

Hypothyroidism, androgen excess, diabetes/obesity, starvation

How do each of these methods help evaluate a woman's ovulatory function?

A **menstrual cycle history** that reveals amenorrhea indicates anovulation and a cause of infertility, whereas a normal monthly menstrual cycle is a strong indicator of normal ovulation.

A **basal-body-temperature chart** that indicates normal ovulation is reflected by a biphasic curve during ovulation, with a rise in temperature by 0.5°F to 1.0°F during the luteal phase (because of an increased level of progesterone). The highest temperature in one menstrual cycle occurs during ovulation.

Urinary LH kits. Over-the-counter monitors that detect the LH surge in the urine. This method allows for appropriate timing of intercourse.

Measurement of a **serum progesterone level in the mid-luteal phase** (18-24 days after the onset of menses) is the definitive confirmation for ovulation. Normal levels are between 6 and 25 mg/mL.

Sonogram and/or endometrial biopsy shows secretory glands, may be used to evaluate whether the endometrium is optimal for normal implantation of the egg.

If a female's ovulatory function is intact, what other factors may cause female factor infertility and what is their relative frequency?

Tubal damage (14%)

Endometriosis (9%)

Coital problems (5%)

Cervical factor (3%)

What is the major cause of tubal infertility and by what method may tubal abnormalities and/or other uterine cavity abnormalities be evaluated?

Pelvic inflammatory disease (PID)

Hysterosalpingogram should be obtained for evaluation

What are other causes of tubal infertility?

Prior abdominal or pelvic surgery, ectopic pregnancy, severe endometriosis

When should laparoscopy be used?

It should be considered for couples with otherwise unexplained infertility or in women with known or suspected endometriosis and/or pelvic adhesions.

How should a woman who presents with infertility and early stage endometriosis be treated for fertility?

Surgical resection of endometriosis lesions and other pelvic adhesions, followed by a trial of clomiphene or gonadotropin plus IUI (intrauterine insemination)

What is meant by assessing a female's ovarian reserve and what are the most commonly used tests to evaluate this?

This assessment is to determine quantity and possibly quality of remaining oocyte pool. The most commonly used tests are the day 3 FSH test and the clomiphene citrate challenge test (CCCT), and AMH (anti-Müllerian hormone) levels.

TREATMENT OF INFERTILITY

What is the general approach to treatment of infertility?

A stepwise approach, from least to most invasive (and expensive)

Clomiphene citrate → induction with gonadotropins → in vitro fertilization (IVF)

What modifications in lifestyle habits may improve fertility?

Smoking and alcohol cessation, decrease in caffeine consumption, increased frequency of coitus, maintaining a healthy weight and diet

What is clomiphene citrate and in which patients is it used?

It is a selective estrogen receptor modulator (SERM) that ultimately increases gonadotropin release. It is the agent of choice for women less than 36 years of age and in normogonadotrophic normo-estrogenic anovulation.

When is induction with human menopausal gonadotropins (hMG) indicated?

Subcutaneous injection of hMG, specifically FSH, is used in women who have failed with clomiphene and in women with hypothalamic amenorrhea with hypopituitarism.

How is follicle development and ovulation induced in women in hypogonadotropic hypogonadal anovulation with normal pituitary function?

Pulsatile administration of GnRH stimulates endogenous production of FSH and LH.

What agent should be used in women who have anovulation because of hyperprolactinemia?

Dopamine agonists such as bromocriptine or cabergoline

Do these induction agents have an associated risk for ovarian cancer and breast cancer?

Historical evidence has indicated an association between clomiphene use and ovarian cancer, more recent studies do not support this association. However, it is recommended that induction with clomiphene be limited to 12 cycles. There has been no reported risk between fertility drugs and breast cancer.

What is intrauterine insemination (IUI)?

It consists of collecting a specimen of sperm, followed by washing and concentration of the sperm. The concentrated sperm is then injected trans-cervically into the upper uterine cavity using a small catheter.

ASSISTED REPRODUCTIVE TECHNOLOGIES

What are the different modalities of assisted reproductive technologies (ARTs)?

In vitro fertilization-embryo transfer (IVF-ET)

Intracytoplasmic sperm injection (ICSI)

Gamete intrafallopian tube transfer (GIFT)

Zygote intrafallopian tube transfer (ZIFT)

Oocyte donation

What is the mechanism of each of the following technologies and their success rate of pregnancy?

IVF-ET: the ovary is hyperstimulated by daily FSH injections. Multiple mature eggs are collected by a transvaginal procedure and combined with sperm in the laboratory. After fertilization, selected embryos are placed in the uterus. Pregnancy is achieved 28% of the time and 82% result in one or more births.

ICSI: involves taking a single sperm from the male partner and injecting it directly into the cytoplasm of the egg in the laboratory. It is commonly used as treatment for male infertility factor. Overall fertilization rate is 60%.

OSTEOPOROSIS

What is osteoporosis?

A disorder of the skeleton that involves **low bone mass** and **microarchitectural disruption**, both of which lead to skeletal fragility and increased fracture risk.

What is the prevalence of osteoporosis?

Over 30% of women over 50 years have radiographic evidence of osteoporosis; over 44 million men and women are currently diagnosed with osteoporosis in the United States.

Who does osteoporosis affect?

Predominately **thin**, **postmenopausal** women and more often Caucasian and **Asian** women

Why does osteoporosis affect women more than men?

Women have a **lower peak bone mass** and have **accelerated bone loss** after menopause.

When does bone mass peak?

At the age of 30 to 35 years

What is the pathogenesis of osteoporosis?

Bone loss, which is a result of a mismatch between bone resorption and bone formation. Most is a result of either age-related or menopause-related bone loss.

How does osteoporosis typically present?

Often with **hip fracture**, a **vertebral compression fracture** (leading to kyphosis), or a **wrist fracture** after minimal trauma

What is the differential diagnosis of osteoporosis?

Osteomalacia

Hyperparathyroidism

Multiple myeloma

Pathological fracture secondary to metastatic cancer

What is "high turnover" osteoporosis and what are the causes?

Osteoporosis primarily secondary to **increased bone resorption**

Caused by e**strogen deficiency**, hyperparathyroidism, hyperthyroidism, hypogonadism, cyclosporine, heparin

What is "low turnover" osteoporosis and what are the causes?

Osteoporosis primarily secondary to **decreased bone formation**

Caused by **advanced age**, liver disease, heparin

What drug causes both decreased formation and increased resorption of bone, leading to osteoporosis?

Glucocorticoids

What drugs are known to cause osteoporosis?

Glucocorticoids; heparin; medroxyprogesterone acetate; vitamin A; certain retinoids

Describe age-related bone loss:

Loss of both the cortical and trabecular bone that begins around age 30 to 40 years, in both men and women; partially because of **decreased calcium absorption**

Describe menopause-related bone loss:

Loss of all but especially trabecular bone that occurs for 10 years beginning after the onset of menopause because of the **decline in estrogen levels**

Can hormone replacement therapy be used to prevent menopause-related bone loss?

Yes, however it is not first-line therapy because of its cardiovascular and breast cancer risks.

What is the relationship between lactation and bone loss?

Lactation is associated with a 1% to 4% bone loss; however, it is regained after lactation is completed. There is no association between osteoporosis and lactation earlier in life.

What is the relationship between calcium and osteoporosis?

Calcium has been shown to reduce bone loss when a, 1000 to 1500 mg supplement is taken by postmenopausal women daily.

How is osteoporosis diagnosed?

Either by the **presence of a fragility fracture** or by testing for **bone mineral density** (BMD) with a dual-energy x-ray absorptiometry (**DEXA**) scan of the spine and/or hip. Osteoporosis is defined as a BMD of less than 2.5 standard deviations below the mean.

Are there any abnormal lab tests in osteoporosis?

No

What is osteopenia?

Decreased BMD; diagnosed on a DEXA scan as a BMD between 1 and 2.5 standard deviations below the mean

Who should be screened for osteoporosis using a DEXA scan?

Women under 65 years who have one or more risk factors for osteoporosis

All women over 65 years of age

In women with osteoporosis, what are risk factors for fracture?

Medical history: **previous fracture or fracture in first-degree relative,** inflammatory bowel disease (IBD), celiac disease, cystic fibrosis, history of hyperthyroidism, use of anxiolytic, anticonvulsant, or neuroleptic drugs, type II diabetes, dementia

Social history: **cigarette smoking,** consumption of lots of caffeine, sedentary lifestyle, inadequate calcium intake

Physical examination: **low body weight,** tall stature

What are the categories of treatment for osteoporosis?

Reduce risk of falls; nonpharmacologic therapies; drug therapies

What types of nonpharmacologic therapies are useful for the treatment of osteoporosis?

Diet: adequate calcium/vitamin D intake

Exercise: any weight-bearing exercise (including walking) at least 30 minutes three times per week

Cessation of smoking

Avoidance of drugs that increase bone loss

Who should be considered for pharmacologic therapy?

Postmenopausal women with diagnosed osteoporosis or with high risk for its development

What types of drugs are available?

Bisphosphonates; selective estrogen receptor modulators (SERMs); estrogen; calcitonin; vitamin D

How do bisphosphonates work?

They **increase bone mass** and **reduce the incidence of fracture by inhibiting resorption of bone.** They are **first-line therapy** for osteoporosis treatment.

What are the side effects of bisphosphonates?

Pill-induced **esophagitis, osteonecrosis of the jaw** (rare)

How do SERMs work?

They **increase BMD** and **reduce the risk of vertebral fractures.**

What other benefits do SERMs confer?

Lower risk of breast cancer; decrease total cholesterol and LDL

What are the side effects of SERMs?

Increased risk of venous thromboembolism

What are the indications for estrogen/progesterone therapy?

Persistent menopausal symptoms

Inability to tolerate other antiresorptive medications

How does parathyroid hormone (PTH) work and how is it administered?

If given intermittently, PTH stimulates bone formation more than it causes resorption.

When is calcitonin used?

Not a first-line treatment; used in women with pain secondary to a fracture because it offers analgesia in addition to its antiosteoporotic effects

What are the potential side effects of calcitriol that limit its use?

Hypercalcemia, hypercalciuria, and renal insufficiency

How are thiazide diuretics used in the prevention of osteoporosis?

Used in postmenopausal women with hypertension because they decrease bone loss slightly and increase calcium absorption

What is tibolone and how is it used in osteoporosis?

A **synthetic steroid** that metabolizes to have the effects of estrogens, androgens, and progestins. It **improves BMD;** however, it may increase the risk of stroke.

PERIMENOPAUSE AND MENOPAUSE

How is menopause defined?

12 months of amenorrhea after the final menstrual period because of a loss of ovarian activity

What is the average age of menopause in the United States?

51 and a half years

What are some factors that cause an earlier age of onset for menopause?	Smoking Genetic factors Nulliparity Hysterectomy Living at higher altitudes
What is premature menopause?	Also known as premature ovarian failure; the **spontaneous cessation of menses before the age of 40 years**
What are the other phases of menopause?	**Perimenopause**: the phase preceding menopause; reflected by menstrual cycle irregularities **Postmenopause**: phase of life that follows menopause
When does perimenopause begin?	Between 5 and 10 years before menopause
How does the menstrual cycle length change in the perimenopause?	Early phase: the menstrual cycle remains regular but is shortened by 7 days or more Late phase: more menstrual cycle variability; may skip two or more cycles
How do the following hormones change during the perimenopausal state?	
FSH/LH:	**Increases**
Estrogen:	**Remains normal** (until follicular growth stops)
Progesterone:	**Decreases**
Why does FSH change during perimenopause?	The decline in the number of follicles and the irregular maturation of follicles leads to a **decreased concentration of inhibin** (which normally inhibits FSH secretion). This causes the rise in FSH levels.
What are the symptoms of perimenopause?	Hot flashes Sleep disturbances

How do the following hormones change at menopause?

    Androstenedione: Decreases

    FSH/LH: Markedly increases

    Testosterone: Increases

    Estrogen: Decreases

Why do estrogen levels change during menopause?   Because of the loss of ovarian follicles

Compare the changes in the levels of FSH and LH during menopause   Both increase; however **FSH increases more than LH**

Why does FSH increase more than LH?   Renal clearance of FSH is less than that of LH.

What disorder presents with the same hormonal abnormalities as menopause (increased serum FSH > LH)?   **Primary ovarian failure**, which can be seen in Turner syndrome

What are the chief complaints from women going through menopause?

Hot flashes

Hair/skin changes

Atrophic urogenital system (symptoms of urinary tract infection, dyspareunia)

Vaginitis (atrophic)

Variable moods

Osteoporosis

Coronary artery disease

Note: **Can be remembered by the mnemonic "**menopause causes HHAVVOC**"**

Describe the pathophysiology and the treatment for each of the symptoms of menopause: See Table 7.1

What complaint is often associated with hot flashes?   Insomnia (because symptoms often occur at night)

What are the clinical manifestations of an atrophic urogenital system?   Symptoms similar to those seen in UTIs (including urinary frequency, urgency, dysuria, pyuria, and urge incontinence)

Where does menopause-associated osteoporosis typically begin?   In the spine

Table 7.1 The Pathophysiology and Treatment for Symptoms of Menopause

Symptom/Condition	Pathophysiology	Treatment
Hot flashes	Estrogen withdrawal → thermoregulatory dysfunction	Short-term estrogen replacement therapy
Hair and skin changes	Decreased collagen → wrinkles	Estrogen replacement therapy
	Decreased estrogen, no change in testosterone → male growth patterns	
Atrophic urogenital system	Decreased estrogen → atrophy of urethral epithelium → loss of urethral tone, shrinkage of the uterus, cervix, vagina, ovaries, and bladder	Estrogen replacement therapy
Vaginitis (atrophic)	Decreased estrogen → epithelial atrophy → soreness, burning, dyspareunia, sexual dysfunction	Lubricants (mild) vaginal estrogen (severe)
Variable moods	Hormonal/life changes → nervousness, anxiety, depression	Estrogen replacement therapy
Osteoporosis and joint pain	↑ Bone resorption phase and ↑ osteoclasts; ↓ bone formation phase and ↓ osteoblasts	Raloxifene or bisphosphonates
Coronary heart disease	↑ LDL, ↓ HDL → increased atherosclerosis	Hormone replacement therapy does not have any benefit
Cognitive decline	Change in areas important for memory → memory loss, possible link to Alzheimer disease	Estrogen or combined hormonal therapy has no benefit

What is the rate of bone loss associated with osteoporosis?

Before menopause, bone loss occurs at a rate of 0.5% per year; after menopause it increases to over 1% per year

What type of bone is most sensitive to the changes in estrogen levels associated with menopause?

Trabecular bone

What are the two most commonly used hormone replacement therapies?

Unopposed estrogen therapy

Continuous combined therapy with conjugated estrogen and medroxyprogesterone acetate

Is there cardiovascular benefit to using unopposed estrogen therapy (ET) and continuous combined oral estrogen-progestin therapy (CCE-MPA)?

According to data from the Women's Health Initiative (WHI) study, there is no benefit from estrogen therapy and a slight increased risk with combined therapy.

What is the risk of breast cancer when using unopposed estrogen therapy or combined estrogen-progestin HRT?

In the WHI **unopposed estrogen trial, there is no increase in risk of breast cancer** in 10,000 women who had a hysterectomy. In the **combined estrogen-progestin group, there was significant increase in the risk of breast cancer.**

What are the relative risks of endometrial cancer when using unopposed estrogen therapy versus combined estrogen-progestin hormone therapy?

Treatment with estrogen alone greatly increases the risk of endometrial hyperplasia and cancer.

Adding a progestin diminishes this excess risk of endometrial hyperplasia and carcinoma.

When is estrogen replacement therapy (ERT)/hormone replacement therapy (HRT) contraindicated?

Women who have abnormal vaginal bleeding

History of breast cancer

History of coronary heart disease (CHD)

History of estrogen-dependent neoplasia

History of DVTs or thromboembolic event

History of liver dysfunction/disease

What are complications of estrogen replacement therapy?

Endometrial cancer

Breast cancer

Thromboembolic disease

Stroke

Uterine bleeding

Gallbladder disease

Hirsutism, Virilization, and Polycystic Ovarian Syndrome

HIRSUTISM AND VIRILIZATION

What is hirsutism?

Excessive growth of **androgen-dependent** hair (eg, on the upper lip, chest, chin)

What is virilization?

Excessive androgen-induced changes n addition to hirsutism. These include clitoromegaly, voice deepening, increasing muscle mass, and other masculinizing signs.

What is hypertrichosis?

It is a rare disease that refers to **diffusely increased androgen-independent** fine body hair, usually caused by drugs or systemic illnesses. It does not represent hirsutism.

How does the clinical presentation of hirsutism differ from that of virilization?

Hirsutism manifests with **increased "midline" hair** on the upper lip, chin, ear, cheeks, lower abdomen, chest, back, and upper arms. Amenorrhea is seen in severe cases. *Virilization* is excess hair and additional characteristics such as **deepening of he voice, acne, breast atrophy, clitoromegaly, balding, and increased strength.**

Which androgens cause and are elevated in hirsutism?

Testosterone and dehydroepiandrosterone sulfate (DHEAS)

What two organs may be involved in hirsutism and what steroid does each mainly secrete?

1. **Ovary:** testosterone
2. **Adrenal gland:** DHEAS

What is the role of 17OH progesterone in the development of hirsutism?

17OH progesterone is a precursor to the biosynthesis of cortisol and can be converted peripherally into androgens if found in excess.

What is the most common disorder that causes hirsutism?

Polycystic ovarian syndrome (PCOS)

What other underlying diseases may cause hirsutism?

Congenital adrenal hyperplasia (CAH; 21-hydroxylase deficiency)

Androgen-secreting ovarian tumors (Sertoli-Leydig or granulosa-theca tumors)

Adrenal tumors

Cushing syndrome

Exogenous androgens (danazol)

Hyperprolactinemia

Other rare disorders (hyperthecosis)

What is idiopathic hirsutism?

It is a diagnosis given to women with hirsutism without adrenal or ovarian dysfunction, normal serum androgen concentrations, normal menstrual cycles, and no other identifiable cause of their hirsutism. There is often a positive family history.

How may the presenting signs and symptoms of a patient help specify the disorder causing hirsutism?

Ovarian tumor: pelvic mass, sudden onset of amenorrhea, virilization

PCOS: obesity, acne, long history of irregular menses, slow onset of hirsutism beginning at puberty, acanthosis nigricans

Theca-lutein cysts: hirsutism develops during pregnancy

CAH: gradual onset of anovulation, positive family history

Adrenal tumor: rapid onset, virilization, abdominal-flank mass

Cushing syndrome: moon facies, buffalo hump, centripetal obesity, striae, extremity wasting

Hyperprolactinemia: galactorrhea or visual changes with menstrual irregularities

What laboratory studies assist in the diagnosis of the etiology of hirsutism?

Testosterone greater than 200 ng/mL → androgen-secreting ovarian tumor

DHEAS greater than 700 µg/dL → androgen-secreting adrenal tumor

17α-hydroxyprogesterone greater than 200 ng/dL → 21-hydroxylase deficiency

LH:FSH ratio greater than or equal to 3 → PCOS

Prolactin greater than 200 µg/dL → Prolactinoma

24-hour urinary free cortisol greater than 100 ng/24 h → Cushing syndrome

What imaging studies are warranted?

Pelvic ultrasound may reveal polycystic ovaries or ovarian tumors/cysts

CT/MRI of the abdomen to look for an adrenal mass when DHEAS levels are elevated

How is hirsutism generally treated?

Treat the underlying disorder. The most common medications are **oral contraceptives (OCPs)**, GnRH analogs, and antiandrogens (first-line spironolactone, second-line flutamide, finasteride).

What are the specific treatments for each of the following causes of hirsutism?

Ovarian tumor: surgical removal

PCOS: combination OCPs

CAH: continuous corticosteroid replacement

Adrenal tumor: surgical removal

Idiopathic hirsutism: spironolactone

How do combination OCPs work as antiandrogens?

They suppress LH stimulation of the theca cells and they increase sex hormone-binding globulin (SHBG) (thus decreasing free testosterone).

How does spironolactone act as an antiandrogen?

It is an androgen receptor blocker and it suppresses 5α-reductase in hair follicles.

POLYCYSTIC OVARIAN SYNDROME (STEIN-LEVENTHAL SYNDROME)

Describe polycystic ovarian syndrome (PCOS):

Persistent anovulation, which leads to **secondary amenorrhea** and other menstrual irregularities, and **androgen excess,** which may cause hirsutism and virilization

What is the pathophysiology behind PCOS?

It is a **dysfunction of the hypothalamic-pituitary axis. Increased pulsatile secretions of GnRH** → **excess production of LH** → excess production and secretion of androgens → virilization.

How does PCOS lead to anovulation?

Some of the excess androgens are converted to estrogen. High estrogen levels increase LH (by blocking the inhibitory feedback mechanism of progesterone on the pituitary). High LH levels stimulate the immature follicles to produce more androgens, which then become converted to estrogen. The cycle then repeats.

FSH is inhibited by high estrogen levels. This allows the early growth of multiple follicles, but **failure of the development of the mature follicle and its ovulation.**

What are the two most common presenting complaints of patients with PCOS?

Hirsutism and infertility

What other clinical manifestations are associated with PCOS?

Chronic anovulation

Obesity

Insulin resistance

Irregular bleeding (from a chronically estrogen-stimulated endometrium)

What dermatologic condition may be associated with PCOS?

Acanthosis nigricans

How is the diagnosis of PCOS made?

It is suspected in the presence of menstrual irregularity (anovulation), evidence of androgen excess, and exclusion of other causes of menstrual irregularities and hyperandrogenism.

What test should be ruled out first in a woman who presents with secondary amenorrhea?

Pregnancy test (β-hCG)

How do polycystic ovaries appear on pelvic ultrasound?

They appear with eight or more, small (2-8 mm), subcapsular fluid-filled follicle cysts that look like a **"black pearl necklace."**

How is infertility in PCOS patients treated?

Weight loss is recommended first. Ovulation induction with **clomiphene citrate** can be used. **Metformin** can be added in cases of insulin resistance.

| How is hirsutism treated in PCOS patients? | Combination OCPs are first-line (for women who do not desire pregnancy) |
| | Antiandrogen therapy (spironolactone, flutamide, finasteride) |

| What are complications associated with PCOS? | Increased risk of early onset of type II diabetes mellitus |
| | Increased risk of endometrial hyperplasia and endometrial cancer because of unopposed estrogen stimulation |

| What is HAIR-AN syndrome? | It is a variant of PCOS that leads to hyperandrogenism, insulin resistance, and acanthosis nigricans. |

CLINICAL VIGNETTES

A 67-year-old woman comes for follow-up evaluation of her osteoporosis. She was first diagnosed with osteoporosis after she presented with a vertebral fracture. For the past 3 years, she has been taking adequate doses of calcium and vitamin D. Alendronate, 70 mg once weekly, was added to her regimen a year ago. She is adherent to her therapy. A follow-up bone density was recently performed and the results show T-scores of −3.1 in the spine and −3.5 in the hip, compared to scores of −2.8 and −3.2, respectively, 3 years ago. Her vitamin D level, PTH, calcium, phosphorus, TSH levels are normal. Which of the following is the best next step in management?

a. Discontinue alendronate and start intravenous zoledronate.
b. Increase her dose of ergocalciferol.
c. Add teriparatide.
d. Discontinue alendronate and add teriparatide.

Answer: d

The patient has adequate calcium and vitamin D intake; therefore her bisphosphonate is not adequately effective. Teriparatide (recombinant human parathyroid hormone [1-34]) stimulates new bone formation and is given subcutaneously for 1 to 2 years. It has been shown to decrease the incidence of both vertebral and nonvertebral fractures. Teriparatide should be considered in patients who are intolerant of other medications, are not responding to first-line therapy, or have the greatest fracture risk. There has been no benefit shown of concurrent teriparatide and bisphosphonate therapy, so adding teriparatide to her current regimen is inappropriate. Concomitant treatment with alendronate may decrease the effectiveness of teriparatide by unknown mechanisms, thus adding teriparatide to her existing regimen (choice c) would be inappropriate. Her vitamin D level is normal and therefore she does not require increased doses of ergocalciferol (vitamin D₂) (choice b). There is no evidence that the patient is not properly absorbing alendronate or not adhering to her therapy; therefore, changing to intravenous bisphosphonate is not indicated nor beneficial.

A 52-year-old obese female was begun on combined monophasic estrogen/progesterone hormone replacement therapy (HRT) 8 months earlier for treatment of severe hot flashes and now returns to you with a complaint of intermittent vaginal bleeding. What is your next step in management?

a. She should be referred for a pelvic ultrasound.
b. She should be reassured that this is a normal side effect of HRT.
c. She should have the dosage of her therapy decreased.
d. She should have a pelvic examination and Pap smear.

Answer: a

Vaginal bleeding occurs in 40% of individuals started on monophasic estrogen/progesterone hormone replacement. While considered normal in the first 3 to 6 months of therapy, patients who have vaginal bleeding for more than 6 months or longer than 10 days after initiation of HRT should undergo referral for pelvic ultrasound (choice a) to evaluate the endometrial stripe. If the endometrial stripe is thickened, endometrial biopsy is indicated.

A 45-year-old woman reports that her last period was about 9 months ago. She reports hot flashes occurring frequently throughout the day that cause her to stop working until they pass, as well as disturbed sleep patterns. She asks you about the benefits of hormone replacement therapy. Which of the following statements would you use when counseling her?

a. HRT can be prescribed for her to reduce her risk of coronary disease.
b. HRT with estrogen + progesterone decreases the risk of breast cancer.
c. HRT with estrogen + progesterone decreases the risk of ovarian cancer.
d. HRT with estrogen alone does not increase the risk of venous thromboembolism.

Answer: c

HRT with estrogen + progesterone decreases the risk of ovarian cancer (choice c). It increases the risk of breast cancer (choice b) and venous thromboembolism (choice d). HRT with estrogen + progesterone is not effective for either primary or secondary prevention of CAD (choice a).

SECTION III

Topics in Obstetrics

CHAPTER 8

General Obstetrics

Maternal-Fetal Physiologic Adaptation to Pregnancy

EMBRYOLOGY

What are the developmental stages of early pregnancy?

Fertilization and cleavage result in a **zygote** (an 8-cell mass) which then divides to form the **morula** (a 16-cell mass) 3 days after fertilization. A blastocyst develops and implantation occurs approximately 10 days after fertilization. An **embryonic disk** develops after the first week and a **yolk sac** after 5 weeks.

What are the placental membranes and uterine layers (fetal to maternal)?

Amnion

Chorion (with villi composed of syncytial trophoblasts and cytotrophoblasts)

Decidua parietalis (endometrium)

Myometrium

Serosa (See Fig. 8.1)

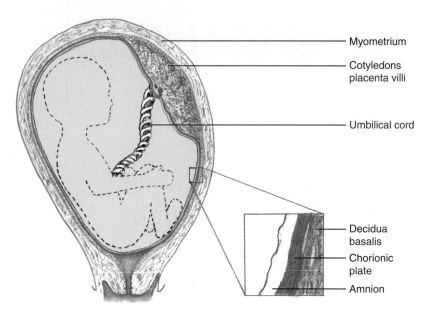

Figure 8.1   Embryologic layers of the human fetus at 3 months.

How does the timing of division affect the development of monozygotic twins?	Division in less than 72 hours: two embryos, two amnions, two chorions ("di-di")
	Division between 4 and 7 days: two embryos, two amnions, one chorion ("mono-di")
	Division after 7 days: one shared amnion and chorion ("mono-mono")
	Division after the embryonic disk has developed: conjoined twins

FETAL CIRCULATION

What are the major shunts involved with fetal circulation?	Ductus venosus
	Foramen ovale
	Ductus arteriosus

What are the patterns of fetal blood flow (starting from the umbilical vein)?

1. Umbilical vein → ductus venosus and liver → inferior vena cava → right atrium → foramen ovale → left atrium → left ventricle → cephalic/systemic circulation → internal iliac artery → umbilical arteries → placenta

2. Superior vena cava → right atrium → right ventricle → pulmonary artery → ductus arteriosis (mostly) and fetal lungs (small amount) → descending aorta → hypogastric arteries → umbilical arteries (see Fig. 8.2)

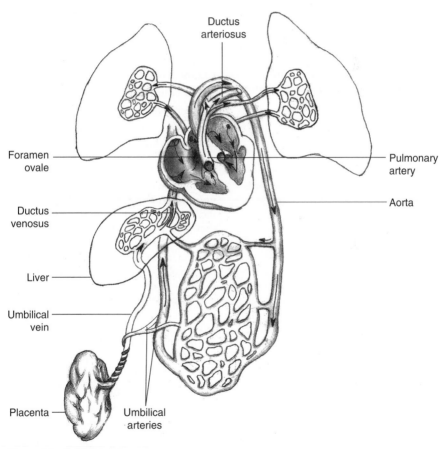

Figure 8.2 Fetal circulation.

Do each of the following vessels carry oxygenated or deoxygenated blood?

Umbilical artery:

Deoxygenated

Umbilical vein:

Oxygenated

What are the embryologic remnants associated with each of the following?

Umbilical vein:

Ligamentum hepatis

Ductus venosus:

Ligamentum venosum

Ductus arteriosus:

Ligamentum arteriosum

Umbilical arteries:

Medial umbilical ligaments

CARDIOVASCULAR

How does pregnancy affect cardiac output (CO), blood volume, and blood pressure (BP)?

CO increases up to 50% (1.8 L/min).

Blood volume increases by 50%.

BP decreases.

These changes **peak during the second trimester** and remain relatively constant until delivery.

Pregnancy affects which components of CO?

Remember, CO = SV × HR. Both stroke volume (SV) and heart rate (HR) increase; however, SV increases more than HR.

How does pregnancy affect SV?

Preload is increased with an increase in blood volume; afterload is reduced by the low-resistance uteroplacental circulation and by peripheral vasodilatation.

What percentage of CO goes to the uterus during pregnancy?

Up to 20% at term (compared to < 1% in the nonpregnant state)

How does the cardiac examination change during pregnancy?

Heart sounds are **louder** and **split**

Often a **systolic murmur** and an **S3**

Slight left axis deviation on EKG

Mild cardiomegaly on chest x-ray (CXR)

(A **diastolic murmur is never normal** and should be evaluated.)

Describe positional changes that affect CO in pregnancy:

In the supine position the inferior vena cava is compressed, which may decrease CO by up to 30%. Maximum venous return and CO is maintained in the left lateral decubitus (LLD) position.

Describe the hematologic changes of pregnancy:

Red blood cell mass **increases** by 15% to 30% (because of increased erythropoietin).

Plasma volume **increases** by 30% to 50% (because of increased aldosterone).

Hct and Hb **decrease**, causing the physiologic "anemia of pregnancy" (because of increased plasma volume).

Note: **An Hb less than 11 is never normal and must be evaluated** for iron/folate deficiency or a hemoglobinopathy.

When does the anemia of pregnancy reach its nadir?

Around 24 weeks

What is the effect of pregnancy on BP?

BP decreases in the first trimester, nadirs at approximately 24 weeks, and then almost normalizes by term. Diastolic is affected more than systolic.

RESPIRATORY

How does pregnancy affect pulmonary function tests (PFTs)?

Tidal volume increases by 40%.

Minute ventilation increases by 50%.

Functional residual capacity decreases by 20%.

Total lung capacity slightly decreases.

Expiratory reserve volume and total lung capacity decrease.

Forced expiratory volume (FEV1) does not change.

Respiratory rate does not change.

What hormone mediates these effects?

Progesterone

How is the acid base equilibrium affected during pregnancy?	**Respiratory alkalosis** with metabolic compensation (pH between 7.40 and 7.45)
What is the effect of pregnancy on oxygen consumption?	Increases by over 20% owing to the placenta, fetus, and maternal organs

RENAL/URINARY

What is the effect of pregnancy on renal function?	Glomerular filtration rate (GFR) **increases** by 50% (because of the increase in glomerular plasma flow). Renal blood flow **increases**. Plasma creatinine, BUN, and uric acid levels decrease (because of the increased GFR). Normal Cr, BUN, or UA may indicate underlying pathology (preeclampsia, renal insufficiency).
Why is the pregnant woman at increased risk for urinary tract infections?	**Progesterone** reduces ureteral tone and peristalsis, and relaxes the bladder wall allowing reflux through the incompetent vesico-ureteral valves. This results in stasis of urine, dilated ureters, increased pressure in the renal pelvis, and bacterial proliferation.
What are the common causes of bacteriuria in pregnancy?	**Escherichia coli** >> Klebsiella > Proteus > Group B streptococcus (GBS) > Enterococci > Staphylococci
Where does hydronephrosis in pregnancy most commonly occur?	On the **right** side (because of right uterine dextrorotation and right ureter compression)
What happens to plasma osmolality during pregnancy?	The increase in intravascular fluid decreases plasma osmolality.
What is the clinical affect of this change in plasma osmolality?	**Pitting edema** in gravity-dependent areas
What is the significance of trace protein or glucose in the second or third trimester?	It is **normal**, because of increased GFR.

GASTROINTESTINAL

When does morning sickness occur?	During the **first trimester,** as levels of hCG are rapidly rising. After hCG levels peak (~10 weeks), morning sickness decreases.
What is hyperemesis gravidarum?	An idiopathic, noninfectious, **severe nausea and vomiting** that causes dehydration, ketone formation, weight loss, hypokalemia, and metabolic alkalosis.
How does progesterone affect the GI tract?	Lower esophageal sphincter tone decreases (can lead to **GERD**) Small bowel and colon transit decreases (can lead to bloating and **constipation**) Venous congestion (can lead to **hemorrhoids**) Biliary tract peristalsis decreases (increases risk of cholelithiasis and cholecystitis)
How do liver function tests (LFTs) change in pregnancy?	**Alkaline phosphatase is increased** (because of placental production). Other enzymes are within normal limits. (Abnormalities may suggest pathology: hepatitis, HELLP, acute fatty liver of pregnancy, cholestasis of pregnancy, or other pathologies)
How does pregnancy affect the risk of pancreatitis?	Increases the risk (because of increased risks of cholelithiasis and hyperlipidemia)
Why is the mortality associated with appendicitis higher in pregnancy?	Because of the gravid uterus, the appendix is pushed higher leading to a delay in the diagnosis.

HEMATOLOGIC

How is the coagulation system affected by pregnancy?	Decreased protein S Resistance to protein C Increased factor I (fibrinogen), II, V, VII, VIII, X, and XII Because of these, **pregnancy is a hypercoagulable state**

What are the potential complications of this hypercoagulable state?	**Venous thrombosis** (occurs 0.7 per 1000 women in pregnancy) and subsequent **pulmonary embolism**. Both occur predominantly in the **third trimester**.
What is the effect of pregnancy on immunity?	Cell-mediated immunity is weakened but humoral immunity is strengthened.

ENDOCRINE

What is hCG and where is it formed?	Human chorionic gonadotropin; in the **syncytiotrophoblast** of the placenta
hCG is structurally related to what other glycoprotein hormones?	Luteinizing hormone (**LH**), follicle-stimulating hormone (**FSH**), and thyroid-stimulating hormone (**TSH**) (they all have the same α subunit but different β subunits)
How does hCG promote pregnancy?	**Maintains the corpus luteum for first trimester** Causes sexual differentiation in the male fetus Ensures adequate T_3 and T_4 production Increases relaxin secretion by the corpus luteum (leading to decreased vascular resistance)
What are the three major types of estrogen and where are they predominately produced?	1. **Estrone: adrenals** (dehydroepiandrosterone [DHEA] is the precursor) 2. **Estriol** (least bioactive): **placenta** 3. **Estradiol** (most bioactive): **ovaries**
What happens to the adrenal hormones during pregnancy?	Adrenocorticotropic hormone (ACTH), corticotropin-releasing hormone (CRH), and cortisol all increase
What is oxytocin?	A hormone produced by the hypothalamus and released by the posterior pituitary. Concentrations rise throughout gestation, during labor, and with lactation or nipple stimulation.
What are the major actions of oxytocin?	**Contraction of uterine myometrium**, ductal myoepithelial contraction (milk expression), orgasm, and bonding

What peptide is similar to oxytocin and what are the clinical consequences?

Antidiuretic hormone (ADH)

Induction/augmentation of labor with oxytocin may cause severe fluid retention and pulmonary edema.

What happens to thyroid hormone levels during pregnancy?

TBG increases

Total T_3 and T_4 levels increase but free **T_3 and T_4 levels** (and thus thyroid function) **remain unchanged,** TSH does not change.

What mediates these thyroid hormone changes?

hCG stimulates TSH to increase total T_4 and T_3 levels. Estrogen increases the hepatic production of TBG.

What is hPL and where is it formed?

Human placental lactogen; in the **syncytiotrophoblast** of the placenta

What is the function of hPL?

It **antagonizes insulin** and **increases lypolysis** to ensure adequate glucose delivery to the fetus

How does maternal glucose metabolism change during pregnancy?

hPL causes mild maternal **insulin resistance** and can lead to the development of gestational diabetes.

Why does gestational diabetes mellitus (GDM) occur?

There is insufficient maternal insulin to counter the hyperglycemic effects of placental hPL. It occurs most commonly in the third trimester, when hPL levels are highest.

DERMATOLOGY

What are striae distensae or striae gravidarum?

Stretch marks; caused from a diminution of elastin fibers and fibrillin microfibrils

What other skin changes occur during pregnancy?

Chloasma or **melasma** (hyperpigmentation of the face)

Linea nigra (darkening of the linea alba from the pubic symphysis to the xiphoid process)

Hyperpigmentation of the axilla, genitalia, perineum, anus, inner thighs, neck, scars, nevi, and lentigo

Palmar erythema and **telangiectasias Hirsutism** and **acne**

REPRODUCTIVE

What is Chadwick sign?	**Bluish color** of vulvar and vaginal membranes because of venous congestion; a normal finding in pregnancy
What other vaginal changes occur in pregnancy?	Increased vascularity and distensibility; increased vaginal discharge (because of increased capillary permeability and desquamation)
What changes occur to the cervix and uterus during pregnancy?	**Hegar sign (softening of the lower uterine segment** that occurs in early pregnancy) Increased eversion of the cervical columnar epithelium
What breast changes occur in pregnancy?	Enlargement, increase in cystic components, darkening of areolae, hypertrophy of sebaceous glands, colostrum production (in late pregnancy)

Prenatal Care

DIAGNOSIS AND TERMINOLOGY

When should prenatal care begin?	Preconception or as soon as pregnancy is suspected.
What are the major goals of preconceptive counseling?	Minimize unplanned pregnancies Optimize chronic medical disorders (diabetes mellitus [DM], epilepsy, hypothyroid, cardiovascular disorders) Promote healthy behaviors Counsel regarding adequate diet, exercise, and nutritional supplements (folic acid and iron) Offer appropriate vaccinations (rubella, diphtheria, hepatitis B virus) Screen for genetic or chromosomal abnormalities Improve patient's readiness for pregnancy and parenting

What does folic acid supplementation help prevent?	Neural tube (NT) defects
Who should take folic acid supplementation?	All women of reproductive age; the NT closes 26 days after fertilization (often before a woman is aware of pregnancy) therefore they need to begin supplementation before becoming pregnant.
How much folic acid should healthy women of reproductive age consume?	A balanced diet plus 0.4 mg daily
What are the early signs and symptoms of pregnancy?	Amenorrhea or irregular bleeding Nausea/vomiting Breast tenderness Urinary frequency
How is pregnancy diagnosed?	**β-hCG**
When does β-hCG become positive?	Serum tests become positive following implantation (about 10 days after fertilization). Urine tests become positive 2 to 3 weeks after fertilization or around on the first day of a missed period.
Where is hCG formed?	In the **placental trophoblasts**
What is the primary function of hCG?	To **maintain the corpus luteum** and to produce **progesterone**.
Why is the β subunit of hCG measured?	β subunit of hCG differentiates it from LH, FSH, and TSH, which all share the same β subunit.
What are some reasons that β-hCG may be abnormally elevated?	Multiple gestations Trophoblastic disease Molar pregnancy Choriocarcinoma
At what rate does serum β-hCG increase?	Serum concentrations **double every 48 hours during the first trimester** and peak at 100,000 IU/L; levels then regress to 30,000 IU/L from the 20th week until term

A woman with a positive pregnancy test presents to the ER with vaginal bleeding. She has been trying to become pregnant and cannot remember her last menstrual period (LMP). Her serum β-hCG is 200 IU/L and no gestational sac is visualized on transvaginal ultrasound. What is your next step in management?

Ask the patient to return in 2 days to recheck the β-hCG. If it is not doubling appropriately she may have an ectopic pregnancy or a spontaneous abortion. A gestational sac should be visualized with a β-hCG greater than 1500 IU/L.

What is the estimated gestational age (EGA)?

Duration of the pregnancy **dated from first day of the LMP**. The EGA of a normal pregnancy at term is 40 weeks.

What is the developmental age (DA) of a pregnancy?

Duration of the pregnancy **dated from fertilization**; typically 14 days less than the EGA (such that the DA of a normal pregnancy at term is 38 weeks)

What is the estimated date of confinement (EDC)?

The "due date" when the pregnancy is full term

What is Naegele rule?

For women with a regular 28-day menstrual cycle:

EDC = LMP – 3 months + 7 days + 1 year

What gestational ages are defined by the following terms?

First trimester: less than 14 weeks

Second trimester: 14 to 28 weeks

Third trimester: more than 28 weeks

Viability: 24 weeks

Prematurity: 24 to 36 weeks

Term: 37 to 42 weeks

Post dates: more than 40 weeks

Post term: more than 42 weeks (increased risk of perinatal morbidity and mortality)

What ages are defined by the following terms?

Neonate: birth to 28 days of life

Infant: birth until 1 year of life

What are the patient's Gs and Ps?

Gravidity: total number of pregnancies

Parity: all viable and nonviable pregnancies, including spontaneous, therapeutic, and voluntary abortions

What are the four numbers that follow parity?

1. **T** (term): deliveries more than 37 weeks EGA
2. **P** (preterm): deliveries between 20 and 37 weeks
3. **A** (abortuses): deliveries prior to 20 weeks (such as abortions or ectopic pregnancies)
4. **L** (living): living children (including twins or adoptions)

What are the Gs and Ps for a mother of three with a history of an normal spontaneous vaginal delivery (NSVD) at term, preterm twins, a fetal demise at 23 weeks, and an ectopic pregnancy at 6 weeks?

G4 P1213

How is pregnancy dating confirmed?

Ultrasound (most accurate in the first trimester) and **fundal height** on physical examination

What size-date discrepancy* would require further evaluation?

1. Ultrasound should be within 1 week of the EGA during the first trimester, within 10 days during the second trimester, and within 3 weeks in the third trimester.
2. FH should be within 3 weeks of the EGA (determined by LMP).

*A size-date discrepancy suggests either underlying pathology or an error in dating (requiring the EDC to be changed).

In what circumstances is fundal height greater than dates?

Twins, polyhydramnios, macrosomia, fibroids, hydatidiform mole (molar pregnancy)

To what EGA does each fundal height correspond?

12 weeks EGA

Symphysis pubis:

20 weeks EGA

Umbilicus:

Fundal height in centimeters above the symphysis pubis corresponds to EGA after 20 weeks

With each of the following tools, when can fetal cardiac activity be detected?

Transvaginal ultrasound:	6 weeks EGA
Abdominal ultrasound:	10 weeks EGA
Doppler fetal heart monitor:	12 weeks EGA
Ascultation:	20 weeks EGA

What fetal parameters are measured on ultrasound to assess EGA?

First trimester: crown-rump length

Second/third trimesters: femur length, abdominal circumference, biparietal diameter, and head circumference

Why is dating important?

Monitoring growth, appropriate timing of screening markers (quad screen, gestational diabetes mellitus [GDM]), delivery planning (fetal lung maturity, postdates)

A woman presents to the emergency room with abdominal pain. Her period is 1 week late and her serum β-hCG measures 2000 IU/L. Transvaginal ultrasound (TVUS) visualizes thickened endometrial tissue and fluid in the cul-de-sac. What is the greatest concern?

Ruptured ectopic pregnancy. TVUS can visualize a gestational sac at 5 weeks EGA, which corresponds to a serum β-hCG level of 1500 to 2000 IU/L.

MANAGEMENT

What are relevant aspects of a patient's past obstetrical history (ObHx)?

For each prior pregnancy:

Date of delivery

Mode of delivery or outcome

Gestational age and weight at delivery

Anesthesia complications

Any history of infertility

Type of uterine incision with prior C-sections

Year and EGA of all abortions and procedures

What are relevant aspects of a patient's past gynecologic history (GynHx)?

Gyn triad: age of menarche/cycle length/duration of menstruation

History of cysts, fibroids, abnormal Pap smears, gyn surgeries

STIs

Prior use of contraception

What are relevant aspects of a patient's genetic & family history (FHx)?

Relatives with pregnancy-related disorders (eg, pregnancy losses)

Family history of chronic medical conditions (diabetes, thyroid disorders, hemoglobinopathies)

Consanguinity

Twins

Congenital, chromosomal, or metabolic abnormalities (blood disorders, mental retardation) Ethnicity of the mother and father (for possible screening tests)

How much weight should a woman be advised to gain in pregnancy?

Average women should gain **between 25 and 35 lbs** (underweight women should gain more and overweight women should gain less).

When does a fetus experience the most rapid weight gain?

In the third trimester; the fetus gains approximately ½ lb/wk

What is the recommended daily nutritional intake during pregnancy?

Calories: an **additional 300 kcal/d** for each fetus

Protein: increase daily intake by 5 to 6 g

Iron: requirements double to 30 mg/d

Calcium: increases by 1000 mg in the third trimester during fetal bone calcification

Daily intakes of copper (2 mg), folate (0.4 mg), vitamin C (50 mg), vitamin D (10 mcg or 400 IU), and vitamin B_{12} (2 mcg) should continue

Which substances and foods should be limited or avoided?

Tobacco, alcohol, street drugs

Herbal medications

Caffeine more than 500 mg or more than 4 cups a day (can cause SAB or growth restriction)

Iodine (can cause fetal goiter)

Large amounts of vitamins A, D, E, and K

Unpasteurized dairy

Methylmercury (in raw fish, shark, swordfish, king mackerel, and tilefish)

Should exercise change during pregnancy?

Activity can be maintained at the same intensity prior to pregnancy, in the absence of obstetric or medical complications. If a patient does not, she should be encouraged to begin light exercise.

How often are prenatal care visits scheduled?

Every 4 weeks during the first and second trimesters

Every 2 weeks in the third trimester (28-36 weeks)

Once a week near term (36-40 weeks)

Postdates will require more involved monitoring.

(Adequate prenatal care requires more than nine visits, with the first visit during the first trimester)

What are the four cardinal questions asked during each prenatal care visit?

1. Do you have any **contractions?**
2. Do you have any **leakage of fluid**?
3. Do you have any **vaginal bleeding**?
4. Do you feel **fetal movement** (after 20 weeks)?

What are important parameters in evaluating the pelvic shape?

Pelvic inlet (diagonal conjugate = distance from the pubic symphysis to the sacral promontory)

Prominence of ischial spines

Pelvic sidewalls (convergent vs parallel)

Shape of sacrum

What measurements are taken during each standard prenatal care visit?

Weight

Blood pressure

Urine dip (protein, glucose, leukocytes)

Fundal height

Abdominal doppler fetal heart rate (after 12 weeks)

Which vaccines should be offered to pregnant women?

Any required inactivated vaccines and the **influenza vaccine** (in the second or third trimester)

Do not give vaccines that contain active viral components (measles, mumps, oral polio vaccine, or rubella)

What is advanced maternal age (AMA)?

More than 35 years of age at the time of delivery

What symptoms must a patient be educated about? What do each signify?	**Vaginal bleeding** (SAB in first trimester, placental abruption or placenta previa in second or third trimester) **Edema, headache, blurry vision, right upper quadrant pain, epigastric pain** (preeclampsia) **Dysuria, fever, chills** (pylonephritis)
What are the signs and symptoms of preterm labor?	Any of the following symptoms between 20 and 37 weeks EGA: Abdominal, vaginal, or lower back pain or pressure that does not improve after hydration/rest Uterine contractions every 10 minutes for more than 1 hour A sudden thinning or increase in vaginal discharge Bleeding from the vagina
What is round ligament pain?	As the gravid uterus increases rapidly during the second and third trimester, tension on the round ligament may cause sharp shooting inguinal and groin pain. Rest, warm compresses, and acetaminophen may relieve the pain.
What is the prevalence of domestic violence (DV) among pregnant women?	DV affects approximately 1 in 6 women (more prevalent among pregnant than nonpregnant women).

SCREENING

What are routine intake prenatal labs?	**Hematology**: blood type and screen (T&S), hemoglobin and hematocrit Rubella status (immune or nonimmune) HIV HBV (HBsAg) Syphilis (RPR or VDRL) Chlamydia and gonorrhea cervical cultures Tuberculosis (PPD) Urine culture Pap smear

What are some appropriate screening tests for the following groups?

Mediterranean or Asian descent Hgb electrophoresis for thalassemia

African descent Hgb electrophoresis for sickle cell and thalassemia

Ashkenazi Jews descent Hexosaminidase A leukocyte assay for Tay-Sachs

DNA analysis for: Canavan disease, Bloom syndrome, cystic fibrosis, familial dysautonomia, Fanconi anemia, Gaucher disease, mucolipidosis Type IV, Niemann Pick disease, or Tay-Sachs disease

Caucasian descent Delta F 508 mutations for cystic fibrosis (autosomal recessive)

Serum phenylalanine level for phenylketonuria

In an Rh(–) pregnant woman with an Rh(+) father of the baby, would her first or second child be at greatest risk?

Her **second child,** because of isoimmunization and the development of anti-Rh antibodies. The first Rh(+) fetus will only be mildly affected, if at all.

What is the major complication associated with isoimmunization?

Hemolytic disease of the newborn (with possible hydrops, anasarca, or death)

How is Rh isoimmunization prevented?

With Rh immune globulin (RhoGAM)— an antibody to the D antigen

Who is given RhoGAM?

All Rh(–) mothers with a possible Rh(+) fetus

When is RhoGAM given?

At 28 weeks EGA

At delivery

Within 72 hours of an abortion or vaginal bleeding at any gestational age

Following all invasive procedures (CVS or amniocentesis)

Name some additional screening and diagnostic tests. At what EGA are these routinely completed:

Genetic Screening

> First trimester: nuchal translucency screen (with serum free β-hCG and PAPP-A) is done between 11 and 13 weeks.

> Second trimester: quad or triple screen is done between 15 and 18 weeks.

Anatomic survey with ultrasound (to assess for fetal anomalies): 18 to 20 weeks.

Glucose challenge test (GCT): 24 to 28 weeks.

Streptococcus group B (perineal and rectal culture): 36 weeks.

Repeat Hgb, Hct, and syphilis: third trimester.

In sexually high risk women, what tests should be repeated? At what EGA?

Gonorrhea, Chlamydia, and HIV after 28 weeks (third trimester)

What is the nuchal translucency?

A cystic space dorsal to the cervical spine measured by ultrasound at 11 to 13 weeks

It is a **sensitive indicator of chromosomal abnormalities** — a large diameter signifies a greater risk of aneuploidy and poor fetal outcome.

What other tests enhance the sensitivity of a nuchal translucency?

Maternal serum free β-hCG and plasma protein A (**PAPP-A**) measurements

What is measured in the triple screen?

α-fetoprotein (AFP)

β-hCG

Estriol (E3)

In the quad screen?

Quad screen: all of above plus **inhibin A**

When are these tests employed and what do they assess?

Between 16 and 20 weeks

Abnormal values correlate with various chromosomal, genetic, and developmental disorders

How should an abnormal triple/quad screen be followed-up?

With a detailed ultrasound and possibly an amniocentesis

What do the following triple screen results suggest?

↓ AFP, ↑ hCG, ↓ E3:   Trisomy 21

↓ AFP, ↓ hCG, ↓ E3:   Trisomy 18

An elevated AFP may indicate what fetal conditions?

Neural tube defects

Gastroschisis/Omphalocele (abdominal wall defects)

Fetal death

Placental abnormalities

A decreased AFP may indicate what fetal condition?

Down syndrome

What are the most common neural tube defects (NTDs)?

Anencephaly and spina bifida

What is a glucose challenge test (GCT)?

A screening test for gestational diabetes. The patient drinks 50 g of glucose and her blood sugar is tested 1 hour later.

What is the cutoff for the GCT?

Serum glucose greater than 130 to 140 mg/dL

What should be done if a patient has an abnormal GCT?

A diagnostic test called the glucose tolerance test (GTT)

What is a Glucose tolerance test (GTT)?

After an overnight fast, blood sugar is tested. 100 g glucose is then given and blood sugar is checked every hour for 3 hours.

What are the normal values for a GTT?

Fasting < 95 mg/dL

1 hour < 180 mg/dL
2 hours < 155 mg/dL
3 hours < 140 mg/dL

When is gestational diabetes diagnosed?

If there are **two or more abnormal values** on the GTT

What is a level I ultrasound?

An ultrasound done routinely on women between 18 and 22 weeks gestation that looks at the following:

1. Estimated gestational age of fetus
2. Size of fetus
3. Number of fetuses
4. Location of the placenta
5. Fetal cardiac activity
6. Amount of amniotic fluid
7. Basic anatomical structures (including the brain, spine, stomach, kidneys, bladder, and the four chambers of the heart)

What is a level II ultrasound?

A more detailed and targeted ultrasound done for high-risk women or women with a suspected fetal anomaly on their level I ultrasound.

What is chorionic villus sampling (CVS)?

A diagnostic procedure for genetic anomalies that involves transvaginal or transabdominal aspiration of placental cells at **10 to 13 weeks** EGA.

What is the risk of CVS?

There is a 1/200 risk of adverse fetal outcome (such as limb deformaties) or demise. This is minimally higher than an amniocentesis.

What is an amniocentesis?

A diagnostic procedure done **after 14 weeks** EGA that can detect chromosomal/genetic abnormalities, amniotic infection, inflammation, and fetal lung maturity. It involves transabdominal aspiration of the amniotic fluid from the uterine cavity.

What is the risk of amniocentesis?

There is less than 1/300 risk of adverse fetal outcome (chorioamnionitis, preterm labor, ruptured membranes) or fetal demise.

PRENATAL TESTING AND MONITORING OF THE FETUS

What is quickening and when does it occur?

The mother's first **perception of fetal movement (FM)**; it usually occurs **between 16 and 20 weeks** (may be earlier in a multipara).

What is a "kick count"?

After 26 to 32 weeks, fetal well-being can be assessed by asking the mother to count FM, "kick counts," which should occur at least eight times every 2 hours.

What are the commonly used tests of fetal well-being and when are they used?

Nonstress test (**NST**).

Biophysical profile (**BPP**).

Modified biophysical profile.

They are used most commonly for reassurance in high risk pregnancies or in the complaint of **decreased fetal movement.**

What is an NST?

Placement of an external fetal monitor to trace the fetal heart rate for 20 minutes. A tocodynamometer monitor is also placed to assess for uterine contractions (see Fig. 8.3).

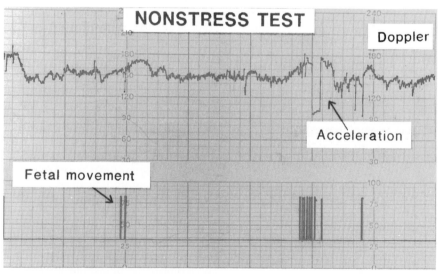

Figure 8.3   Reactive nonstress test. (*Reproduced with permission, from Cunningham FG et al. Williams Obstetrics. 22nd ed. New York, NY: McGraw-Hill; 2005:279.*)

What is a reactive NST?

Two accelerations above the baseline of **15 beats per minute (bpm) for 15** seconds within 20 minutes

What does a reactive NST indicate?

Reassuring fetal status

What is fetal tachycardia?

A baseline FHR **more than 160 bpm**

What is the most common cause of fetal tachycardia?

Maternal tachycardia

What are some other causes of fetal tachycardia?

Maternal fever

Anemia

Asphyxia

Infection

Autoimmune disorders

Adrenergic medications

Cardiac anomalies (eg, SVT)

What is fetal bradycardia?

A baseline FHR **less than 110 bpm**

What are some causes of fetal bradycardia?

Physiologic (short episodes because of transient compression of the fetal head/ umbilical cord)

Maternal hypotension

Local anesthesia (eg, paracervical block)

Uteroplacental insufficiency (eg, placental abruption, uterine rupture, cord prolapse)

Cardiac anomalies

How is fetal heart rate variability assessed?

10 minutes of fetal heart tracing is reviewed to assess peak-to-trough differences in heart rate. Variability may be:

Absent

Minimal (< 5 bpm)

Moderate (normal = 6-25 bpm)

Marked (> 25 bpm)

What is suggested by a sinusoidal pattern on EFM?

Severe fetal anemia, hypoxia, or exposure to sedative hypnotics

What are the five components of the biophysical profile (BPP)?

1. **Breathing**: 30 seconds after 30 minutes of observation (seen as rhythmic deflection of fetal chest wall and diaphragm).
2. **Movement**: three gross body movements in 30 minutes.
3. **Tone**: extension and flexion of an extremity.
4. **Amniotic** fluid: vertical pocket is more than 2 cm or normal amniotic fluid index (AFI).
5. **Reactive NST.**

Each is worth 2 points for 10 possible points. The fetus is given 30 minutes to demonstrate each variable.

What do each of the following BPP scores signify?

8 to 10: reassuring fetal status with an intact CNS

6: equivocal test; repeat within 24 hours

4: high risk of fetal hypoxia; consider delivery

0 to 2: fetal hypoxia; delivery immediately regardless of EGA

Other than fetal hypoxia, what are some other causes of a low BPP?

Fetal sleep cycle

Transplacental sedatives

Corticosteroids

Which of the BPP elements are lost first as the fetus becomes progressively more hypoxic?

Breathing is lost early, then FHR accelerations, movement, tone, and finally amniotic fluid

How is chronic fetal stress manifested?

Oligohydramnios (AFI < 5 cm or vertical pocket < 2 cm), because of several days of decreased renal perfusion.

During hypoxic stress, where is fetal blood preferentially shunted?

Brain, heart, and adrenals

What are umbilical artery Dopplers?

A measurement of the ratio of systolic to diastolic flow (S/D) through the umbilical artery.

What is a normal S/D ratio?

Less than 3.0 in the third trimester because of low placental resistance; this ratio is dependent on gestational age

When should umbilical artery dopplers be done?	Only in cases of **intrauterine growth restriction**
Before the development of NST/BPP, what test was performed to assess uteroplacental insufficiency?	A **contraction stress test** (CST). Nipple stimulation or oxytocin was administered to induce three contractions (ctx) every 10 minutes with concurrent FHM. A normal test has no late decelerations. This is rarely performed today.
What are the three types of decelerations?	1. Early 2. Late 3. Variable
Describe early decelerations:	A gradual decrease from baseline that mirrors a contraction
What do early decelerations signify?	A vagal response from **compression of the fetal head** during uterine ctx; they are **normal.**
Describe variable decelerations:	A **rapid decline** of more than 15 beats from the baseline that is **unrelated to uterine ctx.**
What do variable decelerations signify?	Usually **cord compression** (can be relieved by changing the mother's position)
Describe late decelerations:	A gradual decrease from baseline that **starts after the ctx starts, peaks after the ctx peaks,** and **returns to baseline after the contraction has finished.**
What do late decelerations signify?	Uteroplacental insufficiency
Fetal metabolic acidosis and hypoxia are suggested by what findings on a fetal heart tracing?	Recurrent, prolonged, and **late decelerations** Minimal (> 5 bpm), **decreased** or **absent long-term variability** **Tachycardia** (> 160 bpm), which may also be associated with infection or maternal fever

What is the significance of irregular contractions in the third trimester?	If the fetal status is reassuring, there is no cervical change, and ctxs are less than 4 per hour they are likely insignificant **Braxton Hicks contractions.** If the contractions are painful, the patient may be in latent labor.
What is fetal fibronectin?	A glycoprotein that is normally present in maternal circulation and amniotic fluid. If it is present in the cervicovaginal secretions, it suggests that the **cervix is undergoing structural change** and the patient may go into labor in the next 2 weeks.
How is fetal fibronectin used clinically?	It has a **high negative predictive value**, so it is used to rule out preterm labor.

Labor and Delivery

DIAGNOSIS AND DEFINITIONS

How is labor defined?	**Regular uterine contractions** that result in **cervical effacement** and **dilation**
How is labor diagnosed?	With **tocodynamometry** and **serial cervical examinations**
What are some of the signs of labor?	**Painful contractions** **Bloody show** **Spontaneous rupture of membranes** (SROM)
What is bloody show?	Vaginal passage of blood-tinged mucus
What are the four characteristics of cervical change?	Change in **consistency** (from firm to soft) Change in **position** (from posterior to anterior) Progressive **effacement** (cervix becomes shorter and thinner) **Dilation** of the internal os (from 0-10 cm)

The following terms refer to rupture of fetal membranes (ROM) under what conditions?

SROM: spontaneous rupture of membranes (at ≥ 37 weeks)

PPROM: preterm, premature rupture of membranes (EGA < 37 weeks with rupture)

Prolonged PROM: rupture of membranes more than 18 hours without the onset of labor

What are the four signs and symptoms of spontaneous rupture of membranes?

Initial gush with **continued loss of fluid**

Pooling of vaginal fluid on sterile speculum examination

Positive **nitrazine** blue test (indicating that the vaginal fluid is alkaline, with a pH > 6)

Ferning of dried fluid under low power magnification (because of fetal urine salt crystals in the amniotic fluid)

What can cause a false-positive nitrazine blue test?

Anything that causes the vagina to become more alkaline, such as:

Sperm

Blood

Infection

Douching

What is the pH of amniotic fluid?

7.0

Describe the following terms:

Nulligravida: a woman who never conceived

Nullipara: a woman who never carried a fetus to viability

Primipara: a woman who has delivered a viable fetus in the past, regardless of the outcome of the fetus

Multigravida: a woman who has carried more than one fetus to viability, regardless of the outcome of the fetus

Grand multiparity: given birth five or more times

What is the term for a difficult delivery, protracted labor, or arrest of labor?

Labor dystocia

How does labor affect the shape of the fetal head (in cephalic presentation)?

The fetal calvarium undergoes **molding**, where the bones of the skull shift to minimize the diameter that must pass through the bony pelvis

On vaginal examination, the presenting fetal vertex is noted to be soft without any identifiable sutures or fontaneles. What is the term for this fetal finding (which often occurs in prolonged labors with slow cervical dilation)?

Caput succedaneum. the tissues overlying the fetal calvarium become edematous and swollen

Why are women in labor predisposed to gastric aspiration?

Increased intraabdominal pressure

Relaxation of the lower esophageal sphincter

Recumbent laboring position

What are some of the consequences of gastric aspiration?

Pneumonia

Bronchospasm

Adult respiratory distress syndrome (ARDS)

What precaution is taken in labor to minimize this risk?

Oral intake is restricted to clear liquids

What is a pudendal block?

A method of administering local anesthesia to the pudendal nerve (sacral nerve roots 2, 3, and 4), with subsequent decreased vulvar sensation.

How is a pudendal block administered?

Transvaginally. The anesthetic is injected medial and inferior to the ischial spines through the sacrospinous ligaments bilaterally.

When can an epidural be placed?

At any point in labor once the patient begins experiencing painful contractions

Where is an epidural catheter placed?

A guide needle is used at the interspinous space between the fourth and fifth lumbar vertebra. The ligamentum flavum is penetrated and the catheter is threaded into the potential epidural space, which consists of lymphatics and venous plexuses. An epidural injection enters the extradural or peridural space — it does not penetrate the dura mater.

Where is a spinal block placed?	It enters the dura and then the subarachnoid space, bathed by cerebral spinal fluid. Only the pia mater separates the cord from the injected substance.
What are the risks associated with epidurals and spinal blocks?	Spinal headache Hypotension Infection Hematoma High spinal blockade (leads to apnea) Cord compression (a surgical emergency)
What advantages does a spinal block offer?	A faster onset and requires a lower dose of anesthetics
What risks are increased with a spinal block?	Hypotension Nausea Compromised placental perfusion Ascending respiratory paralysis (because of anesthesia reaching the cervical nerve roots 3, 4, and 5)
Does regional, local, or general anesthesia increase the rate of cesarean delivery?	No

FETAL POSITION

What is the fetal lie?	The **crown-rump axis** of the fetus **in relation to the longitudinal axis of the uterus**
What types of fetal lie are there?	Longitudinal Transverse Oblique
What is the fetal presentation?	The **fetal part closest to the cervix and pelvic inlet**
What is the most common fetal presentation?	Cephalic, followed by breech

What are the other types of fetal presentation? Describe them:

Types of cephalic presentation:

Vertex

Brow

Mentum

Face (depending on which part is leading through the cervix)

Types of breech presentation (See Fig. 8.4):

Frank breech (flexed hips and extended knees)

Complete breech (flexed hips and knees)

Footling breech (one knee flexed, one knee extended)

Other:

Hand

Shoulder

Funic (cord)

Compound (involves more than one fetal part leading)

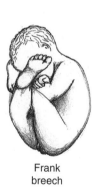

Frank
breech

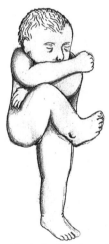

Single footling breech

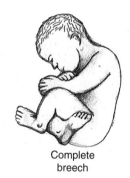

Complete
breech

Figure 8.4 Breech presentation.

What is the incidence of malpresentation (any presentation not cephalic) at the onset of labor?

Less than 4%

Fetal attitude or posture describes what characteristic?

The **degree of flexion of the fetal neck, back, and joints** of the limbs

Describe the fetal postures from most flexed to most extended:

Vertex → Military → Brow (forehead) → Face

What are the risks associated with an extended neck?

The fetus requires a larger leading diameter and thus has less ability to negotiate the birth canal. This can lead to **labor dystocia.**

What are the shapes of the two fetal fontanels and when do they close?

1. The **anterior** fontanel is **diamond shaped** and closes late in infancy (near 13 months).
2. The **posterior** or occipital fontanel is **triangle shaped** and closes early in infancy (near 2 months).

During labor how are the fetal fontanels examined? What is the significance of this examination?

The fetal scalp is examined on sterile vaginal examination (SVE). The **location of the posterior fontanel** is noted with regard to **maternal left/right** and **anterior/posterior/transverse orientation**. This describes the specific **position** of the presenting fetal head. (See Fig. 8.5)

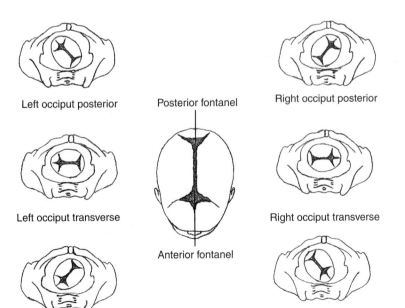

Left occiput posterior

Posterior fontanel

Right occiput posterior

Left occiput transverse

Right occiput transverse

Anterior fontanel

Left occiput anterior

Right occiput anterior

Figure 8.5 Vertex presentations.

Why does the occiput posterior (OP) position frequently cause labor dystocia?

Because the fetal head must be more flexed and rotate more extensively (135° instead of 90°) to pass under the symphysis pubis. Additionally, this position is often associated with brow or face presentations.

What is a normal synclitism?

When the leading sagittal suture is parallel to the pelvic outlet

What is anterior asynclitism?

When the **sagittal suture is deflected toward the sacrum**, allowing more of the parietal bone to be palpated anteriorly

What is posterior asynclitism?

Deflection of the fetal sagittal suture toward the maternal symphysis pubis. It is normal unless the tilt is severe.

How is the position of a fetus described in a face or breech presentation?

The relationship of the fetal mentum (chin) or sacrum are described in relation to maternal right, left, anterior, and posterior.

Leopold maneuvers convey what information about the fetus?

Estimated fetal weight (EFW)

Fetal presenting part

Fetal lie

Engagement

What are the four Leopold maneuvers?

First position: hands are placed at the cephalic margins of the fundus to determine the nonpresenting part that occupies the fundus and the fetal lie.

Second position: hands are placed at the right and left margins of the fundus to feel for small fetal parts and to confirm fetal position.

Third position: thumb and finger are placed just above the symphysis pubis to assess engagement of the presenting part.

Fourth position: facing the patient's feet, the examiner's fingers trace the fundus toward the pelvic inlet to identify the anterior shoulder with cephalic presentation and to assess the degree of descent of the presenting part (see Fig. 8.6).

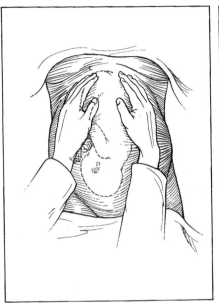

First maneuver

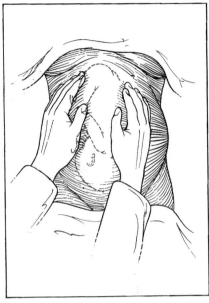

Second maneuver

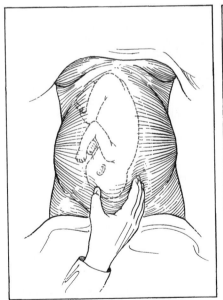

Third maneuver

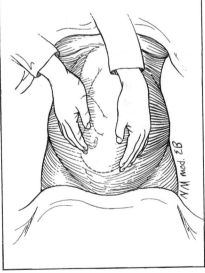

Fourth maneuver

Figure 8.6   Leopold maneuvers. (*Reproduced with permission, from Cunningham FG et al. William Obstetrics. 22nd ed. New York, NY: McGraw-Hill: 2005:416.*)

PELVIMETRY AND VAGINAL EXAMINATION

When is an SVE indicated?	During PNC visits at term
	Upon presentation to labor and delivery with symptoms of labor
	Periodically throughout the course of labor to assess progress
When should a manual pelvic examination *not* be performed?	When there is **bright red blood per vagina.** An ultrasound should be performed first to confirm no placenta previa.
	When the membranes are ruptured, SVEs should be minimized (to reduce risk of infection).
What information is gathered during a manual pelvic examination?	Fetal position
	Cervical dilation/cervicaleffacement/ station of the presenting fetus
	Cervical consistency (firm, soft)
	Cervical position (posterior, anterior)
	Clinical pelvimetry (diagonal conjugate, pelvic sidewalls, interspinous diameter, and a wide pubic arch)
What is the interspinous diameter and what is its significance?	The distance between the ischial spines
	Used to estimate the station of the presenting fetal part
What station is associated with each of the following positions?	
A leading edge that is −3 cm above the ischial spines:	−3 station
A leading edge that is at the level of the spines:	0 station
A leading edge that is 3 cm past the spines:	+3 station
What is zero station (determined on SVE)?	When the **leading fetal edge is at the level of the maternal ischial spines.**
What is its obstetrical significance of zero station?	It represents the **most narrow sagittal obstetric diameter** and so signifies that the largest fetal diameter has engaged the bony pelvis.

What is the significance of pelvic classification and clinical pelvimetry?

Clinical pelvimetry seeks to describe the pelvic inlets, angles, and diameters. However, pelvic type and pelvimetry are not reliable predictors of vaginal delivery, labor dystocia, or cesarean section and so they are rarely employed in contemporary obstetrics.

What is the best indicator of pelvic adequacy?

Prior vaginal delivery, prior progress of labor, or family history ofcephalopelvic disproportion (CPD)

STAGES OF LABOR

What defines the first stage of labor?

The onset of **consistent painful contractions** until the cervix is **completely dilated** (10 cm) and **100% effaced.**

How is the first stage of labor further subdivided?

Into **latent** and **active phase** (See Fig. 8.7)

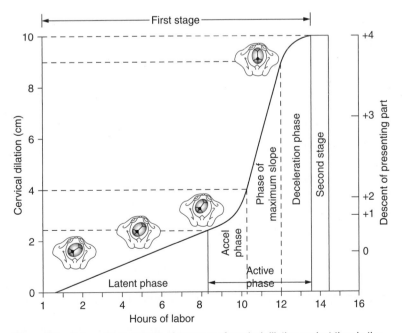

Figure 8.7 Schematic illustration of progress of cervical dilation against time in the successive stages of labor.

Describe the latent phase:

Regular painful contractions that result in **cervical dilation up to 3 to 5 cm**

Describe the active phase:

A **faster rate of cervical dilation** which typically begins after approximately 4 cm dilation and/or full effacement in the presence of regular uterine contractions that **continues through full cervical dilation of 10 cm**

What are minimum adequate rates of cervical dilation during the active phase?

For **multiparas**: at least **1.5 cm/h**
For **nulliparas**: at least **1.2 cm/h**

What are some conditions that slow the active phase?

Uterine dysfunction
Fetal malposition
CPD

How is the active phase of the first stage of labor further subdivided?

Acceleration phase: an increasing rate of dilation from 3 to 5 cm cervical dilatation to 8 cm

Deceleration phase: a slower rate of cervical dilation after 8 cm until full dilation

How is arrest of dilation defined?

More than 2 hours with no cervical change in the presence of adequate contractions

What is the second stage of labor?

From a **fully dilated** and **fully effaced** cervix **until delivery** of the fetus

What is a protracted labor?

When there continues to be some cervical change or descent of the fetus, however it is **progressing slower than would be expected**

Define protraction of the second stage in terms of fetal descent:

In **nulliparas**: fetal head descent **less than 1 cm/h**

In **multiparas**: fetal head descent **less than 2 cm/h**

Define protraction of the second stage in terms of length of labor (with and without an epidural):

In nulliparas:
    2 hours without an epidural
    3 hours with an epidural
In multiparas:
    1 hour without an epidural
    2 hours with an epidural

What is arrest of labor?

Complete cessation of dilation (no change for 2 hours) **or descent** (no change for 1 hour) despite adequate contractions

What are the causes of secondary arrest of labor?

Problems with the three "P"s:

Power (inadequate uterine contractions)

Passage (pelvic disproportion)

Passenger (malpresentation, macrosomia)

Define arrest of descent:

More than 2 hours in a nullipara or **more than 1 hour** in a multipara with no descent of the fetus despite adequate contractions.

If the patient has had an epidural or regional anesthesia she is given 1 additional hour.

When should a woman begin pushing to aid in the descent and delivery of the fetus?

During the **second stage** (after full cervical dilatation)

Why is pushing avoided in the first stage of labor?

To prevent cervical lacerations and maternal exhaustion

A nulliparous patient at term has dilated from 6 to 7 cm over 2 hours. Is this adequate change, protracted dilation, or arrest of dilation?

Protracted dilation (a nullipara should dilate at least 1.2 cm/h during the active phase of labor)

In the above patient, what should be done?

Her contraction pattern should be evaluated (possibly with an IUPC) and her labor can be augmented if her contractions do not appear to be adequate.

A rate of cervical dilation less than 5 cm/h in a nulliparous or 10 cm/h in a multiparous patient is considered what type of labor?

Precipitous labor

What risks are associated with precipitous labor?

An increased risk of fetal hypoxia, brain injury, and maternal morbidity such as hemorrhage and vaginal/cervical lacerations

How is the third stage of labor defined?

It begins **after delivery** of the fetus and continues **until the placenta is delivered.**

What is the acceptable duration of the third stage of labor?	Less than 30 minutes (although some clinicians will wait up to 60 minutes)
What are the three Gs that indicate the placenta has separated and is ready to be delivered?	1. Globular uterus 2. Growing cord 3. Gush of blood
What is the fourth stage of labor?	The acute maternal **hemodynamic adjustment to the fluid shifts** associated with labor that lasts 1 to 2 hours after delivery of the placenta
Why is the woman at increased risk for in the fourth stage of labor?	Postpartum hemorrhage

CARDINAL MOVEMENTS OF LABOR

What are the seven cardinal movements of labor?	The positions that describe the behavior of the fetal head during the second stage of labor. They include: 1. **Engagement** 2. **Descent** 3. **Flexion** 4. **Internal rotation** 5. **Extension** 6. **External rotation** (or restitution) 7. **Expulsion** (See Fig. 8.8)
Define fetal engagement in cephalic presentation:	When the biparietal diameter of the fetal head reaches the pelvic inlet or zero station (when the leading fetal edge has reached the ischial spines)
Why does a fetus flex and rotate during labor?	To negotiate the 90° concave curvature of the pelvic passage
The fetus presents the smallest diameter of its head (suboccipito-bregmatic diameter) by engaging what position?	Tight anterior **flexion** of the head (the inability to flex the head may lead to a dystocia)
How does the fetal head undergo internal rotation?	The fetus rotates so as to turn the saggital suture from a transverse to an anteroposterior position, it is a passive movement.
When does the fetal head undergo extension?	As the fetus is crowning at the introitus and the head has passed under the symphysis pubis

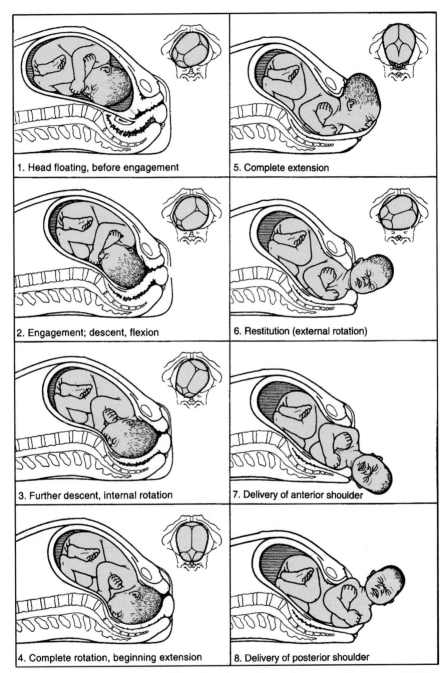

Figure 8.8   Cardinal movements of labor. (*Reproduced with permission, from Cunningham FG et al. Williams Obstetrics. 22nd ed. New York, NY: McGraw-Hill: 2005:418.*)

What cardinal movements occur while the fetal head is at the introitus?

Extension and external rotation

After the fetal head is delivered what subsequent steps should the clinician take?

1. Check for nuchal cord (umbilical cord around the neck).
2. Apply gentle downward pressure to assist the delivery of the anterior shoulder.
3. Gentle upward pressure for the posterior shoulder.
4. Support the subsequent delivery of the fetus's body.

INDUCTION OF LABOR

What are some indications for induction of labor (IOL)?

Prolonged pregnancy (postterm)

Diabetes mellitus

Rh alloimmunization

Preeclampsia

ROM at term

Placental insufficiency

Nonreassuring fetal status

Oligohydramnios

Intrauterine growth restriction

What are some contraindications to IOL?

Previous cesarean with a vertical uterine incision

Prior myomectomy entering the endometrial cavity

Malpresentation (breech)

Active genital herpes

Placenta or vasa previa

What is the Bishop score?

A rating system that evaluates a woman's cervix to **predict the likelihood that she will be able to deliver vaginally following IOL.**

A score of **5 or greater** is favorable.

What are the five cervical components of the Bishop score?

Consistency: firm = 0, medium = 1, soft = 2

Position: posterior = 0, middle = 1, anterior = 2

Effacement: 0%-30% = 0, 40%-50% = 1, 60%-70% = 2, ≥ 80% = 3

Dilation: closed = 0, 1-2 cm = 1, 3-4 cm = 2, 5-6 cm = 3

Station: −3 = 0, −2 = 1, −1 or 0 = 2, +1 or +2 = 3

Mnemonic: "see peds" (C PEDS)

What is the probability of a failed induction of labor with each of the following Bishop scores?

0-4: less than 50%

5-9: less than 10%

10-13: less than 1%

Preinduction cervical ripening can be achieved with what medications?

Prostaglandin PGE1: **misoprostol** (cytotec)

PGE2 or dinoprostone: **prepidil** (cervical gel) and **cervadil** (vaginal insert)

What mechanical techniques are used to ripen the cervix for IOL?

Hygroscopic cervical dilators (laminaria)—seaweed sticks that absorb water and expand

Balloon tipped transcervical catheter or Foley bulb

Membrane stripping or rupture to increase endogenous prostaglandins

INTRAPARTUM ASSESSMENT AND MONITORING

What techniques can be used to count the number of contractions?

Palpation

External tocodynamometry

Intrauterine pressure catheter (IUPC)

Which of these devices is able to assess the force of the contractions?

Only **IUPC**

What are Montevideo units?

Quantifications of intrauterine pressure as determined by IUPC. They are calculated by **multiplying the average peak strength** of the contraction **by the number of contractions** over 10 minutes.

At what target MU are contractions considered adequate?

More than 200

What is uterine tachysystole?

More than five contractions in 10 minutes, averaged over a 30-minute window

What is a tonic contraction?

A contraction that lasts more than 3 minutes (usually in the context of a nonreassuring fetal tracing or fetal decelerations).

Why does uterine hyperstimulation/ tonic contraction compromise placental blood flow?

The pressure in the placental sinuses exceeds maternal systolic BP, resulting in insufficient perfusion and fetal hypoxia

What aspects of the fetus can impact labor (passenger)?

Size (macrosomic > 4000 g)

Lie, presentation, attitude, position, asynclitism

Number of fetuses

Anatomic anomalies (sacrococcygeal teratoma)

Fetal scalp electrode (FSE) monitoring offers what benefits to electronic fetal monitoring (EFM)?

Continuous monitoring of the fetal heart rate in an obese patient or difficult to monitor fetus

How is the FSE applied?

Placental membranes must be ruptured and the electrode is adhered to the fetal calvarium

In what clinical setting is fetal blood sampling (fetal scalp pH) performed?

To acutely assess hypoxemia in the setting of nonreassuring FHR tracing, meconium, or other signs of fetal distress

What is suggested by the following range of fetal scalp pHs?

pH greater than 7.25: reassuring; a low probability of hypoxic-ischemic encephalopathy

pH 7.20 to 7.24: indeterminate; should be repeated in 30 minutes

pH greater than 7.20: a nonreassuring pH; delivery should be expedited with operative intervention

What other clinical information can be utilized to improve the predictive value of a low scalp pH?

FHR variability

MANAGEMENT

What can be used to augment latent labor or prolonged early labor?

Cervical ripening agents (prostaglandins)

Intravenous oxytocin

An amniotomy

What is the effect of oxytocin (Pitocin) on labor?

It **increases the frequency** and **force of uterine contractions.**

What is the half-life of oxytocin?

3 to 5 minutes

A nulliparous patient is receiving 15 mU/min of intravenous oxytocin to augment her labor. Mother and fetus are tolerating labor well. There is no evidence of CPD, and an IUPC indicates 140 MU over a 10 minute interval. What is the next step in management?

Increase the oxytocin; the goal is to achieve more than 200 MU.

What are the risks involved with prolonged high-dose oxytocin administration?

Maternal SIADH and excessive fluid retention (pulmonary edema)

Hyperstimulation of the uterus

Postpartum atony and hemorrhage

Hyperbilirubinemia of the infant

Why is an amniotomy or assisted rupture of membranes (AROM) performed?

To induce or augment labor

To assess for meconium in the amniotic fluid

To place an IUPC or FSE

If the fetal head is not engaged in the pelvis or well applied to the cervix why is an amniotomy contraindicated?

Because of the risk of **umbilical cord prolapse**, compression by the presenting fetal part, and subsequent fetal hypoxia

A woman at 37 weeks EGA presents with painful uterine contractions, reassuring fetal status, no signs or symptoms of ROM, and an unchanged SVE after 3 hours. The cervix remains long, closed, and high. Irregular contractions occur at 15 to 20 minute intervals. What is your diagnosis?

Braxton Hicks contractions (prodromal or false labor)

How should the above woman be managed?

She should be **hydrated**, scheduled for **close clinical follow-up**, and advised to **go home** with labor precautions.

In the presence of a nonreassuring fetal heart rate what initial interventions should be tried?

Position the mother in left lateral decubitus position with flexed knees

Supplemental oxygen with a face mask

Refrain from active pushing

Turn off the oxytocin and consider tocolytics (if tachysystole)

What is tocolysis?

Relaxation of the uterine smooth muscle

What substances are commonly used for uterine relaxation during tachysystole?

Terbutaline (or less often nitrous oxide)

What are the risks of applying traction on the cord during the third stage of labor?

Avulsion of the cord or **uterine inversion**

How can this risk be reduced?

By **applying suprapubic pressure** when applying gentle traction to the cord (fundal pressure should not be applied).

The placenta and uterus should be examined to ensure that no membranes or accessory lobes are retained.

After delivery of the placenta what is given to prevent postpartum hemorrhage?

20 units of **oxytocin** in 1 L of lactated ringers

What are the four classifications of vaginal and perineal lacerations?

First degree limited to vaginal mucosa and skin of the introitus

Second degree extends to the fascia and muscles of the perineal body.

Third degree trauma involves the anal sphincter.

Fourth degree extends into the rectal lumen, through the rectal mucosa.

What are the indications for an episiotomy?

To expedite delivery in the setting of nonreassuring fetal heart tracing or maternal exhaustion

Why is an episiotomy only performed with clear indication?	Third and fourth degree lacerations and anal incontinence of stool or flatus are more common with an episiotomy than with a spontaneous laceration.
What are advantages of midline episiotomies when compared with mediolateral episiotomies?	They are associated with fewer infections, faster healing, less pain, less blood loss, less dyspareunia, and better anatomical results.
What is the one advantage of the mediolateral episiotomy?	Decreased risk of extension to a third or fourth degree laceration
What muscles are affected by second degree lacerations?	Bulbocavernous and ischiocavernous laterally superficial transverse perineal muscle

OPERATIVE VAGINAL DELIVERY

What are the two major types of operative vaginal delivery?	1. Forceps 2. Vacuum
What is required for operative vaginal delivery?	Fully dilated cervix Ruptured membranes Engaged fetal head (at or below zero station) Known absence of CPD Known position of the fetal head Experienced operator The capability to perform an emergency cesarean delivery if necessary
What are the various types of forceps deliveries?	**Outlet:** fetal scalp is visible at the introitus and rotation does not exceed 45°. **Low:** +2 station and may require more than 45° of rotation to AP orientation. **Mid-pelvic:** head is engaged at or below 0 station (but above +2 station), rotation is often required to mimic the cardinal movements of labor. **High:** above 0 station.

Operative vaginal delivery is appropriate or indicated in what context?

Fetal distress

Maternal exhaustion

Arrest of descent or prolonged 2nd stage

Contraindications to pushing

What are the most common maternal morbidities involved with forceps delivery?

Increased perineal trauma (third and fourth degree extensions)

Increased need for blood transfusion (these risks are increased with more rotation or at a higher station).

Vacuum delivery confers what advantages over forceps?

Can be achieved with minimal analgesia

What are some contraindications to vacuum-assisted delivery?

Low birth weight fetus (estimated fetal weight < 2500 g)

Prematurity less than 34 weeks

Suspected fetal coagulopathy

Recent scalp blood sampling

Face or breech presentation

An inability for the mother to engage in expulsive efforts

Cessation of contractions (vacuum traction must be coordinated with maternal effort)

What are the fetal morbidities involved with forceps and vacuum delivery?

Scalp lacerations, bruising, subgaleal hematomas, cephalohematomas, intracranial hemorrhage, neonatal jaundice, subconjunctival hemorrhage, clavicular fracture, shoulder dystocia, facial nerve injury, Erb palsy, retinal hemorrhage, and fetal death

Which operative vaginal delivery is associated with more trauma to the fetus?

Vacuum delivery — there is an increased risk of cephalohematoma and retinal hemorrhage when compared with forceps delivery.

Which operative vaginal delivery method is associated with more maternal trauma to the perineum?

Forceps

CESAREAN DELIVERY

What are some indications for scheduled cesarean delivery?

Previous classical uterine incision

Prior myomectomy that entered the endometrial cavity

EFW is more than 5000 g (or > 4500 g in a diabetic)

Severe fetal hydrocephalus

Malpresentation (breech)

Active genital herpes

Placenta previa

What percentage of deliveries in the United States are cesarean deliveries?

Over 20%

What is the risk of a trial of labor in a woman with a prior classical uterine incision?

A 12% risk of **uterine rupture**, which is associated with fetal compromise, maternal shock, and a 10% maternal mortality rate.

What is the risk of uterine rupture in a laboring patient with a prior lower uterine segment incision?

Less than 1%

What are the signs and symptoms of uterine rupture?

Severe abdominal pain/uterine tenderness

Nonreassuring fetal heart rate tracing

Loss of fetal station

At what EGA is a cesarean section scheduled?

After 39 weeks in a patient with accurate dating of her pregnancy.

Fetal lung maturity tests should be performed if delivery is planned earlier or if the dating method is not adequate.

What is the lower uterine segment and what are the advantages of using this in a C-section?

The region of the uterus just superior to the cervix. The myometrium is **significantly thinner** than the uterine fundus (especially during labor) and is associated with a **lower risk of uterine rupture** in a future pregnancy.

What are the layers (from exterior to interior) that are incised with a Pfannenstiel or low transverse abdominal incision?

Skin → subcutaneous fat → superficial fascia (Camper's and Scarpa's) → anterior rectus sheath (fascia) → rectus abdominus muscle → preperitoneal fat → parietal peritoneum → visceral (vesico-uterine) peritoneum → uterus

What percentage of VBACs (vaginal births after cesarean) are successful?	60% to 80% are successful (depending on the indication for prior cesarean)
What term describes a pathologically thin lower uterine segment through which fetal membranes or fetal parts can be visualized prior to uterine incision?	A **uterine window**
What are some indications for a vertical lower uterine incision?	Premature breech fetus
	Poorly developed lower uterine segment
	Extensive fibrosis of lower uterine segment (following multiple cesareans)
Can the type of previous uterine incision be determined from the skin incision?	No

Postpartum Care

PUERPERIUM MANAGEMENT

What is the duration of the postpartum period, also known as the puerperium?	6 to 8 weeks following delivery, when maternal physiology returns to the pre-pregnancy state
What is uterine involution?	The uterus returning to its pre-pregnancy size via contraction of the myometrium with subsequent atrophy. This constricts vessels and prevents hemorrhage
When is a pregnant woman at highest risk of developing venous thrombosis?	During the immediate puerperium period because of vessel trauma, immobility, increased fibrinogen, factor VII, VIII, IX, X, and platelets
	Approximately 0.7 per 1000 women experience a venous thrombosis during pregnancy or postpartum.
During delivery, which nerve can be injured that leads to urinary retention?	The pudendal nerve; the neuropathy normally resolves within 2 months

Following a 300-minute second stage of labor, a G1P1 is unable to flex her hips against tension and has difficulty walking. What type of neuropathy is likely responsible?

Femoral nerve compression, secondary to hyperflexion of the hips during a prolonged second stage

Which episiotomy is associated with perineal or pelvic hematoma?

Mediolateral episiotomies

How soon should an Rh(D-) mother be given Rhogam (anti-D immune globulin), following delivery of an Rh+ fetus?

Within 72 hours of delivery

Where is the fundus during the postpartum period?

Immediately after delivery: near the umbilicus

After 24 hours: below the umbilicus

1 week: near the symphysis pubis

2 weeks: in the pelvis

6 to 8 weeks: it has assumed its nonpregnant size

What is lochia?

A combination of blood, serous exudate, erythrocytes, leukocytes, necrotic decidua, epithelial cells, and bacteria

What is the progression of the various types of lochia?

Lochia **rubra** (red): blood from the placental bed, mixed with tissue, lasting 3 to 5 days.

Lochia **serosa** (brown): older blood mixed with serous drainage, leukocytes, and cervical mucus, ending by the 10th day after delivery.

Lochia **alba** (yellow-white): lasts from the second to sixth week after delivery and has a small amount of blood, combined with leukocytes, epithelial cells, cholesterol, fat, and mucus.

How long does a woman shed lochia?

4 to 6 weeks; however, it should not be red for more than 2 weeks

What is suggested if a woman continues to have lochia rubra for over 2 weeks?

Retained products of conception (POC) must be considered

Her uterus, cervix, and vagina should be examined with possible dilation and curettage.

How much lochia is shed during the puerperium?

Initially it may be as heavy as a period and should gradually subside daily

The total amount lost is approximately 500 mL.

What is the management of a vaginal wound dehiscence?

Dehiscence of a vaginal laceration repair should be evaluated for infection, irrigated, and debrided of necrotic tissue. Sitz baths should be used liberally.

If discovered in the first 2 to 3 days after delivery, the wound can be resutured; however, if the tissue is friable or has evidence of infection, a secondary repair should be delayed for 6 to 8 weeks.

Antibiotics should be utilized if infection is noted.

What are some signs and symptoms of endometritis?

Elevated temperature (> 100.4°F or > 38°C)

Uterine tenderness

Purulent vaginal discharge

Leukocytosis

When does endometritis usually occur?

Usually within the first 3 to 5 days after delivery

It occurs in 4% of all vaginal deliveries and up to 10% of cesarean deliveries.

What are risk factors for the development of endometritis?

Prolonged ROM

Prolonged labor

Multiple internal examinations

Internal monitoring (FSE or IUPC)

Retained POC

Lower socioeconomic status

Poor nutrition

Concurrent genital tract infection

What is the treatment for endometritis?

It is a polymicrobial infection, with a mixture of aerobic and anerobic bacteria found. Treatment usually consists of **gentamicin and clindamycin** until the patient is afebrile for 24 to 36 hours.

What are other common causes of puerperal fever (postpartum or postcesarean-section fever)?

Wind (atelectasis or aspiration PNA)

Water (cystitis or UTI)

Wound (surgical site infection or laceration)

Walking (PE or a DVT)

Wonder drugs (medication side effect or adverse reaction)

Womb (endometritis)

Wet nurse (engorgement or mastitis: infection often with *S. aureus* or *Streptococcus*)

Phlebitis or septic pelvic thrombophlebitis

BREASTFEEDING AND INFANT CARE

What are the five components of the Apgar score at 1, 5, and 10 minutes?

Appearance (blue, acrocyanosis, pink)

Pulse (absent, < 100, > 100)

Grimace (none, present, vigorous)

Activity (flaccid, flexed, moving)

Respirations (absent, slow, crying)

Each component is given 0, 1, or 2 points

Silver nitrate, erythromycin, or tetracycline ointments are applied to the newborn's eyes to prevent what ocular infection?

Chlamydia and gonorrhea

How does an infant benefit from skin-to-skin contact at birth?

Better temperature and glucose control, as well as an increased likelihood of maternal breastfeeding

Which vitamin is absent from human breast milk?

Vitamin K.

Infants are given a vitamin K shot at birth to prevent hemorrhagic disease of the newborn.

How does prolactin impact breastfeeding?

Stimulates milk production by the terminal exocrine glands

Nipple stimulation also increases oxytocin release from the posterior pituitary. How does this impact breastfeeding?

It causes contraction of the myoepithelial cells of the lactiferous ducts, allowing milk letdown.

How does breastfeeding prevent ovulation?

Prolactin inhibits the pulsatile gonadotropin releasing hormone from the hypothalamus.

What is colostrum?

Thick yellow breast secretions that contain plasma exudates, immunoglobulins (IgA), lactoferrin, albumin, and electrolytes. It is secreted during the first 2 days postpartum.

Why is an ELISA or Western blot repeated at 6 months and 1 year following delivery of an infant to an HIV+ mother?

Maternal transplacental IgG persists for several months in the infant's serum.

The above tests check for antibodies to HIV, not the actual virus.

When does a breastfeeding woman's milk "come in"?

3 to 5 days postpartum

Are mothers who are seropositive for the following conditions advised to breastfeed?

Hepatitis A: yes

Hepatitis B: yes, with vaccination and hepatitis B IgG administration to the infant at birth

Hepatitis C: yes

HIV: no

Are mothers who are exposed to the following substances advised to breastfeed?

Alcohol:	No
Street drugs:	No
Tobacco:	Yes
Hepatitis B vaccination:	Yes
Rubella vaccination:	Yes
Tetracyclines:	No
Sulfa drugs:	No, because they displace bilirubin and increase risk of kernicterus
Quinolones:	No
Chemotherapy:	No
Radiation:	No
Lithium or heavy metals:	No

Is previous mammoplasty (reduction or implantation) a contraindication to breastfeeding?	No. If the integrity of the nipple ducts are preserved, a woman can breastfeed; however, the surgical technique and subsequent scarring may make this difficult.
What is the caloric demand of lactation?	640 kcal/d
How much should breastfeeding women increase their daily caloric intake?	300 to 500 kcal
How much calcium should a breastfeeding woman consume?	1200 mg/d of calcium
A mother does not want to breastfeed although her breasts are extremely tender 5 days postpartum. What is appropriate management?	Tight-fitting bras, avoidance of nipple stimulation, cool compresses, acetaminophen or ibuprofen

PHYSIOLOGIC CHANGES AND RESOLUTION

How is cardiac output (CO) affected during the first day postpartum?	A 60% to 80% increase in CO occurs with the autotransfusion of uteroplacental blood to the intravascular space and decompression of the vena cava.
A leukocytosis less than 25,000 and low-grade fevers less than 101 are considered normal or abnormal 24 hours postpartum?	Normal
Over what time period does the CO and systemic vascular resistance gradually return to nonpregnant levels?	3 to 4 months, with concurrent reduction in left ventricular size and contractility
How does a prepartum cervix (cx) differ from a parous cx?	The prepartum cervical os can be described as a "pinpoint." Over several weeks following delivery, the cx slowly contracts, with the cervical os appearing as a transverse, stellate slit.
Why is a woman who has delivered vaginally at risk for pelvic relaxation, cytocele, rectocele, or incontinence?	Connective tissue and fascial stretching may not return to the pregravid state, resulting in persistent trauma or changes.

What is a persistent defect of the abdominal wall musculature caused by the gravid uterus known as?	Diastasis recti
How much weight is lost following delivery?	Almost half of the gestational weight gain is lost following delivery (13 lbs), with the additional weight loss occurring over the next 6 months (15 lbs).
Do women typically gain weight following pregnancy?	Most women maintain 10% of their gestational weight following the postpartum period
Why do some women note increased alopecia postpartum?	Scalp hair shifts from the predominant anagen phase (growing) during pregnancy to a predominant telogen phase (resting). This **telogen effluvium** typically resolves within 5 months.
What is the condition in which a woman displays hypopituitarism following a delivery with postpartum hemorrhage?	Sheehan's syndrome, because of infarction and necrosis of the pituitary
When does serum human chorionic gonadotropin (HCG) return to normal (nondetectable levels)?	Within 4 to 6 weeks of delivery or abortion
What is suggested by a rising HCG postpartum?	Gestational trophoblastic disease
Why do some women note vaginal atrophy in the puerperium?	Prolactin inhibition of systemic estrogens
How is the thyroid affected postpartum?	Hormone levels are within normal limits by 4 weeks and the thyroid gland decreases to prepregnancy size over 3 months

FERTILITY AND CONTRACEPTION

When does ovulation and menstruation begin in a postpartum nonlactating woman?	Ovulation typically resumes within 45 days to 4 weeks. Average duration to menstruation is 8 weeks postpartum.

When does ovulation and menstruation begin in a postpartum breastfeeding woman?

A woman who is breastfeeding more than 5 times a day can remain anovulatory for the duration of breastfeeding.

How long should the woman maintain "pelvic rest," by refraining from coitus or inserting anything in the vagina?

6 weeks postpartum, so as to decrease the risk of an infection ascending through the patent cervical os, and to reduce the risk of infection or trauma to healing lacerations

What type of birth control will not affect breastfeeding?

IUD

Barrier methods

Progestin only pills (mini pill)

Depo-Provera

Why do oral contraceptive pills (OCPs) and Norplant affect breastfeeding?

Estrogen decreases breast milk production. It can be safely started 6 weeks after delivery if milk production is adequate.

Why do some clinicians recommend that women obtain an IUD 6 weeks postpartum instead of insertion at the time of delivery?

Decreased risk of expulsion because of patent os and uterine cramping

CLINICAL VIGNETTES

A 28-year-old G1P0 at 39 weeks gestation presents to L&D after leakage of fluid. She is ruled in for SROM with positive ferning, pooling, and nitrazine. She is contracting every 4 to 5 minutes and is admitted in latent labor. On the monitor, the fetal heart tones are 140 bpm with moderate variability, positive accelerations, but frequent brief spiky decelerations unrelated to contractions. What is the etiology of the variable decelerations?
   a. Oligohydramnios
   b. Uteroplacental insufficiency
   c. Umbilical cord compression
   d. Fetal head compression

Answer: c

What is being described are variable decelerations. These are thought to be caused by cord compression and do not signify fetal distress. Oligohydramnios increases the risk of cord compression, however it does not cause compression. Uteroplacental insufficiency leads to late decelerations which follow the onset of contractions and return to baseline after the contraction is complete. Fetal head compression leads to early decelerations, which begin and end with the contraction due to fetal vagal nerve stimulation.

A 32-year-old G2P1 at 30 weeks gestation presents to the hospital with left sided pelvic pain. It is cramping in nature but does not radiate. There are no associated fevers, no dysuria, and no hematuria. On examination she has no costovertebral angle tenderness. Her WBC is 10,000/mL. Her UA is negative for infection or blood. A renal US is performed with the finding of mild right hydronephrosis. What is the likely etiology of this finding?

a. Ureterolithiasis
b. Pyelonephritis
c. Compression of the right ureter by the uterus and right ovarian vein
d. Progesterone-related smooth muscle relaxation
e. c and d

Answer: e

Without evidence of stone on US, ureterolithiasis is unlikely. While pyelonephritis is more common in pregnancy, without a fever, CVAT, or infection on the UA this diagnosis is effectively excluded. Mild to moderate hydronephrosis in pregnancy is common, especially on the right, as a result of compression by the uterus and ovarian vein as well as by progesterone-mediated smooth muscle relaxation.

A 26-year-old G5P3013 at 12 weeks gestation calls with symptoms of shakiness, vomiting, and a 5 lb weight loss over the past 2 weeks. These symptoms developed 8 weeks ago, but have worsened. You call her in to your office and draw labs. Which of the following would you expect to see on TFTs?

a. Increased total thyroxine
b. Normal total thyroxine
c. Decreased total thyroxine
d. Decreased free thyroxine
e. Decreased thyronine binding globulin (TBG)

Answer: a

This patient has symptoms of hyperthyroidism. Total thyroxine (T_4) is increased in this patient as a result of this condition. Furthermore, in pregnancy TBG levels are increased. This leads to an increase in total thyroxine.

A 42-year-old G1P0 at 14 weeks gestation presents to your office for routine obstetrical care. She has no medical history and no notable family history. She asks about risk of genetic abnormalities. You discuss amniocentesis, however she does not want such an invasive test. Which of the following tests would be indicated?

a. Maternal alpha fetoprotein (AFP)
b. Fetal nuchal translucency
c. Fetal nuchal translucency with maternal serum PAPP-A and β-hCG
d. Maternal serum AFP, hCG, estriol, and inhibin-A

Answer: d

If this patient declines diagnostic genetic testing (amniocentesis or CVS), genetic screening should be offered. The most sensitive test is an integrated or sequential test, which includes early nuchal translucency combined with maternal serum testing in the first and second trimesters. However this patient is presented too late for that option. In the second trimester, the triple or quad screen (answer d) is the only available tests.

A 27-year-old G1P0 at 41 weeks gestational age presents to L&D with painful contractions. Her cervix changes from 2/2/-2 to 5/0.5/-1 over 2 hours and she is admitted in labor. Fetal heart tones are reactive and she is contracting every 1 to 2 minutes. As an IV is being placed there is a large gush of blood and followed by difficulty in tracing the fetal heart tones. Her heart rate is 82 bpm and her BP is 108/64. What is the immediate next step in management?

a. Emergency cesarean section
b. Type, cross and transfuse two units of packed red blood cells
c. Place an intrauterine pressure catheter (IUPC)
d. Place an internal fetal scalp electrode (FSE)

Answer: d

A gush of blood may be indicative of placental abruption and thus continuous fetal monitoring is imperative. When fetal heart tones are difficult to trace externally, an internal monitor (FSE) can be quickly placed to monitor the fetal heart rate. There is no need for emergent delivery until fetal distress or significant maternal hemorrhage is evident. She is hemodynamically stable and does not need a transfusion. An IUPC is used to monitor contraction intensity and is not indicated.

A 28-year-old G3P2 presents to L&D at 38 weeks gestational age in active labor. She began contracting 5 hours ago and her cervical examination on admission was 8 cm dilated. She is expectantly managed for 2 hours when the nurse calls to ask you to evaluate the fetal heart rate tracing. The baseline is 130 bpm with moderate variability and decelerations that begin and end with each contraction. What is the physiologic etiology of this fetal heart rate pattern?

a. Oligohydramnios
b. Uteroplacental insufficiency
c. Umbilical cord compression
d. Fetal head compression

Answer: d

This patient is in active labor and is likely completely dilated. Decelerations and begin and end with a contraction are early decelerations and are a consequence of fetal head compression. Oligohydramnios in and of itself does not cause decelerations. Umbilical cord compression leads to variable decelerations which appear as decelerations unrelated to contractions (variable in morphology and timing).

A 19-year-old G1P0 presents to L&D at 38 weeks gestational age with painful contractions. She was 2 cm dilated and progressed to 5 cm within 2 hours. She is admitted to L&D and expectantly managed, contracting every 3 to 4 minutes. Four hours later, spontaneous rupture of membranes occurs and she is found to have an unchanged examination. The estimated fetal weight by Leopolds is 7 lbs and clinical pelvimetry deems her to have an adequate pelvis. Fetal heart tones are reassuring and contractions are occurring every 4 to 5 minutes. What is the next step in management?

a. Cesarean delivery
b. Ambulation and reexamination in 2 to 4 hours
c. Begin labor augmentation with oxytocin
d. Discharge the patient home

Answer: c

This patient is in arrested active labor. Arrested labor is defined as no cervical change, whereas protracted labor is defined as cervical change of less than 1.5 cm/h in a multiparous patient or less than 1.2 cm/h in a nulliparous patient. Either can be initially managed with oxytocin augmentation. Cesarean delivery is not indicated at this time. Expectant management does not facilitate delivery and may increase the risk of chorioamnionitis in this patient who has ruptured membranes. Rupture of membranes requires delivery, and thus discharging this patient would not be indicated.

A 34-year-old G2P1 presents for routine prenatal care. Her prior OB history is notable for a low transverse cesarean section for arrest of descent. She delivered a healthy 3800 g infant. She wants to avoid another cesarean section and asks about TOLAC (trial of labor after cesarean). Which of the following statements is true?

a. She should be induced at 37 weeks to minimize the risk of cephalo-pelvic disproportion.
b. The risk of uterine rupture is under 1%.
c. Current guidelines recommend a repeat cesarean section.
d. Her risk of repeat cesarean is decreased because of her prior cesarean indication.

Answer: b

TOLAC is an option for women with one or two prior low transverse cesarean sections. Risks include uterine rupture which occurs in less than 1% of cases. If this occurs, there is an approximately 10% risk of a severe adverse neonatal outcome. Induction increases the risk of uterine rupture and thus spontaneous labor is desired. Women that have a history of a nonrecurring indication for cesarean (such as placenta previa or breech presentation) are more likely to have a lower risk of a repeat cesarean.

CHAPTER 9

Complications of Pregnancy

Early Complications

CONGENITAL ANOMALIES

What is the prevalence of major congenital anomalies in the United States?

Between 2% and 4%

What are the causes of congenital anomalies and what are their relative frequencies?

Single gene disorders (15%-20%)

Chromosomal abnormalities (5%)

Teratogens (either maternal illness, infection, drugs, or chemicals 10%)

Unknown (60%-70%)

What is the overall incidence of chromosomal anomalies in the United States?

0.7% of all live births

More common among abortuses and stillbirths (up to 50%)

What happens to most fetuses with chromosomal abnormalities?

Most do not survive to term.

If they do, they are often with congenital abnormalities (with multiple organ system involvement), growth deficiency, and mental retardation.

Do the same cytogenetic abnormalities produce the same phenotype in each fetus?

No. While it will produce the same pattern of malformations, there is significant variability.

What are the genetic etiologies of chromosomal abnormalities?

Nondisjunction

Unequal recombination

Inversion

Deletions/duplications

Translocations

What is the most common etiology of chromosomal abnormality?

Nondisjunction—the loss or gain of a chromosome resulting in trisomy or monosomy

What is the major risk factor for nondisjunction?

Advanced maternal age

Describe the syndrome associated with trisomy 21:

Known as **Down syndrome**, it is the most common chromosomal abnormality found in live births. It is associated with mental retardation, hypotonia, a single palmar crease, early-onset Alzheimer disease, and other serious congenital features such as duodenal atresia, congenital heart disease, and leukemia.

What is the cytogenetic etiology of trisomy 21 and what are the relative frequencies?

True trisomy (94%)

Robertsonian translocation (3%-4%)

Trisomy mosaicism (2%-3%)

What are the risk factors for trisomy 21?

Advanced maternal age

Describe the syndrome associated with trisomy 18 (Edwards syndrome):

Major features include:

Severe mental retardation

Prominent occiput

Micrognathia

Flexed fingers

Congenital heart disease

Horseshoe kidney

Meckel diverticulum or malrotation

Most of trisomy 18 infants die before term 1 week of life and the vast majority die within 1 year

Describe the syndrome associated with trisomy 13 (Patau syndrome):

It primarily includes malformations of the midface, eyes, and brain. However, omphalocele, genitourinary (GU) anomalies, hemangiomas, polydactyly, rocker-bottom feet, and congenital heart defects are also often found.

80% die within the first month and the vast majority die within the first 6 months.

What is genomic imprinting?

Differential expression of genetic information, depending on whether it is paternally or maternally derived.

It is the basis of diseases such as Prader-Willi syndrome and Angelman syndrome, which involve the same microdeletion on chromosome 15 but result in a different phenotype depending on which parent the deletion came from.

Describe the following sex chromosome abnormalities:

Turner syndrome (45, X)

Characterized by short stature, streak gonads, mild MR, and other abnormalities such as webbed neck, lymphedema, pigmented nevi, and congenital heart defects (eg, coarctation of the aorta)

Klinefelter syndrome (47, XXY)

Characterized by tall stature, microorchidism, and azospermia

What is a teratogen?

Any agent that can lead to abnormalities in a developing fetus.

They can be from maternal illness, microbial infections, drugs, or other chemicals in the environment.

What types of birth defects are associated with the following maternal illnesses?

Diabetes mellitus:

Congenital heart disease, spina bifida, caudal regression, focal femoral hypoplasia

Phenylketonuria:

Microcephaly, mental retardation, congenital heart disease

Adrenal/ovarian tumors:

Virilization of female fetuses (if they secrete androgens)

Autoimmune disease:

A similar disease in fetus as in the mother if the antibodies cross the placenta, congenital heart block (complete AV block)

Obesity:

Neural tube defects

SPONTANEOUS ABORTIONS

What is a spontaneous abortion?	Also called a **miscarriage**, it is a pregnancy that spontaneously ends **prior to 20 weeks of gestation** or **before the fetus has reached 500 g** resulting in expulsion of all or any part of the products of conception.
How common is spontaneous abortion?	It occurs in 8% to 20% of known pregnancies under 20 weeks and in an even higher percentage of subclinical pregnancies.
When do most spontaneous abortions occur?	80% occur prior to 12 weeks.
Chromosomal abnormalities (aneuploidy) are the most common cause of spontaneous abortion in the first trimester. What are the two most common genetic abnormalities that cause this?	1. Autosomal trisomies 2. Monosomy X
Are there any therapeutic interventions that prevent first trimester pregnancy loss?	No, nothing has been proven in randomized controlled trials to prevent this.
What are some causes of second trimester spontaneous abortion?	Cervical insufficiency Infection Chromosomal or structural malformation Maternal thrombophilia
What increases the risk of spontaneous abortion?	**Advanced maternal age** **Prior spontaneous abortion** **Heavy cigarette use** Short interpregnancy interval Maternal medical disease Heavy alcohol or caffeine intake Trauma Increased parity Advanced paternal age

What are the three most common
symptoms of a spontaneous abortion?

1. History of amenorrhea
2. Vaginal bleeding
3. Pelvic pain

Describe each of the following types
of spontaneous abortions:

Complete abortion:

Uterine bleeding with complete
expulsion of the product of conception
(POC) and closed cervical os

Inevitable abortion:

Uterine bleeding with cervical dilation
but without expulsion of any POC

Incomplete abortion:

Uterine bleeding with cervical dilation
but with incomplete expulsion of
the POC

Missed abortion:

Embryonic demise without expulsion of
POC and with closed cervical os

Septic abortion:

Embryonic demise with evidence of
infected products of conception
(eg, fever, uterine tenderness)

Threatened abortion:

Uterine bleeding with closed cervical os
and normal cardiac activity

What percentage of women exhibit
signs of threatened abortion during
their pregnancy? What percentage of
these women will spontaneously
abort?

Approximately 25% and 50%,
respectively

What must be considered in the
differential diagnosis of a threatened
abortion?

Ectopic pregnancy

Cervical, vaginal, or uterine pathology

Bleeding related to implantation

What is the first diagnostic test you
should perform in a woman with a
known intrauterine pregnancy who
presents with vaginal bleeding?

Ultrasound

How is vaginal bleeding in the first trimester evaluated?

Via history, physical examination, hCG levels, and ultrasound. The following algorithm (Fig. 9.1) can be used:

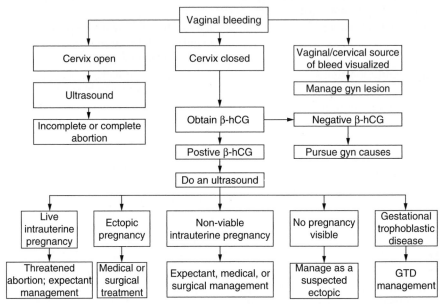

Figure 9.1   Evaluation of vaginal bleeding in the first trimester. *(Adapted, with permission, from uptodateonline.com Clinical manifestations, diagnosis, and management of ectopic pregnancy by Togas Tulandi).*

What are the ultrasonographic criteria for diagnosis of a nonviable intrauterine pregnancy?

Absence of fetal cardiac activity in an embryo with a crown-rump length more than 5 mm

Or,

Absence of a fetal pole when the mean sac diameter more than 20 mm

What are the treatment options for an incomplete, inevitable, or a missed abortion?

Surgical, medical, or expectant management

What are the advantages and disadvantages surgical, medical, or expectant management?

See Table 9.1

Table 9.1 Treatment Options for Abortion

	Advantages	Disadvantages
Surgical Management	Greatest efficacy; quickest evacuation	Invasive; procedural/ anesthesia risks
Medical Management	Less invasive; avoids anesthesia; patient can do it in the privacy of her own home	Requires more than two visits; less quick
Expectant Management	Least invasive	Timing is unpredictable; risk of needing an unplanned procedure

Why is it imperative that spontaneous abortions be evacuated?

Because after several weeks-months, the trophoblastic tissue might enter the maternal bloodstream, triggering the coagulation cascade and causing a **coagulopathy**

What laboratory tests must be done after a spontaneous abortion?

Type and screen (because Rh immunoglobulin must be given to Rh[–] women)

Can a woman do anything to prevent a spontaneous abortion?

Typically no, and so all women need to be reassured that it is not their fault.

Should a woman who has had a spontaneous abortion undergo an evaluation for the cause?

No. These are fairly common and are often sporadic.

What is recurrent pregnancy loss (RPL)?

Three or more consecutive losses of pregnancy prior to 20 weeks

What is the incidence of RPL?

Approximately 0.5% to 1%

What is the risk of spontaneous abortion?

After one prior loss: 10% to 20%

After two consecutive losses: 25% to 45%

What does the diagnostic workup of RPL consist of?	A complete medical, surgical, genetic, and family history
	A physical examination with attention to signs of **endocrinopathies** or **pelvic organ anomalies**
	Laboratory evaluation including: **uterine assessment** (HSG)
	Antiphospholipid labs (anticardiolipin antibodies and lupus anticoagulant)
	Evaluation of ovarian reserve
	Possibly other tests (eg, evaluation for inherited thrombophilias, thyroid function tests [TFTs], and a karyotype)
What is the treatment for RPL?	It is dependent on the etiology; however, it can include:
	Surgery (for pelvic organ abnormalities)
	Low molecular weight heparin or aspirin (for antiphospholipid syndrome)
	Synthroid (for hypothyroidism)

Late Complications

HYPERTENSIVE DISORDERS OF PREGNANCY

Hypertensive disorders in pregnancy are defined by blood pressures that are persistently elevated above what values?	Systolic greater than 140 mm Hg or diastolic greater than 90 mm Hg
What percentage of United States pregnancies are complicated by hypertensive disorders?	10% to 20%
What are the various hypertensive disorders observed during pregnancy?	Chronic hypertension (cHTN)
	Gestational hypertension (gHTN)
	Preeclampsia
	Eclampsia
If a woman at 18 weeks estimated gestational age (EGA) presents with a BP of 146/82. What is her probable diagnosis?	Chronic hypertension (cHTN), because it was likely present and undiagnosed prior to pregnancy

What anti-hypertensives are used to lower the BP of a pregnant woman?

Methyldopa, labetolol, or nifedipine

Does anti-hypertensive therapy improve fetal outcomes?

No. It is used only to reduce maternal complications associated with hypertension (eg, stroke, MI).

How is gHTN diagnosed (dx)?

The onset of two BPs more than 140/90, separated by 6 hours after 20 weeks EGA

What is the difference between gHTN and preeclampsia?

Proteinuria is present in preeclampsia and it is absent in gHTN.

What are risk factors for preeclampsia?

Extremes of age

A history of preeclampsia

Multifetal gestations

Diabetes mellitus

Chronic or gestational hypertension

Nephropathy

Antiphospholipid antibody syndrome

Collagen vascular disease

Obesity

African-American race

Note: **smoking is not a risk factor**

What percentage of women with gHTN develop preeclampsia?

50%

Do gHTN and preeclampsia resolve postpartum?

Yes, but women are at increased risk of developing chronic hypertension.

How is preeclampsia diagnosed?

The new onset of hypertension (> 140/90) and proteinuria (≥ 0.3 g protein in a 24-hour urine specimen or persistent 1+ on dipstick) after 20 weeks of gestation

The hypertension should be documented on two separate occasions, at least 6 hours apart.

What is the cure for preeclampsia?

Delivery, though a woman remains at risk for the development of eclampsia postpartum

Once preeclampsia is suspected, why is 24-hour urine collected to assess protein excretion?

Single dipstick UA values do not correlate well with the degree of end-organ pathology present.

24-hour urine collection offers a more accurate reflection of the volume of protein lost by the kidneys.

Proteinuria is defined as more than 300 mg/24 h.

In the setting of cHTN, how is preeclampsia diagnosed?

With the onset of proteinuria, rising blood pressures, or other signs/symptoms of end-organ disease

What are the two types of preeclampsia?

1. Mild
2. Severe

What percent of cases are mild in the United States?

75%

What are the systemic and clinical features of severe preeclampsia?

Endothelial damage

Severe hypertension more than 160 mm Hg systolic or more than 110 mm Hg diastolic

Pulmonary edema because of capillary leak

Liver abnormalities

Elevated transaminases

Epigastric or RUQ pain (hepatic congestion and pressure on the liver capsule)

Hematologic abnormalities

Hemoconcentration

Thrombocytopenia

Microangiopathic hemolysis (schistocytes and helmet cells, increased serum lactate dehydrogenase)

CNS manifestations

Brisk deep tendon reflexes

Persistent headache (which does not resolve with tylenol, hydration, or rest)

Visual changes (scotoma, blurring, cortical blindness)

Renal dysfunction

Nephritic range proteinuria (> 5 g/d) because of the impaired integrity of the glomerular barrier

Oliguria (< 500 mL in 24 hours)

Uteroplacental insufficiency

Intrauterine growth restriction

What percentage of women with a history of preeclampsia have a recurrence in subsequent pregnancies?

25% to 65% with severe disease

5% to 7% with mild disease

What are some serious maternal complications of preeclampsia?

Cerebral hemorrhage

Disseminated intravascular coagulation (DIC)

Eclamptic seizure

Pulmonary edema

Oliguria and renal failure

Rupture of the hepatic capsule

What is considered to be the most severe manifestation of preeclampsia, without the onset of eclampsia (without seizures)?

HELLP syndrome (hemolysis, elevated liver function tests, low platelets)

How many women with preeclampsia develop HELLP?

2% of patients

Can a woman develop HELLP without a prior diagnosis of preeclampsia?

Yes, a small percentage of women do not exhibit hypertension or proteinuria

What laboratory abnormalities are associated with HELLP?

Lactate dehydrogenase greater than 600 IU/mL

Bilirubin greater than 1.2 mg/dL

Platelets less than 150

Elevated alanine and aspartate aminotransferase (AST and ALT)

What is the appropriate management of severe preeclampsia, HELLP, or eclampsia?

Delivery and anticonvulsant prophylaxis.

If the fetus is preterm, it is reasonable to attempt to administer steroids for fetal lung maturity (48 hours) before delivery.

What is eclampsia?

Generalized tonic-clonic seizures, which are not attributed to any other pathology

What is the most common symptom prior to the onset of seizures?

Intense headache, which does not resolve with medication, hydration, or rest

Do all women who develop eclampsia have proteinuria?	No, 10% lack proteinuria. However, they typically have other clinical and histologic manifestations.
How often do women with mild or severe preeclampsia progress to eclampsia?	Approximately 1 in 200 mild preeclamptics and 2% of severe PEC patients seize if they are not treated with anticonvulsant prophylaxis.
What percentage of seizures occur antepartum, intrapartum, and within 48 hours postpartum?	25%, 50%, and 25%, respectively
What medication is used to prevent seizures in a preeclamptic?	Magnesium sulfate ($MgSO_4$)
What medication is used to treat eclamptic seizures?	Magnesium sulfate ($MgSO_4$) is the primary treatment. Barbiturates, benzodiazepines (diazepam), and antiepileptics have also been used but are less effective.
What are the signs and symptoms of magnesium toxicity (in order of progression)?	Decreased deep tendon reflexes (first sign) Lethargic and blunted mental status Respiratory depression Pulmonary edema Chest pain and cardiac arrest (at levels of 30 mg/L)
Why is urine output monitored during magnesium treatment?	Magnesium is renally excreted. Blood levels may quickly become toxic if the patient becomes oliguric.
How is magnesium toxicity managed?	**Calcium gluconate** (to stabilize cardiac membranes), hydration, respiratory, and cardiac support

ABNORMAL PLACENTATION

What is a velamentous insertion of the cord or a velamentous umbilical cord?	Umbilical vessels that are surrounded only by fetal membranes, with no Wharton jelly
Is a velementous cord more common in twins?	Yes, it occurs in 10% of twins and 1% of singleton gestations.

What is placenta previa?

The edge of the placenta is in close proximity to or overlies the internal os of the cervix.

What is the incidence of placenta previa?

1 in 200 births

What are the various types of placenta previa?

Complete previa: the placenta covers the internal os of the cervix

Partial previa: the placental edge partially covers the internal os

Marginal previa: the placenta is adjacent but not covering the cervical os

Low-lying placenta: the placenta lies 2 to 3 cm from the cervical os

(see Fig. 9.2)

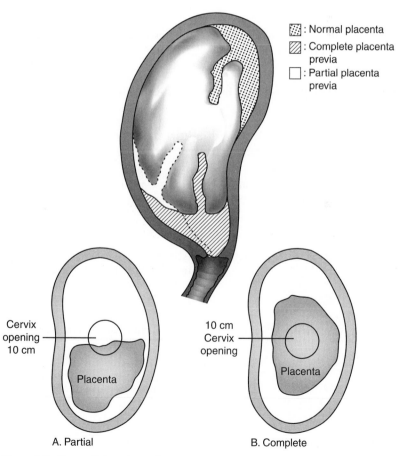

Figure 9.2   Types of placenta previa.

Can placenta previa diagnosed early in pregnancy resolve during the course of the pregnancy?	Yes, as the lower uterine segment enlarges and the placenta grows. 90% will resolve by term.
What are risk factors for placenta previa?	Endometrial scarring Increasing maternal age Prior cesarean section Prior curettages Maternal smoking or cocaine abuse Multiple gestation
What are some of the complications associated with placenta previa?	Hemorrhage Placenta accreta (10%) Malpresentation Preterm premature rupture of the membranes (PPROM)
Are women with a history of placenta previa at risk for previa in subsequent pregnancies?	Yes, the recurrence rate is 4% to 8%
What type of delivery is indicated in previa?	Cesarean delivery
What is a vasa previa?	Velamentous fetal vessels that cross the internal os
Rupture of membranes (ROM) or vaginal manipulation in vasa previa is associated with what risk?	Fetal exsanguination (seen as a concomitant finding of nonreassuring fetal heart rate such as a sinusoidal pattern)
What is a placenta accreta? Percreta? Increta?	Accreta: abnormal placental implantation through the endometrium to the myometrium that results in a placenta that is abnormally adherent to the uterus Increta: chorionic villi invade into the myomentrium Percreta: chorionic villi invade to or through the serosa (can invade surrounding organs)

What are risk factors for placenta accreta?

Placenta previa in current pregnancy

Previous cesarean delivery

Previous myomectomy

Asherman syndrome

Submucous leiomyoma

Maternal age greater than 35 years

Are there any tools that can diagnose placenta accreta?

Though ultrasonography and color doppler studies may help in the diagnosis, they are not definitive for placenta accreta.

Aside from hemorrhage, what is another consequence of placenta accreta that is life-threatening?

Uterine rupture

What abnormal placentation may cause increased risk of preterm delivery?

Circumvallata placenta, which is more common in older, multiparous patients

THIRD TRIMESTER BLEEDING

Antepartum hemorrhage refers to what type of bleeding?

Vaginal bleeding after 20 weeks EGA that is caused by some process other than labor.

What are the major causes of antepartum bleeding?

Placental abruption 30%

Placenta previa 20%

Uterine rupture

Vasa previa

Other causes such as infection, trauma, polyps, neoplasia, or bloody show

How often is antepartum hemorrhage observed in the third trimester?

4% of pregnancies

What is placental abruption?   Premature separation of the placenta from the uterine wall (secondary to decidual hemorrhage). See Fig. 9.3.

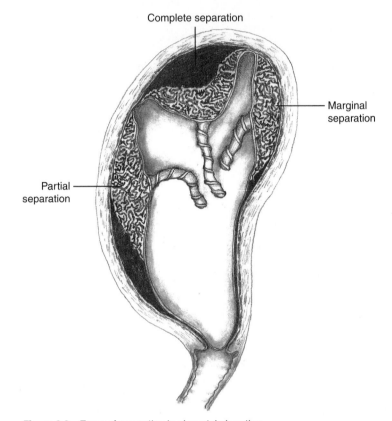

Complete separation

Marginal separation

Partial separation

Figure 9.3   Types of separation in placental abruption.

What are risk factors for placental abruption?

Trauma

Hypertension

Preterm premature rupture of membranes

Maternal thrombophilia

Drug use (cocaine, tobacco)

History of abruption

What are the classic symptoms of placental abruption?

Vaginal bleeding, abdominal pain/ uterine tenderness, contractions, nonreassuring fetal heart rate tracing

What labs should be ordered for evaluation of abruption?	CBC
	Type and screen
	Coagulation profile (including fibrinogen)
What is the initial management of painless blood per vagina in the third trimester?	Transabdominal ultrasonography is used for initial placental localization.
	A manual examination should *not* be performed until previa is ruled out.
Name some laboratory tests that identify the etiology of the vaginal bleeding (fetal vs maternal):	Apt or Kleihauer-Betke tests (identify fetal cells in maternal circulation)
What is the classic presentation of placenta previa?	**Painless blood per vagina** after 20 weeks EGA, which may range from spotting to hemorrhage
How often are painful uterine contractions reported in the setting of vaginal bleeding because of placenta previa?	10% of presentations
	However, vaginal bleeding and painful uterine contractions are more suggestive of abruption, especially in the setting of recent trauma.
Delivery should be expedited in which situations?	Persistent nonreassuring FHR, hemodynamic instability, significant bleeding with known fetal pulmonary maturity (> 34 weeks EGA), or disseminated intravascular coagulopathy (DIC)
In the context of intermittent contractions, third trimester bleeding, and less than 32 weeks EGA, what conditions must be met to allow for 48 hours of corticosteroids with possible tocolysis?	The mother must be hemodynamically stable and uninfected. The fetus should have a reassuring FHR.

PROM AND PPROM

What is the definition of premature rupture of membranes (PROM)?	Rupture of placental membranes (ROM) in a full term pregnancy, with the absence of labor
How prevalent is PROM?	It occurs in 8% of US pregnancies.

What are common other causes of leakage of fluid?

Urinary incontinence (stress incontinence)

Vaginal discharge

Semen (post intercourse)

What physical findings support the diagnosis of ROM?

Pooling of vaginal fluid on speculum examination

Positive **nitrazine** test of the vaginal fluid

Ferning of dried fluid under low power magnification

Ultrasound with decreased amniotic fluid (less specific)

If ROM is uncertain with the above examinations, what is a definitive test that can be performed?

Amnio dye test—pigment is injected into the amniotic fluid and a tampon is examined for leakage of this dye.

Do women who present with PROM go into spontaneous labor?

Yes, 70% will go into labor within 24 hours

What is considered prolonged PROM?

PROM for more than 18 to 24 hours, without the onset of labor

What are the benefits of immediate induction upon presentation to the hospital with PROM?

Reduced fetal and maternal infections, such as chorioamnionitis, endometritis, neonatal sepsis, and intensive care unit admission

What are the risks of induction with a poor Bishop score?

Failed induction, protracted labor, cesarean section

What is the definition of preterm premature rupture of membranes (PPROM)?

ROM in the absence of labor at less than 37 weeks EGA

How prevalent is PPROM?

1% to 3% of US pregnancies

What is the most common risk factors for the development of PPROM?

Genital tract infections

Chorioamnionitis

What are other risk factors for the development of PPROM?

Placenta previa

Smoking

Cervical incompetence

Multiple gestations

Polyhydramnios

Antepartum hemorrhage

Personal history of PPROM

What is the rate of PPROM recurrence in subsequent pregnancies?	13.5%
Is PPROM an indication for hospitalization?	Yes, from the time of diagnosis until delivery
Prior to delivery, what type of adverse outcomes are seen following PPROM?	Intrauterine infection 13% to 60% Placental abruption 4% to 12% Umbilical cord prolapse 1% to 2% Precipitous delivery
How should PPROM at ≥34 weeks EGA be managed?	Immediate delivery has been shown to result in better outcomes, as long as expert neonatal care is available.
What are fetal lung maturity tests?	**Lecithin/sphingomyelin ratio** (L/S) **Phosphatidylglycerol** (PG) **Fluorescence polarization** **Lamellar body count**
What is surfactin?	A phospholipid produced by type II pneumocytes, which decreases surface tension in the alveoli. Insufficient surfactin production will result in RDS.
When and why is betamethasone or dexamethasone used?	They are corticosteroids that cross the placenta and stimulate production of surfactin and lung maturation in the premature fetus. A 48-hour course is given between 24 to 34 weeks if delivery is anticipated.
Other than RDS, what risks of prematurity are attenuated by administration of steroids?	Intraventricular hemorrhage (IVH) Necrotizing enterocolitis (NEC) Neonatal mortality Systemic infection in the 1st 48 hours of life
What is the window of maximal benefit of antenatal steroids?	Within 24 hours to 7 days after administration
What effect does prophylactic antibiotic administration have in the setting of PPROM?	Reduces maternal and neonatal infection. Prolongs the latency period between the time of membrane rupture and the onset of labor.

What antibiotics are typically administered in the setting of PPROM?	Ampicillin and erythromycin for a total of 7 days
What conditions would require immediate delivery of PPROM, regardless of lung maturity?	Advanced labor Placental abruption Intrauterine infection Non-reassuring fetal testing Fetal compromise (severe oligohydramnios or cord prolapse)

PRETERM LABOR AND CERVICAL INSUFFICIENCY

What is the definition of preterm labor (PTL)?	Labor (regular uterine contractions with cervical change) that starts before the 37th week of pregnancy
What is the most significant risk factor for PTL?	Previous history of preterm delivery (PTD)
What are other risk factors for PTL?	Multiple gestations Extremes of maternal age Cervical insufficiency Sexually transmitted infections Maternal infection (eg, pyelonephritis, appendicitis) Uterine malformations or fibroids Substance abuse (eg, cocaine, tobacco) Low socioeconomic status
What is the definition of preterm birth (PTB) or preterm delivery (PTD)?	Birth that occurs before 37 completed weeks EGA
What are the causes of PTD?	Iatrogenic (for maternal or fetal indications) Intrauterine growth restriction Severe preeclampsia Placenta previa Nonreassuring fetal testing PPROM Intra-amniotic infection Other pathology or idiopathic preterm labor

What is the prevalence of PTD in the United States?

12% of all deliveries

2% occur before 32 weeks

What is the impact of PTD on neonatal morbidity and mortality?

In the United States, PTB accounts for 85% of all perinatal morbidity and mortality.

Disability occurs in 60% of survivors of birth at 26 weeks EGA.

Hydration may decrease preterm uterine contractions based on dilution of what hormone?

Antidiuretic hormone (ADH) is increased in the setting of dehydration and it may have some crossreactivity with uterine oxytocin receptors.

Diluting ADH and decreasing the systemic production may decrease preterm uterine irritability.

What class of medications is used to prevent uterine contractions? What are some examples?

Tocolytics

Magnesium sulfate

Calcium channel blockers (nifedipine)

Beta adrenergic agonists (terbutaline, ritodrine)

COX inhibitors (indomethacin)

When should tocolysis be started?

To delay delivery 48 hours in PTL with EGA less than 34 weeks so as to administer corticosteroids

Why is it not advisable to use more than one tocolytic concurrently?

Increased risk of pulmonary edema

What do contraindications to tocolysis include?

Fetal distress, severe oligohydramnios, fetal demise, intrauterine infection

When are the following tocolytics contraindicated?

Magnesium sulfate:

Myasthenia gravis, use cautiously in patients with compromised renal function

Calcium channel blockers:

Heart failure

Beta adrenergic agonists:

Cardiac disease, uncontrolled diabetes or hyperthyroidism

COX inhibitors:

Bleeding disorders, hepatic dysfunction, GI ulcers, renal dysfuncion

What are some of the fetal side effects of indomethacin?

Premature closure of the **ductus arteriosus** (if used longer than 48 hours)

Oligohydramnios

What type of patient has been shown to benefit from progesterone supplementation in randomized controlled trials?

Patients with a history of spontaneous or idiopathic PTL.

Progesterone injections are administered to asymptomatic patients as weekly injections of 17 α-hydroxyprogesterone caproate beginning in the second trimester and continuing through term.

Prophylactic progesterone injections reduce the rate of PTB by what percent?

15% to 70%

A woman who presents with painless cervical dilation and bulging fetal membranes during the second trimester is consistent with what diagnosis?

Cervical insufficiency, formerly known as cervical incompetence

What sonographic findings are consistent with cervical insufficiency?

Short cervical length, dilated internal cervical os, and funneling of the fetal membranes

How prevalent is cervical insufficiency?

2% of all US pregnancies

What treatment may be offered to patients with cervical insufficiency?

Prophylactic or emergent cerclage, the efficacy of this intervention may be specific to certain subgroups; however, it has not been consistently demonstrated in trials.

What are risk factors for cervical insufficiency?

History of cervical conizarion, multiparity, history of cervical trauma

What is considered a highly specific test for PTL?

Fetal fibronectin (fFN) assay because of a false-positive rate of 3% to 4%. Unfortunately, the sensitivity and positive predictive value (41%) are not as impressive.

What is fetal fibronectin?

Fetal fibronectin is a glycoprotein present in maternal circulation and AF, if present in the cervicovaginal secretions more than 50 ng/mL; it suggests that the cervix is undergoing structural change and the patient may go into labor in the next 2 weeks.

What common interventions have *not* proven to prevent PTL?

Bed rest, home uterine monitoring, prophylactic broad-spectrum antibiotic therapy, abstinence from sex, hydration, long-term or prophylactic tocolytic therapy

Medical Conditions of Pregnancy

ENDOCRINE DISORDERS

Gestational Diabetes Mellitus

What is pregestational diabetes mellitus (GDM) and how is it characterized?

It is a **diagnosis of diabetes mellitus prior to pregnancy.** It occurs in 1% of all pregnancies and includes both Type I diabetes and Type II diabetes.

What is GDM and how is it characterized?

It is **defined as glucose intolerance with onset or first recognition during pregnancy.** More than one half of those patients at risk will end up developing diabetes mellitus later in life.

How may pregnancy predispose some women to GDM?

Placental secretion of anti-insulin and diabetogenic hormones that contribute to the diabetic state include:

Human placental lactogen

Growth hormone

Corticotropin-releasing hormone

Prolactin

Progesterone

Tumor necrosis factor-α

Leptin

What are several risk factors for the development of GDM?

Age more than 25 years

Obesity (BMI > 30 in the nonpregnant state)

Prior history of GDM

Family history of diabetes (especially in a first-degree relative)

Previous stillbirth or child with a congenital malformation

Birth of a prior macrosomic infant

Polycystic ovary syndrome

In addition to diabetic retinopathy, nephropathy, and neuropathy, what are several obstetric-related maternal complications associated with GDM?

Preeclampsia

First trimester abortions and stillbirths

Asymptomatic bacteriuria

Higher incidence of cesarean section, vacuum, and forceps deliveries

What are several adverse neonatal outcomes associated with hyperglycemia?

Congenital malformations

Macrosomia (shoulder dystocia)

Intrauterine fetal demise

Hypoglycemia

Hyperbilirubinemia

Higher incidence of neonatal respiratory distress syndrome (delay in the fetal lung maturity)

Preterm birth

Intrauterine growth restriction

Polyhydramnios

Why are neonates of diabetic mothers at risk of hypoglycemia?

In utero, glucose crosses the placenta. In response, the fetus develops a hyperinsulinemic state. Immediately after delivery, it is not exposed to such high blood sugars and these high insulin levels result in hypoglycemia.

With what other endocrine disorders is Type I diabetes mellitus associated?

There is a 5% to 8% incidence of hypothyroid disease as well as approximately 25% risk of developing postpartum thyroid dysfunction

What congenital malformations are associated with pregestational diabetes mellitus?	Heart defects (**transposition of the great vessels**, ventricular septal defect [VSD], atrial septal defect [ASD]) **Neural tube defects** **Caudal regression** (pathognomonic, but very rare) Situs inversus Anal/rectal atresia Renal anomalies (duplex ureter)
How does hyperglycemia cause congenital malformations?	Hyperglycemia is teratogenic during the period of organogenesis (first 8 weeks of pregnancy); therefore, preconceptual glucose control and monitoring is crucial for normal development. Glycosylated hemoglobin (HbA_{1c}) levels correlate directly with the frequency of congenital anomalies as shown in Table 9.2.

Table 9.2 HbA1c and Fetal Malformations

HbA_{1c} Levels (%)	Frequency of Anomalies (%)
5-6	2-3
8.9-9.9	8.1
10	20-25

How does GDM cause fetal macrosomia?	Maternal glucose crosses the placenta. In response, the fetus produces more insulin. Insulin is a potent growth hormone and leads to increased somatic growth, macrosomia, central fat deposition, and enlargement of internal organs.

Which women should be screened for gestational diabetes?

Though controversial, **universal screening of all pregnant women is recommended by ACOG.** However, low-risk women may be exempt from screening. These women should have all of the following characteristics:

Age less than 25 years

Normal BMI before pregnancy

No first-degree relative with diabetes mellitus

No history of abnormal glucose testing

No history of poor obstetric outcome

Member of an ethnic group with a low prevalence of GDM (ie, patient is *not* Hispanic, African, Native American, South or East Asian, Pacific Islander)

When should screening be performed?

If there is a high suspicion of GDM, screening should be done at the first antenatal visit; otherwise, screening can be performed at 24 to 28 weeks of gestation. (If a high-risk patient has a negative screening test at the first antenatal visit, she should be rescreened at 24-28 weeks).

What screening test is recommended for GDM?

A **50 g oral glucose challenge test (GCT)** is given. Plasma or serum glucose level is measured 1 hour later without regard to the time of the prior meal. A value **140 mg/dL** is the most commonly used parameter and is considered abnormal.

If the screening test is positive, what are the next recommended tests for diagnosing gestational diabetes?

A **100 g, 3-hour oral glucose tolerance test (GTT)** performed after an overnight fast. GDM is present if a diagnosis of **two or more** of the following are met or exceeded (see Table 9.3).

Table 9.3 Three-hour Glucose Tolerance Test

Status	Plasma or Serum Glucose Level (mg/dL)	Plasma or Serum Glucose Level (mmol/L)
Fasting	95-105	5.3
1 hour	180	10.0
2 hours	155-165	8.6
3 hours	140	7.8

What is the White Classification of Diabetes?

The White Classification System initially attempted to predict perinatal risk according to the age of onset of diabetes, duration of diabetes, and type of end-organ damage. The American College of Obstetricians and Gynecologists has recommended a single diabetes classification system as shown in Tables 9.4 and 9.5.

Table 9.4 White Classification

Class	Onset	Fasting Plasma Glucose	2-Hour Postprandial Glucose	Therapy
A$_1$	Gestational	< 105 mg/dL	< 120 mg/dL	Diet
A$_2$	Gestational	> 105 mg/dL	> 120 mg/dL	Insulin

Table 9.5 White Classification of Pre-existing Diabetes

Class	Age of Onset (yr)	Duration (yr)	Vascular Disease	Therapy
B	> 20	< 10	None	Insulin
C	10-19	10-19	None	Insulin
D	< 10	≥ 20	Benign retinopathy	Insulin
EF	Any	Any	Neph (**NEF**) ropathy	Insulin
R	Any	Any	Proliferative retinopathy	Insulin
H	Any	Any	Heart disease	Insulin
RT	Any	Any	Renal transplant	Insulin

What are the major components of antenatal maternal care for pregestational diabetics?

Preconceptual counseling for achievement of normal hemoglobin A_{1c} levels before pregnancy

Baseline renal function with serum creatine level and a 24-hour urine collection analysis

Assessment of asymptomatic bacteriuria by urine culture

Thyrotropin and free thyroxine

Comprehensive eye examination by an ophthalmologist

What antepartum fetal assessment is appropriate in women with pregestational or gestational diabetes?

1. An ultrasound assessment for fetal growth and anatomy and a fetal echocardiogram at around 18 to 20 weeks
2. Repeat growth ultrasound(s) in the third trimester
3. Testing for fetal malformations (nuchal translucency and serum screening for neural tube defects and/or second trimester triple or quadruple screening)
4. Starting at 32 weeks, weekly NST/AFIs should be performed increasing to two times a week beginning at 36 weeks

How common is diabetic ketoacidosis (DKA) in women with pregnancy-related diabetes and what is the typical presentation?

It is found in 5% to 10% of all pregnancies complicated with pregestational diabetes mellitus. It is more common in Type I pregestational diabetes mellitus.

The typical presentation includes abdominal pain, nausea and vomiting, altered sensorium, low arterial pH, low serum bicarbonate, serum and urine ketones, and increased anion gap. Recurrent late decelerations may be seen on fetal heart monitoring (improves when maternal ketoacidosis is corrected) and are signs of fetal distress (academia) (see Fig. 9.4).

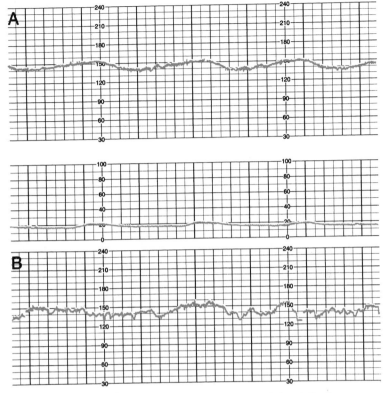

Figure 9.4 Antepartum fetal heart rate tracings at 28 weeks' gestation in woman with diabetic ketoacidosis. A. During maternal and fetal acidemia B. Return of normal accelerations. *(Reproduced, with permission, from Cunnigham FG et al.* Williams Obstetrics, *22nd ed. New York: McGraw-Hill, 2005:378.)*

How is DKA managed in the pregnant woman?	The same as in nonpregnant women. Aggressive hydration and IV insulin is mandatory. Glucose, potassium, and bicarbonate levels should be monitored closely and replenished appropriately.
When is cesarean delivery indicated for women with gestational diabetes?	If the expected fetal weight is greater than 4500 g, to prevent birth trauma from shoulder dystocia.

Thyroid in Pregnancy

What are the two major changes in thyroid function during pregnancy?	1. An increase in serum thyroxine-binding globulin (TBG) concentrations. 2. Stimulation of the thyrotropin (TSH) receptor.

| What two hormones have thyroid-stimulating activity? | 1. Estrogen (increases serum TBG concentration)
2. hCG |
| How do thyroid function test results change in normal pregnancy, and in hyperthyroid and hypothyroid states? | See Table 9.6 |

Table 9.6 TFTs in thyroid disease

Maternal Status	TSH	FT$_4$	TT$_4$	TT$_3$	RT$_3$U
Normal	NC	NC	↑	↑	↓
Hyperthyroid	↓	↑	↑	↑ or NC	↑
Hypothyroid	↑	↓	↓	↓ or NC	↓

TSH: thyroid stimulating hormone; FT4: free thyroxine; FTI: free thyroxine index; TT4: total thyroxine; TT3: total triiodothyronine; RT3U: resin T3 uptake; NC: no change

| Which of the thyroid-related hormones does *not* cross the placenta? | TSH |
| Which thyroid hormones or thyroid-related molecules can cross the placenta? | Thyroid hormone, T$_3$, T$_4$, TRH, iodine, TSH receptor immunoglobulins |

Hyperthyroidism

| What are the clinical manifestations of hyperthyroidism? | Nervousness, tachycardia, palpitations, hypertension, weight loss, tremors, flushing, frequent bowel movements, excessive sweating, and insomnia |
| What are several pregnancy-related complications associated with poorly controlled hyperthyroidism? | Spontaneous abortion or stillbirth
Preeclampsia
Preterm delivery
Placental abruption
Cardiac arrhythmias
Congestive heart failure
Low birth weight
Thyroid storm
Hyperemesis gravidarum |

What are several etiologies of hyperthyroidism?	**Graves' disease (90%)** Toxic nodular goiters Iatrogenic Iodine induced Subacute thyroiditis hCG-mediated
What three syndromes are associated with hCG-mediated hyperthyroidism?	See Table 9.7

Table 9.7 Syndromes Associated with Thyroid Dysfunction in Pregnancy

Syndrome	Description	Treatment
Transient subclinical hyperthyroidism	It occurs in 10% to 20% of normal pregnant women during the period of highest serum hCG concentrations.	None needed
Hyperemesis gravidarum	It is a syndrome that is characterized by nausea and vomiting with weight loss of more than 5% during early pregnancy. Women may have either subclinical or mild overt hyperthyroidism.	IV fluids, anti-emetics, thiamine, and treatment of hyperthyroidism
Trophoblastic hyperthyroidism	It occurs in about 60% of women with a hydatidiform mole or choriocarcinoma.	Removal of the mole or therapy directed against the choriocarcinoma (IV/IM methotrexate + repeat β-hCG until it trends to 0)

What additional clinical manifestations suggest Graves' disease?	Exophthalmos; goiter; pretibial myxedema
How is hyperthyroidism diagnosed?	Elevated levels of serum FT_4 and low serum TSH (< 0.01 mU/L)

What is the management and treatment for pregnant women with hyperthyroidism?

The goal of treatment is to maintain the mother's serum free T_4 concentration in the high-normal range for nonpregnant women using the lowest drug dose.

1. **Radioiodine is absolutely contraindicated.**
2. **Iodine is contraindicated as it can cause fetal goiter.**
3. Propylthiouracil (PTU) 50 mg bid or less is recommended for treatment of moderate to severe hyperthyroidism-complicating pregnancy. If treatment fails, consider methimazole.
4. Beta blockers may be given to ameliorate the symptoms of moderate to severe hyperthyroidism in pregnant women (low-dose atenolol may be appropriate to begin).
5. Thyroidectomy during pregnancy may be necessary in women who cannot tolerate thionamides because of allergy or agranulocytosis (preferably during second trimester).

What percent of neonates born to women with Graves' disease have hyperthyroidism because of transplacental transfer of TSH receptor-stimulating antibodies?

1% to 5%

What are the clinical manifestations of fetal hyperthyroidism?

Fetal tachycardia (> 160 beats/min)

Fetal goiter

Advanced bone age

Poor growth

Craniosynostosis

Cardiac failure

Fetal hydrops

Though rare, what are several manifestations of fetal and neonatal thyrotoxicosis?

Fetal tachycardia and intrauterine growth restriction

What is a thyroid storm?

It is an acute, life-threatening medical emergency characterized by a high metabolic state in patients with thyrotoxicosis.

What is a major consequence of thyroid storm?	Maternal heart failure
What are the clinical signs and symptoms of a thyroid storm?	Fever, tachycardia out of proportion to the fever, changed mental status, confusion, nervousness, nausea and vomiting, seizures, diarrhea, and cardiac arrhythmias
	(It can be initiated by infections, stress, surgery, labor, and/or delivery)
How is a thyroid storm treated?	Transfer to the ICU
	PTU
	IV sodium iodine or supersaturated solution of potassium iodide is given after PTU
	Dexamethasone
	Propranolol
	Phenobarbital for restlessness (if needed)
	Supportive measures (O_2, antipyretics, cooling blankets, IV hydration)

Hypothyroidism

What are the clinical manifestations of maternal hypothyroidism?	Fatigue, constipation, intolerance to cold, dry skin, muscle cramps, hair loss, weight gain, myxedema, carpal tunnel syndrome, and prolonged relaxation of deep tendon reflexes
What are the most common etiologies of hypothyroidism in pregnant or postpartum women?	**Hashimoto disease (most common in developed countries)**
	Iron deficiency (worldwide)
	Subacute thyroiditis
	Thyroidectomy
	Radioactive iodine treatment
What other endocrine disease is associated with hypothyroidism?	Type I diabetes mellitus
What are the several pregnancy-related complications associated with hypothyroidism?	Miscarriage
	Preeclampsia
	Preterm delivery
	Low-birth weight
	Placental abruption
	Postpartum hemorrhage

What is the management and treatment for pregnant women with hypothyroidism?	**Levothyroxine.** TSH levels should be checked 4 weeks later. Levothyroxine doses should be adjusted at 4-week intervals until the TSH level is stable.
What is a significant impact of maternal hypothyroidism on the fetus and/or neonate?	Congenital cretinism Mental retardation Intrauterine growth restriction
What are the signs of congenital cretinism?	Growth failure, mental retardation, floppy baby, macroglossia, other neuropsychologic deficits
How common is congenital hypothyroidism in neonates?	1:4000 births and only 5% of neonates are identified by clinical symptoms at birth
What is the common cause of congenital hypothyroidism in neonates?	75% of hypothyroid infants have some form of thyroid agenesis.
What are the clinical manifestations of hypothyroidism in neonates?	Lethargy and slow movement Hoarse cry Feeding problems Constipation Macroglossia Umbilical hernia Large fontanels Hypotonia Dry skin Hypothermia Prolonged jaundice
Which neonates should be screened for hypothyroidism?	Screening of all newborns is now routine in the United States.

Other Thyroid Disorders

How common is postpartum thyroiditis?	It occurs in 5% to 10% of women during the first year of childbirth or pregnancy loss. It is directly related to increasing serum levels of thyroid autoantibodies.

What are the clinical phases and characterstics of postpartum thyroiditis?

Phase 1 is characterized by thyrotoxicosis-like symptoms (small, painless goiter; fatigue; palpitations) between 1 and 4 months after delivery. Some women return back to a euthyroid state, while others go into **Phase 2—the development of transient hypothyroidism or permanent hypothyroidism** (4-8 months postpartum). See Table 9.8.

Table 9.8 Phases and Characteristics of Postpartum Thyroiditis

Clinical Phase	Onset	Incidence (%)	Mechanism	Symptoms	Treatment	Sequelae
Thyroto-xicosis	1-4 months postpar-tum	4	Destruction-induced hormone release	Painless goiter, fatigue, palpita-tions	β-blocker for symp-toms	Return to euthyroid state or develop hypothy-roidism
Hypo-thyroidism	4-8 months postpar-tum	2-5	Thyroid insuffi-ciency	Goiter, fatigue, depres-sion	Thyroxine for 6-12 months	Transient or perma-nent hypothy-roidism

What laboratory results help make the diagnosis of postpartum thyroiditis?

New-onset abnormal values of TSH and T_4 may be present. The presence of antimicrosomal and/or thyroperoxidase—antithyroid peroxidase antibodies confirm the diagnosis.

Postpartum thyroid dysfunction is seen 25% of the time with what other endocrine disorder?

Type I diabetes mellitus

How is the presence of a thyroid nodule or thyroid cancer assessed and managed during pregnancy?

Fine-needle-aspiration biopsy of the nodule should be done. Benign nodules are followed; if required, surgery is best performed in the second trimester.

Thyroid radionuclide scanning is contraindicated.

Other Endocrine Disorders of Pregnancy

What is Sheehan syndrome?

It is partial or complete pituitary insufficiency because of postpartum necrosis of the anterior pituitary gland following severe intrapartum or early postpartum hemorrhage.

What are the characteristic signs and symptoms of Sheehan syndrome?

Failure of lactation, amenorrhea, breast atrophy, loss of pubic and axillary hair, hypothyroidism, and adrenal cortical insufficiency

GASTROINTESTINAL DISORDERS

Acute Fatty Liver of Pregnancy

What is acute fatty liver of pregnancy (AFLP)?

It is a rare complication of pregnancy (1:5000-16,000) characterized by microvesicular fatty infiltration of hepatocytes.

In which trimester does this disease typically appear?

Third trimester

Deficiency of which enzyme has been associated in the pathogenesis of acute fatty liver of pregnancy?

Long-chain 3-hydroxyacyl-CoA dehydrogenase (LCHAD)

What are the common clinical manifestations of this disease?

Nausea and vomiting (most frequent symptom)

Abdominal pain (commonly epigastric)

Malaise

Anorexia

Jaundice

What laboratory findings may be seen in patients with acute fatty liver of pregnancy?

Elevated AST and ALT

Elevated bilirubin

Prolonged prothrombin time

Low fibrinogen

Low platelets

Elevated serum creatinine

Low glucose levels (30% of patients)

What other major disorder with similar laboratory results must be ruled out and how is this condition characterized?	HELLP syndrome. It is characterized by hemolysis, elevated liver enzymes, and low platelets.
What is the gold standard for diagnosis of acute fatty liver of pregnancy?	**Liver biopsy** revealing microvesicular fatty infiltration of hepatocytes. However, this is rarely performed since it is an invasive procedure.
What is the management and treatment?	Maternal stabilization (fluids, blood products, antibiotics) Supportive care (mechanical ventilation, dialysis) Prompt delivery of the fetus
What should newborns of mothers with acute fatty liver of pregnancy be tested for?	Deficiency of LCHAD
What is the rate of recurrence?	It can recur in future pregnancies but the rate is unclear.

Intrahepatic Cholestasis of Pregnancy

What is intrahepatic cholestasis of pregnancy (ICP)?	It is a condition characterized by jaundice and pruritis secondary to the accumulation of bile acids.
In what trimesters does it usually occur?	Onset is more common in the third trimester, but sometimes occurs in the second.
What hormonal factors may be involved in the pathogenesis of ICP?	High concentrations of estrogen and excess progesterone may be risk factors for ICP.
What is the cardinal clinical manifestation of ICP that helps distinguish this disease from other liver conditions?	**Severe pruritis** (especially on the palms and soles of the feet) Jaundice is present 10% of the time; jaundice without pruritis warrants other causes of liver disease

What do laboratory values reveal in patients with ICP?	Increased serum total bile acids (chenodeoxycholic acid, deoxycholic acid, cholic acid)
	Marked elevation of the cholic/chenodeoxycholic acid ratio
	Elevated alkaline phosphatase
	Elevated total and direct bilirubin
	Elevated AST and ALT
	Normal prothrombin time (usually)
What are the main liver conditions that must be ruled out?	Hepatitis (autoimmune and viral)
	Biliary tract disease
	Acute fatty liver of pregnancy
	HELLP syndrome
What is the treatment of ICP?	Ursodeoxycholic acid has been shown to alleviate pruritis and normalize bile acids and improve liver function test results.
	Early delivery (37 weeks) to reduce risk of IUFD
Can oral contraceptives that contain estrogen be given postpartum?	Yes. Oral contraceptives containing low-dose estrogen can be given after normalization of liver function tests. Women should be advised of a potential recurrence of pruritis.
What are several complications of ICP?	Fetal death
	Spontaneous preterm birth
	Postpartum hemorrhage
	Neonatal respiratory syndrome
	Meconium-stained amniotic fluid
What is the rate of recurrence?	It recurs 60% to 70% in future pregnancies, but may be milder in severity

Hyperemesis Gravidarum

What is hyperemesis gravidarum?	It is persistent vomiting typically in the first trimester that is severe enough to cause weight loss, dehydration, acidosis from starvation, alkalosis from vomiting, and hypokalemia.

What hormones may be associated with hyperemesis?

It may be related to high or rapidly rising levels of serum **estrogen or hCG,** or both.

What is the association between hyperthyroidism and hyperemesis gravidarum?

Although there are biochemical signs of hyperthyroidism (elevated thyroxine levels), this is most likely the effect of hCG on the TSH receptor (seen in 60%-70% of patients).

How is hyperemesis gravidarum treated?

First-line pharmacotherapy consists of vitamin B_6.

Antiemetics and IV fluids should be given until the vomiting is controlled.

What are several life-threatening complications of hyperemesis gravidarum?

Mallory-Weiss tears

Esophageal rupture

Pneumothoraces

Pneumomediastinum

What two vitamin deficiencies are a result of prolonged vomiting and can have severe consequences?

1. Vitamin B_1 (thiamine) deficiency can cause Wernicke encephalopathy
2. Vitamin K deficiency can cause coagulopathy with epistaxis.

What is the effect of hyperemesis gravidarum on the fetus?

IUGR and fetal death may occur in the setting of persistent vomiting and maternal weight loss.

What should mothers be advised regarding recurrence of hyperemesis gravidarum?

It often recurs in subsequent pregnancies.

RENAL AND URINARY TRACT DISORDERS

Urinary Tract Infections

Why do we screen for asymptomatic bacteriuria in pregnancy?

Both hormonal and mechanical changes predispose the pregnant woman with asymptomatic bacteriuria to develop acute pyelonephritis, which is associated with preterm birth and perinatal death. Pyelonephritis in pregnancy will lead to septicemia in 10% to 20% and ARDS in 2% of cases.

How prevalent is asymptomatic bacteriuria in pregnancy?	4% to 7% of pregnant patients. If left untreated, up to 40% of cases will progress to pyelonephritis.
How is this condition detected?	Screening with a urine culture is recommended at the first prenatal visit.
How is asymptomatic bacteriuria treated?	Any FDA category B drug such as **cephalosporins, nitrofurantoin, or trimethoprim-sulfamethoxazole** can be used. Quinolones (FDA category C) are generally not used during pregnancy. Seven-day courses are recommended, along with a follow-up culture to document sterile urine.
	Persistent bacteriuria should be treated based on sensitivities. Suppressive antibiotics (most commonly nitrofurantoin) should then be considered in these patients. See Table 9.9.

Table 9.9 Antimicrobial Used for Treatment of Pregnant Women with Asymptomatic Bacteriuria

7-Day Course (Recommended)
Amoxicillin, 3 g
Ampicillin, 2 g
Cephalosporin, 2 g
Nitrofurantoin, 200 mg
Trimethoprim-sulfamethoxazole, 320/1600 mg

How is symptomatic cystitis treated in pregnancy?	Treatment and follow-up are similar to asymptomatic bacteriuria. Acute pyelonephritis should be treated with IV antibiotics and hospitalization. Suppressive antibiotics should be given following treatment to any pregnant patient treated for acute pyelonephritis.

NEUROLOGIC DISORDERS

Epilepsy and Seizure Disorders

What are the two major pregnancy-related threats to women with epilepsy?

1. Increase in seizure frequency
2. Increased risk of congenital malformations in the fetus

Increased seizure frequency is associated with subtherapeutic anticonvulsant levels and/or a lower seizure threshold. What pregnancy related changes contribute to this?

Pregnancy-related changes such as nausea and vomiting, decreased gastrointestinal motility, increased intravascular volume, increased drug metabolism from induction of hepatic and placental enzymes, antacid use (reduces drug absorption because of abnormal protein binding), and increased glomerular filtration rate decrease anticonvulsant concentrations.

Decreased seizure threshold can be affected by sleep deprivation, and hyperventilation and pain during labor.

What are the maternal and fetal side effects for the following traditional anticonvulsant medications?

See Table 9.10

What is the association between anticonvulsants and folic acid deficiency?

All anticonvulsants interfere with folic acid metabolism and patients on anticonvulsants may become folic acid deficient. Folic acid supplementation (4 mg/d) should be begun before pregnancy if possible.

What are the recommendations regarding management and therapy with anticonvulsants?

Women with epilepsy should have preconception counseling regarding the optimal anticonvulsant during pregnancy, a switch to the least teratogenic drug and the least number of medications prescribed, and the lowest dose needed.

Blood levels of anticonvulsants should be measured every trimester and prior to delivery to maintain a therapeutic range.

Patients should be screened for neural tube defects and other fetal anomalies associated with anticonvulsants.

Table 9.10 Anticonvulsants

Anticonvulsant	Maternal Side Effects	Fetal Side Effects
Phenytoin	Nystagmus, ataxia, hirsutism, gingival hyperplasia, megaloblastic anemia	**Fetal hydantoin syndrome:** craniofacial anomalies (upturned nose, mild midfacial hypoplasia, thin philtrum, facial clefts), fingernail hypoplasia, growth deficiency, developmental delay, cardiac defects
Carbamazepine	Drowsiness, leukopenia, ataxia, mild hepatotoxicity	Fetal hydantoin syndrome, spina bifida, fingernail hypoplasia, IUGR
Valproate	Ataxia, drowsiness, alopecia, hepatotoxicity, thrombocytopenia	Neural-tube defects, heart and kidney malformations, hypospadia, polydactyly
Phenobarbital	Drowsiness, ataxia	Clefts, cardiac anomalies, urinary tract malformations
Primidone	Drowsiness, ataxia, nausea	Possible teratogenesis, coagulopathy, neonatal depression

What is the effect of anticonvulsants on vitamin K levels?

Many of the anticonvulsants, particularly phenytoin, induce a deficiency of vitamin K-dependent clotting factors (II, VI, IX, X). This places the patient and her fetus at risk for hemorrhage. The patient should receive vitamin K supplementation from week 36 until delivery, and the newborn should also receive an IM injection of vitamin K after delivery.

HEMATOLOGIC DISORDERS

Thromboembolism

How does pregnancy increase the risk for venous thromboembolism?

Increased venous capacity, relaxation of vascular smooth muscle, and compression of the pelvic veins by the gravid uterus cause venous stasis. Increased risk for endothelial damage occurs during delivery, especially during cesarean delivery. Lastly, estrogen stimulation of coagulation factors and a decrease in fibrinolytic activity favors coagulation during pregnancy.

What diagnostic test should be ordered?

In order to rule out DVT, a compression Doppler **ultrasound** of the affected extremity should be performed.

Thrombosis of the superficial veins of the saphenous system can occur during pregnancy. What are the clinical manifestations of patients with superficial thrombophlebitis?

Tenderness, pain, or erythema along the vein

What is the treatment for superficial thrombophlebitis?

Treatment consists of compression stockings, ambulation, leg elevation, and analgesics

Does deep venous thrombosis (DVT) commonly occur in the left or right lower extremity?

Greater than 80% of DVTs occurs in the **left lower extremity.** This is because of compression of the left iliac vein by the right iliac vein as it branches off the aorta.

What are the clinical features of DVTs?

Although the presentation is variable, signs include **lower extremity tenderness, erythema, swelling, and a palpable cord.** Homan sign may be present (pain on passive dorsiflexion of the foot).

What is the treatment for DVT that occurs during pregnancy?

Anticoagulation with unfractionated or low-molecular weight heparin for the remainder of the pregnancy. This can be continued postpartum or warfarin can be started postpartum for at least 6 weeks.

Why is Coumadin contraindicated during pregnancy?

Fetal warfarin syndrome (FWS)—characterized by hemorrhage and embryopathy, which includes ventral midline dysplasia, nasal hypoplasia, CNS abnormalities, cardiac and renal anomalies

What is a major complication of DVTs?

If untreated, 24% of DVTs will result in **pulmonary embolus**

What are the clinical manifestations of pulmonary embolism (PE)?

Dyspnea, pleuritic chest pain, cough, syncope, hemoptysis, tachypnea, and tachycardia

How is a pulmonary embolism evaluated and diagnosed in the pregnant woman?

It usually consists of an ABG, EKG, and a spiral CT scan or V/Q scan.

What is the treatment of pulmonary embolism?

Anticoagulation with low molecular weight heparin for at least 4 to 6 months

What is septic pelvic thrombophlebitis?

It is thrombosis in the veins of the pelvis because of infection. About 90% of cases occur after a cesarean delivery. It is a diagnosis of exclusion for postpartum fever.

When should septic pelvic thrombophlebitis be suspected?

Continuous and wide-swinging fevers in the puerperium and which do not respond to antibiotics

How is it diagnosed and treated?

CT or MRI should be considered for diagnosis. Treatment includes a combination of antibiotics and heparin.

What are the most significant complications of septic pelvic thrombophlebitis?

Septic pulmonary emboli

Extension of the venous clot in the pelvis

Renal vein thrombosis

Ureteral obstruction

Death

Thrombophilias

What are the most common inherited thrombophilias?	Factor V Leiden mutation Antithrombin deficiency Prothrombin G20210 mutation Protein C deficiency Protein S deficiency Hyperhomocysteinemia
What is antiphospholipid syndrome?	It is an acquired thrombophilia characterized by the presence of certain clinical historical features (including thromboembolism) and the presence of specified levels of circulating antiphospholipid antibodies.
How is antiphospholipid syndrome diagnosed?	The presence of a clinical thrombotic event combined with positive antiphospholipid antibodies (identified twice at least 6 weeks apart)
What are the antiphospholipid antibodies?	Lupus anticoagulant Anticardiolipin antibodies Beta 2 glycoprotein
What are the most common medical problems associated with antiphospholipid syndrome?	Unexplained venous or arterial thromboses Three consecutive early miscarriages Fetal loss after 10 weeks Preterm delivery before 34 weeks due to severe preeclampsia or placental insufficiency
What are several obstetrical complications associated with antiphospholipid syndrome?	Recurrent spontaneous abortions (most common) Preeclampsia and eclampsia Intrauterine growth restriction Uteroplacental insufficiency Preterm delivery Placental abruption Infertility Intrauterine fetal demise
How is pregnancy managed in a patient with antiphospholipid antibody syndrome?	With anticoagulation antepartum continuing for 6 weeks postpartum

Anemias and Hemoglobinopathies

What is physiologic anemia of pregnancy?

During the course of pregnancy, there is an expansion in plasma volume greater than that of the RBC mass. This reflects in a decrease in hematocrit during pregnancy; however, it is not a true anemia.

How is true anemia in pregnancy defined?

It is generally defined as an Hct less than 30% or a hemoglobin less than 10 g/dL

What are the effects of maternal anemia on pregnancy?

Preterm birth

Fetal growth restriction

What are the two most common causes of anemia during pregnancy?

1. **Iron deficiency anemia**
2. Anemia from acute blood loss

What red cell indices, laboratory results, and characteristics on a peripheral blood smear indicate an iron deficiency anemia?

Mean cell volume (MCV) less than 80 f/L.

Mean corpuscular hemoglobin concentration (MCHC) less than 30%

Serum iron is decreased (< 50 mg/dL).

Total iron-binding capacity (TIBC) is increased.

Serum ferritin is decreased (a level < 15 ug/L is confirmatory of iron deficiency anemia).

Blood smear findings include small, pale erythrocytes (microcytic and hypochromic).

What is the treatment of iron deficiency anemia?

Treatment is iron therapy consisting of ferrous sulfate 325 mg bid. If anemia is severe, IV iron may be used.

What is the most common cause of macrocytic anemia in pregnancy? What red cell indices, laboratory results, and characteristics on a peripheral blood smear indicate this anemia?

Folate acid deficiency

Red cell indices reveal an MCV greater than 100 f/L, folate levels less than 4 ng/mL, and erythrocyte folate activity less than 20 ng/mL.

A smear of peripheral blood demonstrates macrocytes, hypersegmentation of neutrophils, and peripheral nucleated erythrocytes.

What is the recommended folate level in pregnant women and what is the treatment for folate deficiency anemia?

A recommended level of folate during pregnancy is 400 ug/d and treatment is 1 mg of folic acid PO once daily.

What are examples of hereditary hemolytic anemias?

Hereditary spherocytosis, glucose 6-phosphate dehydrogenase deficiency (G6PD), pyruvate-kinase deficiency

What are the most common hemoglobinopathies?

Sickle-cell anemia (SS disease), sickle-cell hemoglobin C disease (SC disease), sickle-cell α-thalassemia disease, β-thalassemia, and α_β-thalassemia

What other infections are patients with sickle-cell hemoglobinopathies at an increased risk for?

Urinary tract infections. Urine cultures should be sent every trimester

What is a significant pulmonary complication in patients with sickle-cell disease?

Acute chest syndrome. It is characterized by pleuritic chest pain, fever, cough, lung infiltrates, and hypoxia which all lead to hypoxemia and acidosis.

Which thalassemia is associated with fetal hydrops, intrauterine death, and preeclampsia?

Hb Bart (α-thalassemia major, absence of both α-globin chains)

PULMONARY DISORDERS

Asthma

What percentage of women experience worsening of their asthma during pregnancy?

40%

Another 40% of women experience no change and 20% of report improvement

What are fetal complications of an acute exacerbation of asthma?

Intrauterine growth restriction, low birth weight, preterm birth, neonatal hypoxia, and increased overall perinatal mortality

How is acute asthma managed in a pregnant woman?

It is similar to that of a nonpregnant woman.

IV fluids and supplemental O_2 (keep O_2 saturation > 95%).

β-agonists and high-dose steroids (IV prednisone 40-60 mg q6h).

Continuous pulse oximetry and electronic fetal monitoring.

Which vaccine is recommended for all pregnant women, especially those with asthma?	Influenza vaccination
Which medications should be avoided in pregnant asthmatics during labor and delivery?	Hemabate (prostagladin $F_{2\alpha}$) can cause bronchospasm

Aspiration Pneumonitis

Why are pregnant women at risk for aspiration of gastric contents?	Elevated intra-abdominal pressure, decreased gastroesophageal sphincter tone, delayed gastric emptying, and diminished laryngeal reflexes during pregnancy increases the risk of aspiration
How common are maternal deaths related to aspiration?	It accounts for 30% to 50% of maternal deaths related to anesthetic complications.
What are symptoms and signs of aspiration?	Dyspnea, bronchospasm, tachycardia, cyanosis, hypoxia, hypercapnea, and acidemia
What restrictions are given to women in labor to prevent aspiration?	Women are restricted to clear liquids only while in labor.

CARDIOVASCULAR DISORDERS

Which heart diseases are associated with the highest maternal morbidity during pregnancy?	Primary pulmonary hypertension Uncorrected tetrology of Fallot Marfan syndrome Eisenmenger syndrome (see Table 9.11)
What are the signs and symptoms indicative of significant cardiovascular disease?	See Table 9.12
What are the potential risks to the fetus of patients with functionally significant cardiac disease?	They are at risk for low-birth weight and prematurity. Congenital heart disease in the fetus is more likely to occur in patients with congenital heart disease (1%-5%)

Table 9.11 New York Heart Association Functional Classification of Heart Disease

Class	Description
Class I	No signs or symptoms of cardiac decompensation
Class II	No symptoms at rest; minor limitation with mild to moderate activity
Class III	No symptoms at rest; marked limitation with less than ordinary activity
Class IV	Symptoms at rest; increased discomfort with any physical activity

Table 9.12 Signs and Symptoms Indicative of Significant Cardiovascular Disease

Symptoms	Progressively worsening shortness of breath
	Cough with frothy pink sputum
	Paroxysmal nocturnal dyspnea
	Chest pain with exertion
	Syncope preceded by palpitations or exertion
	Hemoptysis
Physical examination	Abnormal venous pulsations
	Rarely audible S_1
	Single S_2 or paradoxically split S_2
	Loud systolic murmurs, any diastolic murmur
	Ejection clicks, late systolic clicks, opening snaps
	Friction rub
	Sustained right or left ventricular heave
	Cyanosis or clubbing
Electrocardiogram	Significant arrhythmias
	Heart blocks
Chest radiograph	Cardiomegaly
	Pulmonary edema

Reprinted, with permission, from DeCherney AH et al. *Current Obstetrics & Gynecologic Diagnosis Treatment*, 10th ed. New York: McGraw-Hill, 2007:362.

For the following heart diseases, what are their pregnancy-related complications, associated signs and symptoms, and treatment modalities?

See Table 9.13

Describe the classic patient at increased risk for peripartum cardiomyopathy:

A black, multiparous woman who is over the age of 30, and who has had a multifetal gestation in the past and/or preeclampsia

Which cardiac medications are considered safe during pregnancy? Which are contraindicated during pregnancy?

Acceptable cardiac medications: digoxin, loop diuretics, hydralazine, β-adrenergic blockers, calcium-channel blockers

Contraindicated: nitrates, angiotensin-converting enzyme inhibitors, and angiotensin II receptor blockers

ACUTE ABDOMEN AND ABDOMINAL TRAUMA

List the differential diagnoses for the pregnant woman who presents with acute lower abdominal pain:

Gynecologic etiologies: ruptured corpus luteum cyst; adnexal torsion; ectopic pregnancy; abruptio placentae; early labor; salpingitis

Nongynecologic etiologies: pyelonephritis; cholecystitis; diverticulitis

What is the most consistent clinical symptom encountered in pregnant women with appendicitis?

In pregnancy, the appendix is commonly upwardly displaced. Vague pain on the right side of the abdomen is the most consistent clinical symptom of acute appendicitis in the pregnant woman, and there should be a high index of suspicion for appendicitis with any abdominal pain.

What is the first-line imaging modality in pregnant women with suspected appendicitis?

MRI or CT

Ultrasound is less accurate and can lead to a delay in the diagnosis of appendicitis.

What are potential consequences of a ruptured appendix?

Preterm labor, maternal and fetal sepsis, which may lead to fetal neurologic injury or spontaneous abortion/fetal demise

Table 9.13 Common Heart Diseases Occuring During Pregnancy

Heart Disease	Signs/Symptoms during Decompensation	Complications	Treatment	Comment
Mitral regurgitation	Chest pain, palpitations, tachycardia, anxiety, late systolic murmur with a late systolic click	Generally, pregnancy is well-tolerated and unaffected	β-Blockers (propranol) may aid in control of associated symptoms	May occur in as many as 5% of pregnancies
Mitral stenosis	Dyspnea on exertion and at rest, hemoptysis, loud S1, an opening snap, low diastolic rumble at the apex, right ventricular lift	Pulmonary hypertension, right heart failure, hemoptysis, low cardiac output, atrial fibrillation, CHF during labor	Digitalis, quinidine, β-adrenergic blocking agents, anticoagulation with heparin. Severe mitral stenosis may warrant mitral valvotomy, mitral valve replacement, or balloon valvuloplasty	Most common valvular lesion found in pregnancy. Mitral stenosis with a-fibrillation has a high likelihood of congestive failure
Rheumatic heart disease	Dependent on the affected valve	Patients are at high risk for thromboembolic disease, SBE, cardiac failure, and pulmonary edema; fetal loss is also more common	Corrective surgical procedures, such as balloon valvuloplasty, surgical commissurotomy, and valve replacement	90% of rheumatic heart disease patients have mitral stenosis

(Continued)

Table 9.13 Common Heart Diseases Occuring During Pregnancy (*Continued*)

Heart Disease	Signs/Symptoms during Decompensation	Complications	Treatment	Comment
Peripartum cardiomyopathy	Dyspnea; other frequent symptoms include cough, orthopnea, paroxysmal nocturnal dyspnea, and hemoptysis	Heart failure and death are potential complications	Combination of digoxin, diuretics and sodium, β-blockers, and after-load reducers. Anticoagulants, such as heparin should be considered	Usually affects women in late pregnancy (> 36 weeks) or early puerperium (in first 5 months)
Marfan syndrome	Dyspnea, chest pain, aortic diastolic murmur, and midsystolic clink	Aortic aneurysm and possible rupture	Surgical intervention	25%–50% of maternal mortality and 50% chance that offspring will inherit the disease

How does pregnancy predispose to gallstone formation?	Increased estrogens cause an increase in cholesterol saturation
	Biliary stasis
	Decreased gallbladder contraction
What percentage of pregnancies is complicated by trauma? What types of trauma are the most common?	7%
	Motor vehicle accidents (40%)
	Falls (30%)
	Direct assaults (20%)
What is the most common nonobstetric cause of maternal death during pregnancy?	Automobile accidents
What is the most common cause of fetal death?	Death to the mother
What is the second most common cause of fetal death?	Abruptio placentae
What is the management of pregnant women who experienced abdominal trauma?	Admit for observation
	Monitor for contractions
	Fetal well-being should be verified (nonstress test, BPP, FHR monitor).
	Kleihauer-Betke test to assess fetomaternal hemorrhage.
	For the woman who is Rh negative, administration of anti-D immunoglobulin (RhoGAM) should be considered.

Obstetric Infections

TORCH INFECTIONS

Introduction

What are the TORCH infections?

A group of nonbacterial perinatal infections that lead to significant neonatal morbidity and mortality.

T: **Toxoplasma gondii**

O: **Other** (such as syphilis, VZV, HIV, hepatitis, parvovirus B19)

R: **Rubella**

C: **Cytomegalovirus**

H: **Herpes simplex virus**

How does the fetus become infected with the TORCH diseases?

Usually through **transplacental migration of the infection;** however, infection can also occur via ascending chorioamnionitis, maternal exposure intrapartum, or nosocomial neonatal exposure

What modalities can be used to diagnose these infections?

Direct isolation of the pathogen via amniocentesis with culture or PCR of amniotic fluid

Indirect tests—ultrasound for fetal manifestations, maternal antibody titers (IgM, IgG), or testing of fetal blood for IgM via cordocentesis

What is the difference between IgG and IgM?

IgG: rises slowly and often persists for long periods of time. A marker for **overall exposure** to a disease. Crosses the placenta (starting at 16 weeks) to provide passive immunity.

IgM: rises acutely and disappears from the circulation relatively soon after acute infection. A marker for **recent infection.** Cannot cross the placenta. Synthesized by the fetus to provide primary immunity starting at 9-15 weeks.

Toxoplasmosis

What is toxoplasmosis?	Infection with the **protozoa** *T. gondii* that causes an asymptomatic infection in adults but congenital disease if the primary infection occurs during pregnancy
What is the incidence of toxoplasmosis?	0.01% to 0.1% in the United States
What is the life cycle of *T. gondii*?	The domestic cat is the host and it passes the eggs in its feces. Humans can become infected by exposure to the **cat feces**, which can occur with **gardening** or **handling a cat's litter box.** Alternatively, many animals consume the eggs which are found in soil. Humans can become infected by handling or eating the raw or **undercooked meat** of infected animals.
What is the chance of fetal infection if primary infection occurs during pregnancy?	Approximately 33%
What is the difference between first and third trimester infection?	**First trimester: low (15%) congenital infection rate**. Most of those infected have **severe symptoms** and 5% result in fetal demise. **Third trimester: high (65%) congenital infection rate.** Most infections are **mild.**
What are the symptoms of maternal toxoplasmosis?	Usually none; however, many patients report a syndrome of fevers, fatigue, headache, muscle pains, and lymphadenopathy after exposure
What is the classic triad of congenital toxoplasmosis?	**Chorioretinitis, hydrocephalus,** and **intracranial calcifications**

What are other possible clinical manifestations of toxoplasmosis?

Most infants are asymptomatic at birth. However, if signs are present at birth, they can include:

Low birth weight

Fever

Maculopapular rash

Hepatosplenomegaly

Microcephaly

Seizures

Jaundice

Thrombocytopenia

Generalized lymphadenopathy

What abnormalities can develop after birth in an infected and untreated infant?

Chorioretinitis

Mental retardation

Deafness

Seizures

Spasticity

Is toxoplasmosis screening routinely recommended for pregnant women?

No

What are the options for prenatal diagnosis of toxoplasmosis?

Serology of maternal blood (high IgM titers suggest recent infection)

PCR of amniotic fluid

How is congenital toxoplasmosis prevented?

If suspicion is high for congenital infection, **spiramycin** should be given until amniocentesis can be performed for toxoplasmosis PCR. Spiramycin prevents transplacental transmission of the parasite. Spiramycin, however, does not help treat or lessen the effects of congenital toxoplasmosis.

If PCR of amniotic fluid is positive for Toxoplasma, **pyrimethamine** and **sulfadiazine** should be added. **Leucovorin** is given to avoid the bone marrow suppression associated with sulfadiazine.

If PCR of amniotic fluid is negative for Toxoplasma, spiramycin should be continued, and additional agents are not necessary.

What is the prognosis of congenital toxoplasmosis?	Untreated, there is a poor prognosis. Chorioretinitis can eventually lead to blindness. These infants also suffer from seizures and severe psychomotor retardation.

Rubella

What is rubella?	A single-stranded RNA virus of the togavirus family that is also known as **German measles**. It causes a mild, self-limited infection in adults but leads to severe disease if congenitally acquired.
What is the incidence of congenital rubella?	Because of vaccinations, congenital rubella is extremely rare in the United States.
When is congenital rubella infection most likely to cause serious sequelae?	When maternal infection occurs in the first 8 weeks of pregnancy. Infection after the first trimester has almost no risk of developing anomalies in utero.
How is rubella diagnosed in the pregnant state?	By assessing the development of positive rubella antibody titers (which peak 1 to 3 weeks after the development of symptoms, if there are any)
What is the difference between rubella IgM and IgG?	Both increase after exposure; however, **IgM disappears after 1 to 2 months** and so can distinguish acute infection from prior immunization. IgG is present for life.
What are the signs and symptoms of rubella in adults?	Most are asymptomatic, but many women present with a rash.
What are the major clinical manifestations of congenital rubella and how common are each?	**Sensorineural deafness** (50%-75%) **Cataracts** (20%-50%) **Cardiac malformations** (PDA [20%-50%] or pulmonary arterial hypoplasia [20%-50%]) **Neurologic sequelae** (meningoencephalitis, behavior disorders, or MR [10%-20%]) Growth retardation Hepatosplenomegaly Thrombocytopenia Dermatologic manifestations (purpura, known as "blueberry muffin" lesions) Hyperbilirubinemia

How is congenital rubella prevented?	Through vaccination strategies and by testing all pregnant women for immunity
Should the vaccination be given during pregnancy?	**No, it is a live, attenuated virus.**
How is congenital rubella treated?	Supportively—there is no known treatment for rubella.

Cytomegalovirus

What is cytomegalovirus (CMV)?	A DNA herpes virus that is the **most common cause of perinatal infection** in the developed world.
What is the incidence of CMV?	30% to 60% of Americans are seropositive; 1% to 4% of women seroconvert during pregnancy.
What increases the risk of seroconversion?	Immune compromise
How is CMV transmitted?	Via respiratory droplets, saliva, urine, blood, or sexual contact. It is commonly acquired in **daycare centers.**
How is congenital CMV transmitted?	Transplacentally or through breast milk
What is the risk of transplacental transmission for a woman who was previously seropostive? For a woman who is newly infected during pregnancy?	A woman who was **previously seropositive** is at approximately **1%** risk while one **infected during pregnancy** is approximately **40%** at risk.
How is maternal CMV diagnosed?	With antibody titers—a rise in IgG or the development of IgM antibodies predicts primary infection
How is congenital CMV diagnosed prenatally?	**Amniocentesis for PCR or culture** (preferred method)
	Ultrasound (microcephaly, hepatosplenomegaly, intracranial calcifications)
When is congenital CMV infection most likely to cause serious sequelae?	When infection is acquired **early in pregnancy**

What percentage of infected neonates are symptomatic?	5% to 20%
What is the mortality rate associated with congenital CMV infection?	Almost 30%
What are the clinical symptoms of maternal CMV infection?	Most are **asymptomatic**; however, some women have a mononucleosis-like syndrome
What are the possible clinical manifestations of congenital CMV infection?	Most newborns are asymptomatic at birth, but may eventually develop the following anomalies: Hearing loss Impaired speech Chorioretinitis/visual impairment Mental retardation Microcephaly Seizures Paralysis or paresis Death
How can congenital CMV infection be prevented?	Through good hygiene and proper precautions for health care workers; routine prenatal screening is not recommended

Herpes Simplex Virus

What is the incidence of herpes simplex virus (HSV)?	Over 20% of women are seropositive for HSV
What are the two types of HSV?	1. **HSV-1:** causes most nongenital herpes infections 2. **HSV-2:** causes most genital herpes infections (and most neonatal infections)
What is the incidence of congenital HSV?	0.01% to 0.04%
How is congenital HSV transmitted?	Mostly transplacentally; however, it can also be transmitted through ascending infection.

What is the rate of transmission if the mother has primary infection or a recurrent infection?	In the case of **primary infection** the rate of transmission is **50%** while it is **4%** in the case of **recurrent infection**
What can be done to reduce the risk of transmission of HSV if there is an active lesion when the patient is in labor?	**Cesarean delivery** (reduces transmission from 8%-1%)
What can be done to reduce the risk of needing a cesarean section in a patient with known recurrent HSV?	Prophylaxis with acyclovir from 36 weeks until delivery *or* initiated at an episode of preterm labor or PPROM
What complications of pregnancy can occur as a result of HSV infection?	**Preterm labor** or **spontaneous abortion**
What are the three major groups of clinical manifestations of congenital HSV?	1. **Disease localized to the skin, eyes, and mouth (SEM)** 2. **Disease localized to the CNS** 3. **Disseminated disease**
What are other sequelae of congenital HSV?	Temperature instability Respiratory distress Poor feeding Lethargy Hypotension Jaundice DIC Apnea
When do symptoms of congenital HSV develop?	Most newborns are asymptomatic and symptoms begin within the first 4 weeks of life.
What is the mortality rate associated with neonatal HSV infection?	Close to 60%

OTHER VIRAL INFECTIONS

Syphilis

What is syphilis?	Infection with the **spirochete** *Treponema pallidum*

What is the incidence of congenital syphilis?	Less than 40 per 100,000 live births in the United States
How is the fetus infected with syphilis?	**Transplacental transmission,** typically during the second half of pregnancy. Women with primary or secondary syphilis are the most likely to transmit the disease.
What are the possible sequelae of congenital syphilis?	**Fetal manifestations:**

Fetal manifestations:
   Stillbirth
   Spontaneous abortion
   Hydrops fetalis
   Prematurity

Manifestations before 2 years:
   Lesions on palms and soles
   Hepatosplenomegaly
   Jaundice
   Anemia
   Snuffles

Manifestations after 2 years:
   Congenital anomalies
   Active congenital syphilis
   Hutchinson triad

What is the Hutchinson triad?	Hutchinson teeth (blunted upper incisors), interstitial keratitis, and eighth nerve deafness
How is congenital syphilis prevented?	With adequate screening and then treatment (with penicillin) of infected mothers
How is syphilis treated?	With IV or IM **penicillin** G
How should a PCN-allergic pregnant woman be treated for syphilis?	With desensitization, because alternative drugs are teratogenic
How should a woman be followed up after treatment?	Nontreponemal antibody serologic titers should be checked at 1, 3, and 6 months, 1 year, and 2 years after treatment to ensure proper falls of levels. If they do not fall, she should be treated for reinfection.

What is the Jarisch-Herxheimer reaction?	An **acute febrile reaction** precipitated by treatment of syphilis thought to result from the release of large amounts of treponemal lipopolysaccharide (LPS). It may precipitate **preterm labor, contractions,** or **nonreassuring fetal heart tracings** in pregnant women.

Varicella-Zoster Virus

What is varicella-zoster virus?	A double-stranded, linear, DNA herpes virus that causes both chickenpox (varicella) and shingles (zoster)
What is the incidence of VZV in pregnancy?	1 to 5 cases per 10,000 pregnancies (most women are immune secondary to prior infection)
What are the clinical features of varicella in adults?	It includes a **prodrome of fever,** malaise, and myalgia followed 1 to 4 days later by a **vesicular rash.**
What are the complications of varicella infection?	**Bacterial superinfection of vesicles** **Pneumonia** Arthritis Glomerulonephritis Myocarditis Ocular disease Adrenal insufficiency Death CNS abnormalities
Why is varicella in pregnancy a medical emergency?	Because **varicella pneumonia** can develop and it is **very severe** in pregnancy
What is varicella pneumonia?	An infection that develops within a week of the varicella rash that presents as cough, dyspnea, fever, pleuritic chest pain, and/or hemoptysis. It is very severe in pregnant women as it can rapidly progress to respiratory failure.
What is the incidence of varicella pneumonia during pregnancy?	It occurs in 10% to 30% of all VZV cases in pregnancy.

What are the chest x-ray (CXR) findings of varicella pneumonia?	A **diffuse** or **miliary/nodular infiltrative pattern** usually in a **peribronchial distribution** in both lungs
What is the treatment of varicella pneumonia during pregnancy?	Supportive care and acyclovir. All women with VZV require a CXR to rule out varicella pneumonia.
What is the mortality rate associated with varicella in pregnancy?	Untreated, it carries a 40% mortality rate
What are the features of congenital varicella syndrome?	**Chorioretinitis** **Cortical atrophy** **Dermatologic conditions** **Hypoplastic lower limbs** **Hydronephrosis** Clubbed feet Optic atrophy Failure to thrive Cataracts Horner syndrome Microophthalmos Nystagmus Low birth weight Mental retardation Early death
What is the congenital infection rate if the mother has VZV?	Low (2%) in the first or second trimester 25% to 50% if the mother develops a rash 4 days before or 2 days after birth
How can varicella infection during pregnancy be prevented in a patient with a recent exposure?	By giving **VariZIG**, a purified human varicella zoster immune globulin if she is IgG seronegative (not previously immune)
When should VariZIG be given?	To the mother **within 96 hours** after viral exposure if she is IgG seronegative To the neonate if there is exposure within 4 days prior or 2 days after delivery

How should a patient with varicella be managed if she is more than 5 days from delivery?

With close observation (for any signs/sx of varicella pneumonia) and possibly with acyclovir

How should a pregnant woman exposed to zoster be treated?

Reassurance—it is only contagious from direct contact with open lesions.

Parvovirus B19

What is parvovirus B19?

A single-stranded DNA virus

What is the incidence of parvovirus B19 infection in pregnant women?

3% to 4%

How is parvovirus diagnosed?

Serologic testing of IgM and IgG antibodies

Describe the major manifestations of infection with parvovirus B19:

A self-limited infection known as **erythema infectiosum** or **fifth disease** that consists of:

Dermatologic manifestations—a "slapped cheek" appearance on the face and a "lace-like" erythematous rash on the trunk and extremities

Symmetric arthropathy

Flu-like symptoms

What are the manifestations of parvovirus B19 during pregnancy?

Fetal loss or **hydrops fetalis** may ensue; however, there are no long-term developmental sequelae if a normal pregnancy ensues.

What is the risk of fetal loss?

Infection before 20 weeks: 11%

Infection after 20 weeks: less than 1%

What is hydrops fetalis?

Generalized fetal edema

What is the etiology of hydrops in the setting of congenital parvovirus infection?

Destruction of RBC precursors leading to fetal anemia

Myocarditis leading to fetal myocardial dysfunction

What is the risk of hydrops fetalis?

Less than 4%

What do the following serologic results signify?

Positive IgG and negative IgM: prior maternal immunity

Positive IgM and negative IgG: acute infection

How should an infected pregnant woman be managed?

Prior to 20 weeks, no action is necessary. After 20 weeks, women should receive weekly ultrasounds to look for signs of hydrops for 10 weeks after infection.

What sign on ultrasound indicates severe fetal anemia?

Elevated peak systolic velocity on the fetal middle cerebral artery dopplers

How is severe fetal anemia secondary to parvovirus treated?

With intrauterine fetal blood transfusion

HIV

What is HIV?

An RNA retrovirus that incorporates into the host genome and affects primary T cells leading to immunocompromise

How is HIV infection diagnosed?

Enzyme-linked immunosorbent assay (ELISA) testing followed by a Western blot, if the ELISA is positive

How do most pediatric HIV infections develop?

Through mother-to-child transmission via transplacental infection (50%), peripartum infection (30%), or via breast-feeding (20%)

What is the rate of vertical transmission in an HIV positive woman who is untreated?

25%

What is the rate of vertical transmission in an HIV positive woman on zidovudine (ZDV or AZT) alone?

8%

What is the rate of vertical transmission in an HIV positive woman on HAART (highly active antiretroviral therapy)?

1% to 2%

What increases the risk of vertical HIV transmission?

Preterm birth

Prolonged ROM

Concurrent syphilis infection

Chorioamnionitis

Are adverse pregnancy outcomes more common in HIV infected women?

Yes. Preterm birth and fetal growth restriction are more common, and these rates increase with a decreased CD4 count

Which pregnant patients should be given antiretroviral therapy?

All **pregnant patients**, regardless of CD4 count or viral load, **should be offered antiretroviral therapy** in order to reduce the risk of transmission.

When should CD4 counts be measured during pregnancy?

At least once each trimester

When should the viral load be measured during pregnancy?

4 weeks after any change in therapy, monthly until viral levels are undetectable, every 3 months while the viral load remains undetectable, and then once near term

What are some of the intrapartum precautions that should be taken?

Avoid artificial rupture of membranes (HIV transmission increased with increased time after rupture)

Use labor augmentation sooner (HIV transmission increased with longer interval to delivery)

Give IV zidovudine intrapartum

How should the neonate of an HIV infected mother be treated?

With oral zidovudine

When is a cesarean section indicated to prevent transmission?

When the maternal viral load is elevated (generally > 1000 copies/mL).

How much does cesarean delivery reduce the risk of vertical HIV transmission?

By half

Hepatitis

What are the hepatitis viruses?

A group of both DNA and RNA viruses that **invade hepatocytes**, leading to hepatocellular inflammation, scarring, and sometimes death

What are the symptoms of acute hepatitis infection?	Most are asymptomatic or mild. Symptoms, when present, include:
	  Nausea
	  Vomiting
	  Headache
	  Malaise
	  Fatigue
	  Right upper quadrant (RUQ) pain

What are the signs of hepatitis infection?	Jaundice RUQ tenderness Hepatomegaly
What are the laboratory values which can be associated with hepatitis infection?	Elevated transaminases Elevated bilirubin Coagulation abnormalities—increased PT and PTT (in severe cases) Elevated ammonia (in severe cases)
What are the major differential diagnoses of hepatitis infection in pregnancy?	Acute fatty liver of pregnancy Severe preeclampsia HELLP syndrome

Hepatitis A

What is hepatitis A and how is it transmitted?	An RNA picornavirus that is transmitted by the **fecal–oral spread**. It causes about one-third of hepatitis cases in the United States and leads to infection in 1 in 1000 pregnancies in the United States.
How is hepatitis A diagnosed?	**IgM** antibody suggests **recent infection**; **IgG** antibody suggests **prior exposure**
How is hepatitis A prevented?	Vaccination for high-risk women (it is an inactivated vaccine and so is safe to administer in pregnancy)
How is hepatitis A exposure treated?	With passive immunity via hepatitis A immune globulin
What is the effect of hepatitis A on perinatal outcomes?	Hepatitis A is not teratogenic; however, infection can lead to preterm birth and neonatal cholestasis.

Hepatitis B

What is hepatitis B and how is it transmitted?	A DNA hepadenavirus transmitted through **infected blood or bodily fluids**
What is the relationship between hepatitis B and HIV infection?	There is often coinfection, as they have similar modes of transmission. Coinfection with HIV leads to increased liver-related disease.
What is the prevalence of hepatitis B?	There are 1.2 million carriers in United States and 350 million carriers globally.
What percentage of those exposed to hepatitis B develop chronic infection?	In adults: 5% to 10% In infants: 70% to 90%
How is hepatitis B diagnosed?	Through antibody testing
Describe each of the following hepatitis B antigens:	**HBsAg** Hepatitis B surface antigen; it is on the outer viral shell and circulates in the serum **HBcAg** Hepatitis B core antigen; it is in the middle portion of the virus and does not circulate in serum although it is expressed in infected hepatocytes **HBeAg** Hepatitis B 'e' antigen; it correlates with infectivity
Describe the series of hepatitis B antibody responses:	The first marker of infection in **HBsAg**. Then **HBeAg** is detectable, which also denotes early infection. Both of these resolve within 3 to 6 months after infection. One month after infection, **IgM anti-HBc** begins to develop. It peaks at around 4 months and, within 6 months after exposure, **IgG anti-HBc is detectable**. Around the same time, **anti-HBs** develops. Persistence of HBsAg for more than 6 months is considered to be chronic infection.
How is an acute hepatitis B infection diagnosed serologically?	**Anti-HBc IgM** and **HBSAg**
How is chronic hepatitis B infection diagnosed serologically?	HBsAg without anti-HBc IgM
What are the major sequelae of hepatitis B infection?	Chronic hepatitis, cirrhosis, and hepatocellular carcinoma

What is the percentage of risk of vertical transmission in a patient that is HBeAg positive?	90%
What is the percentage of risk of vertical transmission in a patient that is HBeAg negative?	Less than 10%
How does infection with hepatitis B affect pregnancy?	Increased risk of preterm delivery
How does neonatal infection with hepatitis B occur?	Through **peripartum exposure to infected maternal fluids** and through **breast-feeding**. Transplacental infection is rare.
What is the likelihood of developing disease after neonatal hepatitis B exposure?	Most infected neonates are asymptomatic; however, **85% become chronic carriers.**
How is neonatal infection prevented?	Through **prenatal screening** and administration of **hepatitis B immune globulin** as well as the **hepatitis vaccination** of newborns of infected mothers
Is breast-feeding safe in women with hepatitis B?	There is a theoretic risk of transmission; however, hepatitis B immune globulin and neonatal vaccination should eliminate this risk.

Hepatitis C

What is hepatitis C and how is it transmitted?	A single-stranded Flaviviridae virus that is transmitted though exposure to blood and bodily fluids
What is the incidence of hepatitis C in pregnancy?	Depending on the population studied, it ranges from approximately 1% to 5%.
How is hepatitis C diagnosed?	**Serum antibody testing** (those seropositive for anti-HCV have chronic hepatitis)
How does hepatitis C infection affect pregnancy?	It may increase the risk of cholestatic jaundice.

What is the incidence of vertical transmission of hepatitis C?	Between 3% and 6%
How can vertical transmission be prevented?	There are currently no known methods to prevent transmission at birth.

Hepatitis D

What is hepatitis D?	A defective RNA virus that is only infectious if it coinfects with hepatitis B and is transmitted in a similar manner
What percentage of patients infected with hepatitis B are coinfected with hepatitis D?	Approximately 25%
What are the sequelae of infection with hepatitis B and D?	The same as hepatitis B, however the infection is **more severe** than infection with hepatitis B alone.

Hepatitis E

What is hepatitis E?	An RNA virus transmitted usually via contaminated water (fecal-oral).
What are the effects of hepatitis E infection in pregnancy?	There may be a high rate of vertical transmission and there is some evidence that infection is more severe in pregnancy.

BACTERIAL INFECTIONS

Group B Streptococcus

What is group B *Streptococcus* (GBS)?	*Streptococcus agalactiae*, a gram-positive infection of the GI, upper respiratory and genital tracts. It leads to severe disease in neonates if they are infected right before or during birth.
What percentage of women are asymptomatic carriers of GBS?	Approximately 15% to 30%
Where does colonization typically occur?	Primarily in the **rectum**, with secondary infection in the bladder, vagina, and cervix

What are the symptoms of GBS colonization in women?	Usually none
How does symptomatic GBS infection manifest in pregnant women?	UTI, chorioamnionitis, or postpartum wound infection, bacteremia, or endomyometritis
How is GBS colonization diagnosed?	Via routine screening with urine culture and rectovaginal swab
What is the incidence of invasive neonatal GBS infection?	Because of intrapartum chemoprophylaxis, neonatal GBS affects only approximately 1 in 4000 births in the United States
What is the rate of maternal-neonatal transmission of GBS if left untreated?	35% to 75% depending on the degree of infection
What are the clinical manifestations of neonatal GBS infection?	**Bacteremia, sepsis, pneumonia, respiratory distress, meningitis, shock**, or **death** can ensue. If the neonate survives, 33% have long-term neurodevelopmental problems.
What is the difference between early onset and late onset GBS disease?	Early onset refers to infection before 7 days of age and it carries the highest mortality rate. Late onset disease occurs from 1 week to 3 months after birth.
What is the mortality rate associated with neonatal GBS infection?	5% to 15%
What are the major risk factors for neonatal GBS infection that necessitate treatment in a woman who has not been screened for GBS?	Preterm labor GBS bacteriuria during the pregnancy Prolonged ROM (>18 hours) Having a neonate affected by early-onset GBS infection in a previous pregnancy Maternal fever > 38°C during labor
What is the recommended treatment for GBS colonization?	**IV penicillin** or ampicillin
What are the alternatives for patients allergic to penicillin?	Cefazolin or vancomycin Clindamycin or erythromycin are acceptable alternatives only if culture and sensitivities have demonstrated the bacteria to be sensitive to both (because of high rates of cross-resistance).

Listeria Monocytogenes

What is *Listeria*?

A gram-positive, aerobic bacillus that is transmitted via fecal-oral transmission

What is commonly implicated in *Listeria* infection?

Infected foods such as raw vegetables, milk, smoked fish, soft cheeses, and some processed meats

What are the clinical manifestations of listeriosis in adults?

Can be **asymptomatic** or it can cause a **flu-like illness**

What are the clinical manifestations of fetal infection with *Listeria*?

Disseminated granulomatous lesions with microabscesses

Chorioamnionitis

Sepsis

Spontaneous abortion or stillbirth

What is the difference between early onset and late onset *Listeria* infection?

Early onset disease occurs within the first week of life and it typically presents after a **preterm** delivery with **respiratory distress**, fever, and neurologic abnormalities. **Late onset disease** occurs after the first week, and it typically presents as **meningitis.**

What is the treatment for *Listeria* infection in pregnancy?

Ampicillin or trimethoprim-sulfamethoxazole or vancomycin

Gonorrhea

What is gonorrhea?

Caused by *Neisseria gonorrhoeae*, a gram negative diplococcal STI

What are the possible pregnancy complications that can occur as a consequence of gonorrhea infection?

Spontaneous abortion

Stillbirth

Preterm labor

PROM

Chorioamnionitis

Postpartum infection

How should pregnant women infected with gonorrhea be treated?

With **ceftriaxone, cefixime,** or **spectinomycin** PLUS treatment for *Chlamydia* infection (unless it has been excluded)

What are the possible neonatal effects of gonorrhea infection in pregnancy?	Gonococcal ophthalmia, arthritis, and sepsis
How is gonococcal ophthalmia prevented?	By giving all infants prophylactic **erythromycin** or **silver nitrate** eye drops

Chlamydia

What is *Chlamydia*?	Infection with *Chlamydia trachomatis*, an obligate intracellular bacterium
What are the possible pregnancy complications that can occur as a consequence of chlamydial infection?	Preterm labor, PROM, and/or postpartum endometritis
How should pregnant women infected with *Chlamydia* be treated?	With **erythromycin** or **azithromycin** (tetracycline should be avoided because of teratogenicity)
What are the possible neonatal effects of chlamydial infection in pregnancy?	**Conjunctivitis, pneumonia**, and/or **otitis media**
How is chlamydial ophthalmia prevented?	By giving all infants prophylactic **erythromycin** or **silver nitrate** eye drops

Rhesus (Rh) Alloimmunization

What is alloimmunization of pregnancy?	It is when the fetus inherits a blood group factor from the father which the mother does not possess. Exchange of blood during fetal-maternal bleeding causes the mother to become sensitized to the foreign antigen and stimulates the **formation of maternal antibodies (alloimmunization) during that pregnancy**. These antibodies may enter the fetal circulation of her **next pregnancy** and lead to **hemolytic disease in the fetus** and neonate by sensitizing the fetal RBCs for destruction by macrophages of the fetal spleen (see Fig. 9.5).

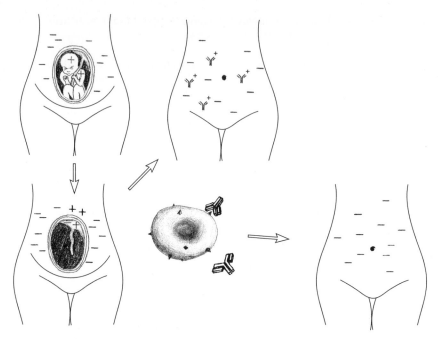

Figure 9.5   Isoimmunization and RHOGAM treatment.

What is erythroblastosis fetalis?

It is when fetal red blood cell destruction far exceeds production and severe anemia occurs. This disease is characterized by extramedullary hematopoiesis, heart failure, edema, ascites, and pericardial effusion. Hemolysis also produces heme and uncomjugated bilirubin, both of which are neurotoxic and may lead to kernicterus.

What is the correct nomenclature for designating a gravida's blood type?

ABO blood type and either Rh(+) or Rh(−)

What is the nomenclature of the Rh blood group system?

The Rh blood system consists of five antigens (C, c, D, E, e).

The D antigen is most commonly implicated in Rh alloimmunization and, therefore, Rh positive usually indicates the presence of the D antigen.

By what mechanisms can Rh alloimmunization occur?

1. **Transplacental fetomaternal hemorrhage during any pregnancy (most common)**
2. Injection with needles contaminated by Rh(+) blood
3. Inadvertent transfusion of Rh(+) blood

What is the most common scenario for fetomaternal hemorrhage?

Uncomplicated vaginal delivery. A minimum volume of 0.1 mL of fetal blood entering the maternal circulation can result in alloimmunization.

What are several less common situations where fetomaternal hemorrhage can occur?

Cesarean delivery, bleeding placenta previa or abruption, manual removal of the placenta, intrauterine manipulation, spontaneous and induced abortion, threatened abortion, ectopic pregnancy, chorionic villus sampling, amniocentesis, and external cephalic version

When should a blood and Rh(D) typing and antibody screen be performed?

Always at the first visit! These tests should also be repeated with every subsequent pregnancy. The American Association of Blood Banks also recommends repeated **antibody screening before administration of anti-D immune globulin at 28 weeks of gestation, postpartum,** and at the time of any event in pregnancy.

What test is the most sensitive test for determining antibody titers and diagnosing Rh(D) alloimmunization? How does it work?

Indirect Coomb's test

Incubation of a known specimen of Rh(+) RBCs with maternal serum is the first step. Maternal anti-Rh antibodies, if present, will adhere to the RBCs. The RBCs are then washed and suspended in serum containing antihuman globulin (Coomb's serum). Red cells coated with maternal anti-Rh will be agglutinated by the antihuman globulin, which is referred to as a positive indirect Coomb's test.

What titer levels are considered critical for significant risk of severe erythroblastosis fetalis and hydrops?

Critical titers may vary from laboratory to laboratory. In general, the critical titer that poses a significant risk for erythroblastosis fetalis and hydrops is 1:16 to 1:32.

What is the direct Coomb's test?

It is done after birth to detect the presence of maternal antibody on the neonate's RBCs. It is performed by placing the infant's RBCs in Coomb's serum; maternal antibody is present if the cells are agglutinated.

Who should be given anti-D immune globulin (RhoGAM)?

To all **Rh(–) women whose fetus is or may be Rh(+) whenever there is a risk of fetomaternal hemorrhage**

How does RhoGAM prevent alloimmunization?

It is an IgG that will attach to the Rh antigen and prevent an immune response by the mother (see Fig. 9.5).

How are sensitized Rh(-) patients evaluated?

There are three options once the gravida reaches the critical titer:

1. **Middle cerebral artery (MCA) doppler** can be performed weekly. MCA doppler is sensitive in diagnosing moderate to severe hemolytic disease.
2. **Amniocentesis** can be performed with two indicated tests: PCR on the fetal amniocytes will determine the fetal blood type. If the fetus is Rh(–), no additional testing is indicated. Indirect measurement of hemolytic disease can be determined by measuring bilirubin concentration in the amniotic fluid using spectrophotometry at a wavelength of **delta-OD 450**. The absorbance measurements indicate the degree of fetal anemia (plotted on a **Liley curve**).
3. **Cordocentesis** can be performed initially to determine fetal blood type and hemoglobin concentration. However, this procedure can have up to a 1% risk of fetal loss.

What should be done once moderate to severe fetal anemia has developed?

Once the fetus reaches a value indicating moderate to severe anemia, cordocentesis with transfusion is indicated.

What is the management of the unsensitized Rh(–) pregnancy (the Rh(–) patient who has a negative antibody screen)?

1. All pregnant women should undergo type and antibody screening for the ABO and Rh group at the first prenatal visit.
2. Another antibody screen is obtained at 28 weeks of gestation to detect women who have become alloimmunized in the interval since the first screen.
3. Anti-D immune globulin should be administered early in the third trimester (300 µg at 28 weeks of gestation).
4. Anti-D immune globulin is effective for 12 weeks, and if the gravida received an injection at 28 weeks' gestation, she should have a repeat injection at 40 weeks' gestation.

What is the Kleihauer-Betke test and when should it be used?

It is a test to quantify the amount of fetal RBCs in the maternal circulation in circumstance where excessive fetomaternal hemorrhage has occurred and Rh sensitization is positive for persistent antibody after initial administration of RhIgG. Additional doses of RhIgG is given according to the amount of excess hemorrhage.

What is the role of postpartum administration of anti-G immune globulin?

It is recommended to administer 300 µg of anti-D immune globulin within 72 hours of delivery of an Rh (+) infant.

What should one do if anti-D immune globulin is inadvertently omitted after delivery?

It is still recommended to give it as soon as possible. Partial protection is afforded with administration within 13 days of the birth, and there may be an effect as late as 28 days after delivery.

How are sensitized Rh(–) patients (positive Rh antibody screen on initial visit) evaluated?

It depends on whether the patient has a history of an affected fetus in a previous pregnancy.

No history of a previous pregnancy affected by Rh isoimmunization:

1. Antibody screen and titers at 0, 20 weeks' EGA, and then every 4 weeks.
2. Determine the paternal Rh type and if Rh(+), determine zygosity.
3. Amniocentesis should be performed if titers reach critical levels.
4. Doppler ultrasound of the MCA should be performed every 2 weeks beginning by 24 weeks. High peak velocity blood flows correlates with severe fetal anemia.

History of a previous pregnancy affected by Rh isoimmunization:

1. Maternal titers are not helpful in following the degree of fetal anemia after the first affected gestation.
2. Determine the paternal Rh type and if Rh(+), determine zygosity.
3. In cases of a heterozygous paternal phenotype, perform amniocentesis at 15 weeks of gestation to determine the fetal Rh(D) status.
4. If the father is a homozygote or the fetus is Rh(+), begin MCA doppler velocity assessment at 18 weeks of gestation. Repeat at 1 to 2 week intervals.

Maternal isoimmunization to which antibodies affect fetal outcome?

Blood cell antigens: C, D (Duffy), E, K (Kell), and Rh

"Duffy dies, Kelly kills, Lewis lives" (L antigen does not have a significant deleterious affect on the fetus)

Fetal Growth Abnormalities

INTRAUTERINE GROWTH RESTRICTION

How is intrauterine growth restriction (IUGR) commonly defined?

An **estimated fetal weight (EFW) at or below the 10th percentile for gestational age**

IUGR is associated with increased perinatal mortality. At what percentile is this risk greatest?

Weights below the third percentile for gestational age

Abnormal fetal growth may be classified as symmetrical or asymmetrical. What is meant by these terms?

In symmetric IUGR, all fetal organs including the brain are proportionally small because of abnormalities in early fetal cellular hyperplasia. There is cellular hypoplasia or a reduction in the total number of cells. This comprises 20% to 30% of all growth-restricted fetuses.

In asymmetrical IUGR, there is a relatively greater decrease in abdominal size compared to head circumference. This is thought to occur from redistribution of blood from nonvital organs (liver, abdominal viscera) to vital organs (heart, brain). There is redistribution away from the kidneys in asymmetrical growth restriction which may lead to oligohydramnios. This comprises 70% to 80% of growth-restricted fetuses.

What are the several causative factors for both symmetric and asymmetric IUGR?

Symmetric: early insults such as chromosomal abnormalities, early teratogenic exposure, and early exposure to TORCH infections

Asymmetric: maternal conditions such as hypertension, vasculopathies, diabetes with vascular disease, and placental abnormalities

What are some genetic syndromes that typically manifest with IUGR?

Trisomy 21 (Down syndrome), Trisomy 18 (Edwards syndrome), Trisomy 13 (Patau syndrome), cri-du-chat syndrome, Turner syndrome, Fanconi syndrome, skeletal dysplasias

Several maternal conditions affect the microcirculation causing fetal hypoxemia, vasoconstriction, or a reduction in fetal perfusion, thus causing IUGR. What are these common maternal etiologies?

Hypertension (chronic and acute)

Cyanotic heart disease

Severe anemia (eg, sickle cell disease)

Renal insufficiency

Systemic lupus erythematosus

Thrombophilias

Pregestational diabetes

What other maternal etiologies cause IUGR?

Infections (rubella, toxoplasmosis, cytomegalovirus, varicella-zoster, malaria)

Teratogens (trimethadione, phenytoin, methotrexate, and warfarin)

Poor nutrition

Substance abuse (cocaine, alcohol)

Socioeconomic factors (race, pregnancy at the extremes of reproductive life, and previous delivery of an IUGR neonate)

What are some neonatal complications associated with IUGR?

Stillbirth, perinatal asphyxia, meconium aspiration syndrome, neonatal hypoglycemia, abnormal neurological development

What are the long-term complications for the child with IUGR?

Lower IQ, learning and behavior problems, major neurologic handicaps

How is the diagnosis of IUGR determined?

Patient history, clinical assessment of fundal height, and sonographic evaluation of the fetus, placenta, and amniotic fluid are necessary

What sonographic measurements are diagnostic and predictive of IUGR?

Estimation of fetal weight using multiple fetal biometric measurements is the best test.

A **lagging abdominal circumference** is highly suggestive of IUGR.

What is oligohydramnios and what role does it have in the diagnosis of IUGR?

Oligohydramnios may be a consequence of IUGR and refers to amniotic fluid volume that is less than expected for gestational age. It occurs when there is diminished fetal urine production, and in IUGR this may be because of hypoxia-induced redistribution of blood flow to vital organs at the expense of less vital organs, such as the kidney. Severe oligohydramnios is associated with high-perinatal mortality.

(15%-80% of fetuses with IUGR do not have decreased amniotic fluid volume)

What are umbilical artery dopplers?

A measurement of blood flow through the umbilical artery. They are read as normal, absent, or reversed end diastolic flow.

When is doppler assessment of the umbilical arteries used?

It is useful as an adjunctive test **in the setting of IUGR** for assessment of fetal status. UA dopplers have no value in normally grown fetuses.

FETAL MACROSOMIA

What is the definition of fetal macrosomia and large-for-gestational age (LGA)?

Macrosomia implies growth beyond 4500 g, regardless of gestational age.

Large-for-gestational age implies a birth weight equal to or greater than the 90th percentile for a given gestational age.

What is the incidence of fetal macrosomia?

9% of infants weigh more than 4000 g

1.5% of all infants weigh more than 4500 g

What are maternal and fetal complications associated with macrosomia?

Maternal: protracted labor, cesarean delivery, genital tract lacerations, postpartum hemorrhage, uterine rupture

Fetal: shoulder dystocia, brachial plexus injuries, fractures of the clavicle, asphyxia

Neonatal: increased risk of depressed 5-minute APGAR scores, increased risk of admission to the NICU, jaundice, hypoglycemia

Long-term: obesity

What pregnancy-related disease is an independent factor for and highly associated with macrosomia?

Pregestational diabetes and gestational diabetes

What are risk factors for macrosomia?

Prior history of macrosomia

Maternal prepregnancy weight

Maternal pregnancy weight gain

Multiparity

Male fetus

Gestational age greater than 40 weeks

Ethnicity

Positive 50 g glucose screen with a negative result on the 3-hour glucose tolerance test

Which genetic and congenital syndromes are associated with macrosomia?

Beckwith-Wiedemann syndrome (pancreatic islet cell hyperplasia)

Fragile X syndrome

Are there any available interventions for treating fetal macrosomia?

For mothers without diabetes, there are no reported interventions

For diabetic mothers, addition of insulin to diet therapy may treat early macrosomia

Is prophylactic cesarean delivery indicated for pregnant women suspected to have macrosomic fetuses?

Prophylactic cesarean delivery to prevent shoulder dystocia may be considered for an EFW more than 5000 g in nondiabetic women and EFW more than 4500 g in women with diabetes (induction of labor for macrosomia is not recommended).

When else should elective cesarean delivery be considered?

For women whose previous delivery was complicated by shoulder dystocia, particularly when a brachial plexus injury occurred.

Multi-fetal Gestation

What is the incidence of *spontaneous* twins and multiple births in the United States?

Twins: 1:80

Triplets: 1:8000

What is the role of maternal age in increased multifetal pregnancy?

The rate of multiples increases with maternal age, most likely as a result of older women undergoing assisted reproductive technology (ART).

What is the significance of multifetal gestation on fetal morbidity and mortality?

It markedly increases the risk of preterm delivery

What is the significance of multifetal gestation on maternal morbidity and mortality?

Women with multiple gestations are six times more likely to be hospitalized with complications. Multifetal gestations contribute to maternal conditions such as preeclampsia, gestational diabetes, and pulmonary embolism.

What is meant by monozygosity and dizygosity?

Monozygotic (identical or maternal) twins form from a fertilization of a single ovum that subsequently divides. Monozygotes can either be monoamnionic/monochorionic or diamnionic/monochorionic depending upon the timing of division of embryos

Dizygotic (nonidentical or fraternal) twins result from fertilization of two separate ova by two separate sperm during a single ovulatory cycle.

When does division of the embryo occur in these types of twins? Describe each:

Conjoined twins: division after 13 days postfertilization (twins share a single cavity and have one placenta, one chorion, one amnion, and one shared umbilical cord).

Monoamnionic/monochorionic placentation: division after amnion formation (between days 8 and 12 postfertilization). These gestations have a single placenta and are at increased risk of cord entanglement during the pregnancy.

Diamnionic/monochorionic placentation: division after trophoblast differentiation and before amnion formation between (days 4 and 8 postfertilization). Twins are in separate cavities and have one placenta, one chorion, two amnions, and two umbilical cords. These gestations are at increased risk for twin-to-twin transfusion syndrome (TTTS) (see Fig. 9.6).

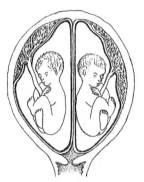

Dichorionic diamniotic

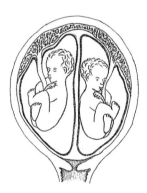

Monochorionic diamniotic

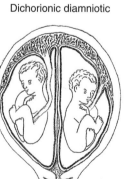

Dichorionic diamniotic

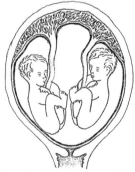

Monochorionic monoamniotic

Figure 9.6 Twin pregnancies.

What percentage of same sex twins with monochorionic placentas are identical?	100%
What is twin-to-twin transfusion syndrome?	A syndrome in which there is unequal flow of blood across the shared placenta, typically resulting in one twin who is smaller (donor twin) and has decreased amniotic fluid and another twin (recipient twin) who is larger with excess amniotic fluid. Perinatal mortality associated with TTTS is high, and twins who survive are at risk of severe cardiac, brain, or developmental disorders.
What is the association between multifetal gestation and cerebral palsy?	There is a three-fold greater risk of cerebral palsy. Causes that may contribute to this risk include low birth weight, congenital anomalies, cord entanglement, preterm delivery, and abnormal vascular connections
What technique is used to reduce the number of fetuses in a multi-fetal gestation?	Fetal reduction or selective fetal termination

Abnormal Labor and Delivery

DYSTOCIA

What is dystocia and what is its incidence?	Abnormal labor; occurs in approximately 25% of nulliparous women
What are the risk factors for abnormal labor?	Advanced maternal age Nonreassuring fetal heart tracing Epidural anesthesia Macrosomia Occiput posterior position Nulliparity Short stature Chorioamnionitis Post-term pregnancy Obesity

What are the three major categories of causes of dystocia?

Problems with the three "P"s:
1. **Power**
2. **Passage**
3. **Passenger**

What is meant by abnormal power?

Inadequate or uncoordinated contractions

What is meant by abnormal passage?

Abnormal size or shape of maternal pelvis leading to **cephalopelvic disproportion** (a disproportion between the fetal head and maternal pelvis)

What is meant by abnormal passenger?

Malposition, malpresentation, macrosomia, or multiple gestations

What are the two major categories of failure to progress?

1. **Protraction disorders**—slower than normal progress
2. **Arrest disorders**—complete cessation of progress

What is uterine hypocontractility?

Uterine activity that is not strong enough or is not coordinated enough to dilate the cervix; quantified as uterine contractions < 200 Montevideo units

What are the criteria for the diagnosis of abnormal labor in each of these categories?

	Nullipara	Multipara
Duration of labor:	> 24.7 hours	> 18.8 hours
Protracted dilation:	< 1.2 cm/h	< 1.5 cm/h
Arrest of descent (with epidural):	> 3 hours	> 2 hours
Arrest of descent (without epidural):	> 2 hours	> 1 hour

When is an arrest of dilation diagnosed?

Cessation of dilation after 4 cm or more despite adequate uterine contractions (> 200 Montevideo units for 2 hours or more)

How is poor progression in the first stage of labor managed?

With an **amniotomy** (if membranes are intact) and/or **oxytocin** (for hypocontractile uterine activity)

If arrest of dilation persists despite these interventions, how should the patient be managed?

Cesarean delivery—she is in active phase arrest

What is a prolonged latent phase?

A latent phase (in the first stage of labor) of over 20 hours for a nullipara or 14 hours for a multipara

What are the risks associated with a prolonged latent phase?

Cesarean delivery

Newborn requiring NICU admission

Thick meconium

Depressed Apgars

What is assisted vaginal delivery?

Also known as operative vaginal delivery, it involves the use of forceps or a vacuum device

What types of abnormal presentations are possible and what are the relative incidences of each?

Face (~1/700)

Brow (~1/1400)

Breech (~1/30)

Compound (~1/1500)

Describe face presentation:

The fetal neck is sharply extended, causing the face to lead into the birth canal

What are the three types of breech presentation?

1. **Frank breech:** fetus has hips flexed and knees extended (feet near head).
2. **Complete breech:** fetus has hips and knees flexed.
3. **Footling/incomplete breech:** fetus has one or both feet present below the buttocks (see Fig. 9.7).

How common is breech presentation?

Approximately 3% to 4% of fetuses at term are breech (increased rates at earlier gestational ages).

What are some of the factors that affect presentation?

Uterine shape (fibroids, placenta previa, poly/oligohydramnios, müllerian anomalies)

Fetal shape (anomalies such as anencephaly)

Fetal mobility (asphyxia, impaired growth, fetal structural malformation, fetal chromosomal anomaly)

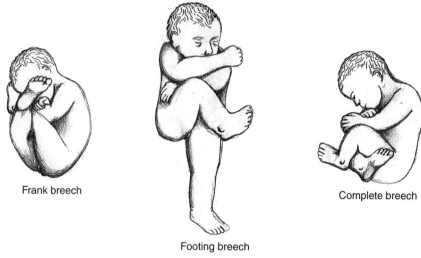

Frank breech

Complete breech

Footing breech

Figure 9-7   Breech presentations.

How is breech presentation diagnosed?	With abdominal palpation and ultrasound
What are the options for management of a breech presentation near term?	External cephalic version Cesarean delivery Vaginal delivery (rarely done)
What is external cephalic version?	A procedure that externally rotates the fetus from the breech presentation to the cephalic presentation
When is external cephalic version done?	After 36 to 37 weeks
What is the success rate of external cephalic version?	Approximately 65%
What is a transverse lie?	When the fetus's longitudinal axis is perpendicular to the long axis of the uterus
What are the two types of transverse lie?	1. Back down: fetal back facing toward the cervix 2. Back up: fetal back facing away from the cervix

What potential problems can be associated with transverse lie?

Placenta previa

Prolapsed umbilical cord

Fetal trauma

Prematurity

MECONIUM

What is meconium?

Fetal feces released into the amniotic fluid

How often is meconium noted before or during delivery?

10% to 15% of births

What are some of the causes of meconium passage in utero?

Placental insufficiency

Cord compression

Infection

How should management of the second stage change in the presence of meconium?

Hand off the neonate to the pediatric team immediately after delivery so that they can suction the oropharynx

What is meconium aspiration syndrome (MAS)?

A **chemical pneumonitis** caused by inhalation of meconium into the fetal tracheobronchial tree during the antepartum or intrapartum period.

What are some of the potential complications of MAS?

Respiratory distress, persistent pulmonary hypertension, death

POST-TERM PREGNANCY

What is the definition of post-term pregnancy?

Also called prolonged pregnancy; a pregnancy **beyond 42 weeks** gestation

What is the incidence of post-term pregnancy?

Approximately 7% to 10% in the United States

What are factors associated with post-term pregnancy?

Incorrect dating

Primiparity

Prior post-term pregnancy

Fetal congenital anomaly

What are the risks to the fetus in post-term pregnancy?

Perinatal death

Intrauterine infection

Macrosomia and associated risks

Asphyxia

Fetoplacental insufficiency

Fetal dysmaturity syndrome

What is fetal dysmaturity syndrome?

Also known as **postmaturity syndrome**, it is placental insufficiency resulting in wrinkly, peeling skin (especially on palms and soles); long, thin body, wasting of subcutaneous tissue; alert appearance with open eyes; long nails.

What are the fetal risks of post-term pregnancy?

Oligohydramnios (and subsequent umbilical cord compression)

Nonreassuring fetal heart tracing

Meconium aspiration

Complications at birth (hypoglycemia, seizures, respiratory insufficiency)

Long-term neurologic sequelae

What are the maternal risks of post-term pregnancy?

Labor dystocia

Macrosomia-related perineal injury

Increased rate of cesarean delivery

How should post-term pregnancies be monitored?

With antenatal fetal monitoring (either via **NST** and **AFI**, **BPP**, or **oxytocin challenge test**) twice weekly beginning at 41 weeks gestation

When should delivery be entertained?

At 41 weeks of gestation if the cervix is favorable

After 42 completed weeks or earlier if there is evidence of **fetal compromise** or **oligohydramnios**

Teratogens

What is the definition of a teratogen?

An agent that acts during the embryonic or fetal development to produce structural abnormalities in the fetus.

What percentage of congenital abnormalities are caused by teratogens?

Approximately 10%

What properties of drugs allow their toxic effects on fetuses to occur?

Lipid-soluble molecules readily cross the placenta compared to water-soluble substances.

Molecules bound to carrier proteins are less likely to cross the placenta.

What is meant by embryopathy versus fetopathy?

Embryopathy refers to exposure to a teratogen within the first 8 weeks, whereas fetopathy refers to exposure after 8 weeks.

What is the general effect of teratogens on each of the three developmental periods of gestation?

Gestation is divided into three periods known as:

1. **Preimplantation period**: the period from fertilization to implantation. An insult causing damage to a large number of cells at this period usually causes death of the embryo (**all or nothing** phenomenon).
2.. **Embryonic period**: the period from the 2nd through the 8th week following conception. This period is the critical stage of organ development (see Fig. 9-8) and is most crucial in regards to structural malformations.
3.. **Fetal period**: the period where maturation and functional development continue after 9 weeks. Certain organs, such as the brain, remain vulnerable toteratogens during this period.

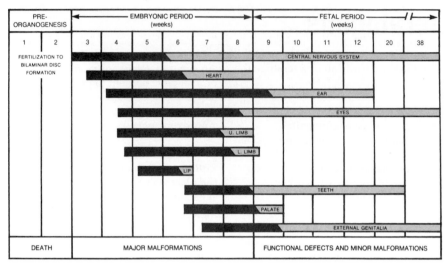

Figure 9-8   Illustrates the critical development period of each organ system.

What are the FDA Pregnancy Drug Categories?

Category A: safety has been established using human studies

Category B: presumed safety based on animal studies

Category C: uncertain safety; though animals studies show an adverse effect, there are no human studies

Category D: unsafe—evidence of risk that may in certain clinical circumstances by justifiable

Category X: highly unsafe—risk outweighs any possible benefit

What are the major abnormalities associated with each known teratogen?

See Table 9.14

Can heparin be used for anticoagulation in pregnant women?

Yes. Heparin does not cross the placenta because of its large negative charge and thus does not have any adverse fetal effects. Low-molecular weight heparins also do not cross the placenta.

Has paternal exposure to these drugs been found to be teratogenic?

There is no evidence for this.

Table 9.14 Teratogens

Teratogen	Syndrome and/or Well-Known Effects of the Teratogen	Other Comments
Alcohol	Fetal alcohol syndrome: congenital heart and brain defects, failure to thrive, developmental delay, mental retardation, ADHD, craniofacial anomalies (absent/hypoplastic philtrum, broad upper lip, micrognathia, microphthalmia, short palpebral tissues, short nose). **Growth restriction** before and after birth	A safe threshold dose for alcohol has not been established
Androgens and testosterone derivatives (ie, danazol)	Virilization of females; advanced genital development in males	Effects are dose-dependent and related to the time of exposure during the developmental period
Phenytoin	**Fetal hydantoin syndrome:** craniofacial anomalies (upturned nose, mild midfacial hypoplasia, thin philtrum, facial clefts), fingernail hypoplasia, growth deficiency, developmental delay, cardiac defects	Syndrome results from accumulation of free oxide radicals in fetal tissues
Carbamazepine	Fetal hydantoin syndrome, spina bifida	
Valproate	Neural-tube defects	Lowers fetal folate levels
Phenobarbital	Clefts, cardiac anomalies, urinary tract malformations	Lowers fetal folate levels
Trimethadione, paramethadione	Cleft palate, V-shaped eyebrows, microcephaly, growth deficiency, mental retardation, speech disturbance, cardiac defects	70% of newborns affected by this drug

(Continued)

Table 9.14 Teratogens (*Continued*)

Teratogen	Syndrome and/or Well-Known Effects of the Teratogen	Other Comments
Warfarin	Exposure between 6-9 weeks: nasal and midface hypoplasia, stippled vertebral and femoral epiphyses Exposure between second and third trimester: hemorrhage, organ scarring, agenesis of the corpus callosum, Dandy-Walker malformation, optic atrophy, blindness, mental retardation	The incidence of spontaneous abortion is 72%
ACE inhibitors	Renal ischemia, renal tubular dysgenesis, anuria, oligohydramnios, lung hypoplasia, limb contractures, hypoperfusion, growth restriction, limb shortening	These changes mostly occur during the fetal period, ACE inhibitor fetopathy. Enalapril is the most teratogenic of the ACE inhibitors
Retinol-vitamin A	Spontaneous abortions, cardiac anomalies, microcephaly	Vitamin A doses higher than 5000 IU should be avoided
Isotretinoin	First trimester use: high rate of fetal loss Strongly associated malformations include bilateral microtia, agenesis or stenosis of the external ear canal, cleft palate, abnormal facial bones/calvarium, cardiac defects, hydrocephalus.	No safe first trimester exposure period or dose
Diethylstilbestrol (DES)	Clear-cell adenocarcinoma of the cervix and vagina and abnormalities of the female genital tract (T-shaped uterus)	
Cyclophosphamide	Absent or hypoplastic digits on the hands and feet, cleft palate, single coronary artery, imperforate anus, fetal growth restriction with microcephaly	Should be avoided in the first trimester but can be given in the second and third trimester

Table 9.14 Teratogens (*Continued*)

Teratogen	Syndrome and/or Well-Known Effects of the Teratogen	Other Comments
Methotrexate	Growth restriction, craniosynostosis, failure of calvarial ossification, hypoplastic supraorbital ridges, micrognathia, and severe limb deformities	Drug alters folate metabolism. Used as an abortifacient. Should not exceed a dose > 10 mg/wk Contraindicated for treatment of psoriasis
Tetracyclines	Yellow-brown discoloration of teeth, hypoplasia of tooth enamel	Effects occur if drug is used in second or third trimester. Should only be used for tx of maternal syphilis in penicillin-allergic women
Aminoglycosides	Nephrotoxicity and ototoxicity in preterm newborns treated with gentamicin or streptomycin	No confirmation regarding congenital defects from prenatal exposure
Streptomycin, kanamycin	Hearing loss, eighth nerve damage	No ototoxicity has been reported with use of gentamicin or vancomycin
Lead	Increased abortion rates, stillbirths	
Tobacco	Dose-dependent intrauterine fetal growth reduction, spontaneous abortion, preterm delivery, placenta previa, cleft lip/palate, hydrocephaly, microcephaly, omphalocele, gastroschisis, and hand abnormalities, sudden infant death syndrome (SIDS)	Cessation of smoking throughout and after pregnancy should be strongly advised

(Continued)

Table 9.14 Teratogens (*Continued*)

Teratogen	Syndrome and/or Well-Known Effects of the Teratogen	Other Comments
Cocaine	Placental abruption, porencephaly, subependymal and periventricular cysts, ileal atresia, cardiac anomalies, urinary tract defects, and visceral infarcts	
Thalidomide	Upper limb reduction, lower limb reduction, gall bladder aplasia, duodenal atresia	Excellent example shows timing of drug exposure and type of birth defect
Methyl mercury	Ranges from developmental delay to microcephaly and severe brain damage	Not a drug but a major pollutant found in fish. Pregnant women should abstain from seafood thought to be exposed to mercury
Marijuana	Possible low birth weight; otherwise, no evidence of association with human anomalies	
Amphetamines	Symmetrical fetal growth restriction, SIDS	
Heroin	Fetal-growth restriction, perinatal death, small head circumference, developmental delays, SIDS	40%-80% of newborns have typical heroin withdrawal symptoms
Lithium	Ebstein anomaly, diabetes insipidus, hypothyroidism, and hypoglycemia	

CLINICAL VIGNETTES

A 21-year-old Southeast Asian G1P0 arrives for her first prenatal visit at 8 weeks gestation. She has no known medical issues. Her hemoglobin is 8.3 g/dL with an MCV of 78.2 (normal 80.8-96.4). She eats a well-balanced diet. She denies any vaginal or rectal bleeding. Her hemoglobin electrophoresis is normal.

What is the most likely diagnosis?

a. Normal
b. Alpha thalassemia minor
c. Hemodilution of pregnancy
d. Sickle cell disease

Answer: b

This patient has microcytic anemia with a normal hemoglobin electrophoresis. This could represent iron deficiency or a hemoglobinopathy. Hemodilution of pregnancy is a result of an increase in plasma volume, which dilutes the hemoglobin but does not lower the MCV (normocytic anemia). Furthermore, this increase in plasma volume reaches its maximum around 34 weeks gestational age and she is merely 8 weeks. Her normal hemoglobin electrophoresis precludes a diagnosis of sickle cell disease. Thus the most likely diagnosis is alpha thalassemia which, in contrast to beta thalassemia most often has a normal hemoglobin electrophoresis.

A 20-year-old G1P0 at 36 weeks gestation is brought to the ER by the paramedics. Her boyfriend woke up to find her having a grand mal seizure on the floor. She was minimally responsive on arrival but with a secure airway. Her BP is 174/108 and she has 3+ protein on a urine dip.

What is the treatment for her underlying condition?

a. Delivery
b. Magnesium sulfate
c. Lorazepam
d. Hydralazine

Answer: a

This case describes an eclamptic seizure. The treatment for eclampsia is delivery and as soon as she is stabilized, this should be pursued. Magnesium sulfate is indicated to prevent recurrent seizures, but magnesium does not treat eclampsia or preeclampsia. Lorazapam can be used if magnesium is ineffective at controlling seizures in eclampsia as a second line agent. Hydralazine is an antihypertensive agent and while this patient does need medication to control her BP, this will not treat her eclampsia.

A 37-year-old G6P4014 at 7 weeks gestation presents for her first antenatal visit. She has a history of 4 prior uncomplicated vaginal deliveries, the last of which was 8 years ago. She has no other significant medical history. On physical examination, she weighs 306 lb and is 62 in tall. Due to her BMI, you order a glucola which returns as 246 mg/dL. A HgA1c is 6.7%.

What does this patient most likely have?

    a. White Class B Diabetes
    b. White Class C Diabetes
    c. Gestational Diabetes Class A1
    d. Gestational Diabetes Class A2
    e. Type I Diabetes

Answer: a

Given this patient's gestational age of 7 weeks and her elevated HgA1c (representing poor glycemic control in the months preceding pregnancy), this is unlikely to represent gestational diabetes. Rather, this patient likely has type 2 diabetes. In the White classification scheme, Class B represents onset at age 20+ or with duration of less than 10 years. Class C represents onset between the ages of 10 to 19 or with a duration of 10 to 19 years.

In the above patient, what complications is she not at risk of?

    a. Preeclampsia
    b. Macrosomia
    c. Fetal growth restriction
    d. Polydyramnios
    e. Birth defects
    f. She is at risk for all of the above

Answer: f

Pre-existing diabetes places a woman at risk for all of the above. Birth defects are not a risk of gestational diabetes but they are a risk of pregestational diabetes.

A 15-year-old Latina G1P0 at 25 weeks gestation returns for her glucola results which revealed a value of 144. The patient underwent a follow up 3 hour glucose tolerance test with the following results: fasting 102, 1 hour 178, 2 hour 160, 3 hour 135 (normal: fasting 95, 1 hour 180, 2 hour 155, 3 hour 140).

What is your next step in her management?

    a. Begin dietary modifications and glucose surveillance
    b. Start oral hypoglycemics
    c. Start insulin therapy
    d. Repeat the glucose tolerance test at 28 weeks gestation

Answer: a

After an abnormal glucola, the appropriate test is a 3 hour glucose tolerance test. This patient had two abnormal results on this test, which translates to a diagnosis of gestational diabetes. These patients are counseled on dietary modifications and their glucose values are recorded. Only if she fails dietary therapy would she potentially require oral agents or insulin.

A 38-year-old G3P2 presents for preconceptual counseling. She has a history of chronic hypertension, epilepsy (that is currently stable on her medical regimen), and a recent history of a DVT. She is currently taking enalapril, methyldopa, oxcarbazepine, and low molecular weight heparin. She wants to know if these medications pose a risk in pregnancy.

Which of these medications should be changed prior to conception due to its teratogenicity?

a. Enalapril
b. Methyldopa
c. Oxcarbazepine
d. Low molecular weight heparin (LMWH)

Answer: a

Enalapril is associated with multiple congenital malformations and should be avoided in pregnancy. Methyldopa is not associated with any teratogenic effects. All anti-epileptics have the potential for teratogenicity. However, aside from valproate, if a patient is stable on an agent it is best to continue that medication. LMWH is not teratogenic and is safe in pregnancy.

A 18-year-old obese G1P0 at 36 weeks gestation presents to L&D from the office after the finding of new onset hypertension. She has had an uneventful antenatal course and has no medical history. On admission, her BP is 150/92 with a repeat value of 142/88. She denies any headaches, blurry vision, or epigastric/RUQ pain. Her UA revealed trace protein and her serum labs (chemistry, CBC) are normal. An US reveals a 2800 g fetus with normal fluid. She is admitted to the antepartum service for serial BPs and a 24 hour urine collection. Her BPs overnight remain 140-50s/80-90s. Her 24 hour urine results the following day with 640 mg of protein.

What is her diagnosis?

a. Mild preeclampsia
b. Severe preeclampsia
c. Chronic hypertension
d. Gestational hypertension

Answer: a

This patient has new onset hypertension as well as proteinuria (defined as protein greater than 300 mg on a 24 hour collection). Thus, she has preeclampsia. She has mild range BPs (< 160 systolic and < 110 diastolic), no symptoms, and normal serum labs which excludes the diagnosis of severe preeclampsia.

16. A 42-year-old G2P1 presents for preconceptual counseling. She had a history of chronic hypertension, hypothyroidism, genital herpes, and depression. She is currently taking labetolol, levothyroxine, acyclovir, and sertraline. She is concerned with potential adverse effects of these medications and asks which are unsafe in pregnancy.

What medication do you advise she stops taking?

a. Labetolol
b. Levothyroxine
c. Acyclovir
d. Sertraline
e. None, all are safe in pregnancy

Answer: e

All of the above medications are considered to be relatively safe in pregnancy. If they are of benefit to maternal health, they should be continued.

A 22-year-old G1P0 at 39 weeks gestation presents to L&D in spontaneous labor. She had not had prenatal care and a rapid HIV test is drawn on admission which is positive.

Which of the following would best decrease the risk for perinatal HIV transmission?

a. **Maternal IV zidovudine throughout labor**
b. **Neonatal oral zidovudine postpartum**
c. **Early amniotomy to facilitate expeditious delivery**
d. **a and b**

Answer: d

All women without records should have a rapid HIV test done on admission. The limited intervention of administration of zidovudine in labor and to the neonate postpartum can reduce transmission from 25% to 8%. Amniotomy should be avoided in this nulliparous woman, as prolonged rupture of membranes increases transmission rates.

An 18-year-old G3P0 at 27 weeks gestation presents to the ED with shortness of breath. She reports having right sided back pain and subjective fevers for the past 2 days, but felt this was normal for pregnancy. On examination, she is febrile to 102.7°F. Her heart rate is 130 bpm, BP is 72/34, and her respiratory rate is 36 with an O_2 saturation of 86% on room air. She has no fundal tenderness but does have marked tenderness along her right flank. Her pulmonary examination is notable for crackles in the lung bases bilaterally.

What is the most likely etiology for this patient's constellation of symptoms?

a. **Pyelonephritis**
b. **Pneumonia**
c. **Pulmonary embolus**
d. **Chorioamnionitis**

Answer: a

This patient has classic symptoms of pyelonephritis (fevers, costovertebral angle tenderness) with associated sepsis and ARDS. ARDS is associated with pyelonephritis in pregnancy likely due to the reduction in plasma oncotic pressure leading to a lower pulmonary capillary pressure at which pulmonary edema can develop. Pneumonia and a pulmonary embolus are important considerations for hypoxia in a pregnant patient, however they do not explain her CVAT on examination. Chorioamnionitis typically presents with fundal tenderness, which this patient does not exhibit.

A 36-year-old G2P0 at 26 weeks gestational age presents to the office with palpitations, anxiety, lack of sleep, and a 10 lb weight loss over the past 2 weeks. She started to develop substernal chest pain this morning. She has no significant medical history. On examination, she is afebrile with a heart rate of 152 and a BP of 158/82. She appears anxious and her eyes are prominently open. Her thyroid is enlarged but nontender. An EKG reveals sinus tachycardia without ST segment changes.

Which of the following is the appropriate immediate first line therapy?

a. Radioactive iodine
b. Propranolol
c. Lorazepam
d. Propylthiouracil (PTU)

Answer: b

This patient is in thyroid storm, which carries with it a maternal mortality rate of 25%. She must be admitted to the hospital for expeditious care. The immediate concern is her symptoms of chest pain and tachycardia, which will respond to beta-blockage with propranolol. She will then need PTU to block production of thyroid hormones. Radioactive iodine is contraindicated in pregnancy because it concentrates in the fetal thyroid gland and can lead to congenital hypothyroidism. Lorazepam is used to treat various anxiety disorders, which this patient does not have.

A 29-year-old G2P1 at 8 weeks gestation presents for her first prenatal appointment. She has no significant medical history and had an uncomplicated pregnancy and NSVD 3 years ago. Her height is 62 in and her weight is 249 lb.

When counseling, you caution her that she is at increased risk of all except which of the following?

a. Gestational diabetes
b. Preeclampsia
c. Cesarean delivery
d. Oligohydramnios
e. All of the above

Answer: d

This patient is obese, with a BMI over 45 kg/m^2. Maternal obesity is associated with marked increased maternal morbidity including an increased risk of gestational diabetes, preeclampsia, fetal macrosomia, cesarean delivery, and multiple postpartum complications. Oligohydramnios has not been associated with maternal obesity.

A 17-year-old G1P0 at 25 weeks gestation presents to the ER with nausea, vomiting, and midline abdominal cramping pain for 6 hours. She has had an uncomplicated antenatal course to date and has no significant medical history. On examination, she is febrile to 101.5°F. Abdominal examination reveals tenderness and guarding to the right of the umbilicus. Fetal heart tones are in the 170s with moderate variability and 10 × 10 accelerations.

What is the next step in management?

a. Urgent delivery for nonreassuring fetal status
b. An abdominal and pelvic ultrasound
c. An x-ray of the pelvis
d. A fetal growth scan to ensure accurate dating

Answer: b

This patient has signs and symptoms suggestive of appendicitis. Remember, the appendix is often displaced due to the gravid uterus and so the diagnosis is often more difficult to make. The first line of imaging is somewhat controversial, however ultrasound is sensitive and specific and it is not associated with radiation exposure. If the ultrasound is inconclusive, then a CT scan can be performed. An x-ray is not an adequate diagnostic tool for appendicitis. Finally, the fetal heart tones are tachycardic as a result of maternal fever, however they are not nonreassuring and will likely improve once the underlying condition has been treated.

A 15-year-old G1P0 at 37 weeks gestational age presents for a routine prenatal visit. She had an uncomplicated antenatal course. She denies any complaints, but her BP is noted to be 142/94 and 140/88 on a repeat reading. A urinalysis is negative for protein. A review of her initial BP at 10 weeks gestation was 100/60 and she has been normotensive throughout this pregnancy. A chemistry panel and CBC are normal.

What is her diagnosis?

a. Mild preeclampsia
b. Severe preeclampsia
c. Chronic hypertension
d. Gestational hypertension

Answer: d

This patient has new onset hypertension after 20 weeks gestation. This meets criteria for gestational hypertension. If she had elevated blood pressures prior to this gestational age, chronic hypertension would be the more likely diagnosis. She does not have any protein in her urine, has no symptoms of preeclampsia, and has normal labs. Thus, she does not have preeclampsia.

A 42-year-old G1P0 at 18 weeks gestation with a twin gestation is undergoing an ultrasound for anatomy. She asks if these are fraternal or identical twins.

Which of the following would suggest a dizygotic twin gestation?

a. Discordant fetal weights
b. Oligohydramnios in twin A with polyhydramnios in twin B
c. A thin dividing membrane (< 1 mm)
d. A twin peak (lambda sign)

Answer: d

Dizygotic gestations have dichorionic placentas, which can be identified with various ultrasound markers including a dividing membrane > 2 mm, discordant gender, two distinct placenta, or a lambda or peak sign. Answers A and B describe signs of twin twin transfusion syndrome which is more common in monochorioic-diamniotic gestations.

A 34-year-old G2P1 at 12 weeks gestation presents for her first prenatal visit. A type and screen is drawn and she is found to have anti-D antibodies. You begin explaining the risk for fetal anemia and the need for surveillance. She is concerned about invasive testing.

What ultrasonographic test is used to assess fetal anemia?

a. Middle cerebral artery (MCA) peak systolic velocity
b. Umbilical artery blood flow
c. Serial fetal growth
d. Biophysical profile (BPP)

Answer: a

Traditionally, amniocentesis (for an assessment of fetal bilirubin and thus hemolysis) was used to assess fetal anemia in Rh sensitized pregnancies. However repeated amniocenteses are associated with increased risk. US assessment of MCA velocity has been shown to be a sensitive and specific marker for fetal anemia. Umbilical artery blood flow is used to risk stratify the growth restricted fetus. Fetal growth scans are used in pregnancies at risk for growth restriction, not anemia. BPPs are a non-specific assessment of general fetal well-being.

A 31-year-old G2P1 at 24 weeks gestation has been followed in your high risk clinic for having anti-D antibodies.

Which of the following findings would you expect to find as a consequence of this pathology?

a. Fetal ascites
b. Oligohydramnios
c. Placenta accreta
d. Placenta previa

Answer: a

This patient has been alloimmunized and is at risk for the development of fetal hydrops. Hydrops is defined as a collection of fluid in two or more body cavities. This can include ascites, thoracic fluid (pericardial or pleural), and/or scalp edema. Oligohydramnios is not a consequence of alloimmunization, rather occasionally polyhydramnios is seen. Finally, alloimmunization does not affect placentation.

CHAPTER 10

Postpartum Complications

POSTPARTUM MOOD DISORDERS

What are postpartum blues?

Emotional lability and associated transient symptoms of mild depression that do not persist

How common are postpartum blues?

50% to 70% of women

When do they occur?

Within 2 weeks of delivery and typically resolve within 2 weeks; they are attributed to dramatic shift in hormones and decreased progesterone

How common is postpartum depression?

4% to 10%

When does a woman present with postpartum depression?

Between 2 weeks and 4 months postpartum. Depression may last 3 to 14 months.

How is postpartum depression diagnosed?

The criteria is similar to major depressive disorder; five of the following symptoms must be present for 2 weeks: SIGECAPS

Sleep changes

Loss of **I**nterest (anhedonia)

Guilt

Decreased **E**nergy

Decreased Ability to **C**oncentrate

Changes in **A**ppetite

Psychomotor Changes

Suicidal ideation

What is postpartum psychosis?	Development of a sense of false reality often with associated mania or withdrawal
How common is postpartum psychosis?	0.1% to 0.2%

POSTPARTUM HEMORRHAGE

How is postpartum hemorrhage defined?	Blood loss greater than 500 mL following a vaginal birth or a blood loss of greater than 1000 mL following cesarean birth
Postpartum hemorrhage is classified as primary or secondary. What is meant by each type?	**Primary:** occurs within the first 24 hours of delivery; occurs in 4% to 6% of pregnancies. **Secondary:** occurs between 6 to 12 weeks postpartum; occurs in about 1% of pregnancies.
What are the etiologies for primary postpartum hemorrhage and secondary postpartum hemorrhage?	**Uterine atony (80%)** Obstetric lacerations Retained placenta Coagulation defects Uterine inversion
What are etiologies for secondary postpartum hemorrhage?	**Subinvolution of placental site** **Retained products of conception** Infection Coagulation defects
What are risk factors for postpartum hemorrhage?	Prolonged labor, augmented labor, rapid labor, history of postpartum hemorrhage, overdistended uterus (macrosomia, twins, hydramnios), episiotomy, operative delivery, chorioamnionitis
In addition to mortality, what major morbidities follow postpartum hemorrhage?	Adult respiratory distress syndrome (ARDS), coagulopathy, shock, loss of fertility, and pituitary necrosis (Sheehan syndrome)

How does Sheehan syndrome clinically manifest?

Failure to lactate, amenorrhea, decreased breast size, loss of pubic and axillary hair, hypothyroidism, and adrenal insufficiency

How should each of the following be evaluated as a cause of excessive bleeding immediately after placental separation? How is each etiology managed?

Uterine atony: pelvic examination reveals a soft, poorly contracted ("boggy") uterus. Uterine massage and administration of uterotonic medications can help.

Obstetric-related lacerations: careful visual assessment of the lower genital tract is necessary. Proper patient positioning, operative assistance, anesthesia, and proper repair of lacerations are indicated.

Genital tract hematomas: patient complains of pelvic pressure and pain; mass enlargement may be visualized. The hematoma may need to be surgically drained.

Retained products of conception: ultrasound can help diagnose a retained placenta. If manual removal is not possible, curettage may be necessary.

Coagulopathy: patient and/or family history of clotting disorders. CBC, PT/PTT, fibrinogen levels, and a type and cross should be ordered. Blood and blood product transfusion may be necessary.

What are proper supportive measures that should be instituted early in women suspected to have postpartum hemorrhage?

IV access, type and cross, early resuscitation with crystalloids infusions, and communication with anesthesiologists

How can uterine atony and subsequent bleeding be prevented?

Administer uterotonic agents, such as oxytocin, immediately after delivery

If uterotonic agents with or without vaginal tamponade measures fail to control bleeding, what procedure is indicated next?

Exploratory laparotomy

What is the definitive measure to control postpartum hemorrhage?	Hysterectomy
Name some common uterotonics.	Oxytocin (pitocin) Carboprost (hemabate, $PGF_{2\alpha}$) Methylergonovine (methergine) Misoprostol (cytotec)
How do each of the uterotonics act?	Oxytocin: increases uterine tone Carboprost: smooth muscle constriction Methylergonovine: vasocontriction Misoprostol (cytotec): increases uterine tone
What are contraindications to the use of each uterotonic?	Oxytocin: pulmonary edema Carboprost: asthma Methylergonovine: hypertension Misoprostol (cytotec): increases uterine tone
What is uterine inversion?	When the uterine corpus/fundus prolapses to (incomplete inversion) and sometimes through (complete inversion) the uterine cervix. It leads to severe hemorrhage.
In addition to postpartum hemorrhage, what is the immediate morbidity associated with uterine inversion?	Endometritis
What are several conditions that predispose to uterine inversion?	Fundal implantation of the placenta Partial placenta accreta Uterine anomalies Weakness of the myometrium Strong traction exerted on the umbilical cord Fundal pressure
What findings on physical examination suggest an inverted uterus?	A bimanual examination may reveal a firm mass at or below the cervix. An abdominal examination will reveal a depression in the location or the absence of the uterine fundus.

If uterine inversion occurs before placental separation, what should *not* be done?

Removal or detachment of the placenta should *not* be performed. This will cause profound hemorrhage.

How should uterine inversion be managed?

Either manual or surgical repositioning of the uterus

POSTPARTUM AND PUERPERAL INFECTIONS

How is puerperal infection defined?

Puerperal infection is used to describe any infection of the genital tract after delivery.

What are several risk factors for puerperal morbidity secondary to infection?

Lower socioeconomic status
Cesarean delivery
Premature rupture of the membranes
Long labors
Multiple pelvic examinations

What are several types of postpartum infections?

Uterine infection (endometritis)
Respiratory Infections (ARDS, aspiration pneumonia, bacterial pneumonia)
Urinary tract infections (pyelonephritis)
Wound infections
Mastitis
Thrombophlebitis

Most postpartum infections are caused by organisms that are present in the female genital tract and which also normally cause female genital tract infections. What are these common bacterial agents?

Gram-positive cocci: group A, B, and D streptococci, *Staphylococcus aureus*
Gram-positive bacilli: Clostridium species
Aerobic gram-negative bacilli: *Escherichia coli, Klebsiella, Proteus* species
Anaerobic gram-negative bacilli: Bacteroides fragilis group
Other: Mycoplasma species, *Chlamydia trachomatis, Neisseria gonorrhoeae*

What does endometritis in the postpartum period refer to?

It refers to infection of the decidua (ie, pregnancy endometrium), and also the myometrium (endomyometritis) and parametrial tissues (parametritis)

What is the most significant risk factor for endometritis?	The route of delivery The risk of infection is 5 to 10 times higher in cesarean delivery compared to vaginal delivery
Which two bacterial agents have been found to be specific for endometritis?	Bacterial vaginosis and group B streptococcus
How is the diagnosis of endometritis determined?	**Fever (> 100.4°F)** Uterine tenderness Foul lochia Leukocytosis Typically presents on postpartum day 2 or 3
What is the "gold-standard" treatment?	IV clindamycin and gentamycin or IV unasyn (ampicillin-sulbactam) Improvement is usually seen 48 to 72 hours after treatment has begun
If the fever has not subsided after 72 hours of antibiotic administration or after a change in antibiotic therapy, what other sources of fever must be considered?	Wound infection Septic pelvic thrombophlebitis Pelvic abscess Drug-induced fever
Are prophylactic antibiotics indicated in women undergoing cesarean delivery?	Yes. Prophylaxis reduces the rate of endometritis by at least two-thirds. Single agents such as **ampicillin** or **first-generation cephalosporins** are ideal prophylactic antibiotics.
In what setting does chronic endometritis occur?	It occurs when there are retained products of conception after spontaneous abortion, pregnancy termination, or delivery.
What are the clinical manifestations of chronic endometritis?	Fever Irregular vaginal bleeding Pelvic pain Malaise A tender, boggy, and enlarged uterus with bloody and/or purulent discharge on physical examination
What is the treatment of chronic endometritis?	Curettage to remove the necrotic material

CLINICAL VIGNETTES

A 17-year-old G1P0 at 37 weeks gestational age is in your clinic for a routine prenatal visit. When discussing her postpartum course, you begin discussion of breast feeding. She is uncertain if she wishes to breastfeed. Which of the following is a contraindication to breast feeding?

a. Maternal use of labetolol
b. Maternal HIV
c. Active mastitis
d. B and C
e. A, B, and C

Answer: b

There are few absolute contraindications of breast feeding. These include maternal HIV, maternal substance abuse, untreated military TB, ongoing radiation therapy or use of certain chemotherapeutic agents, or active herpetic disease on the breast. Labetolol is compatible with breast feeding. Mastitis is not a contraindication to continuing to breast feed.

A 33-year-old G6P5 with a history of 4 vaginal deliveries and one prior low transverse cesarean section (for breech) precipitously delivered a 4508 g new born vaginally without any complications. The placenta delivered spontaneously and was noted to be intact. Immediately after delivery there was rapid vaginal bleeding and 600 mL of blood was lost. What is the most likely cause of her bleeding?

a. Uterine rupture
b. Uterine atony
c. Cervical laceration
d. Uterine inversion
e. Vaginal laceration

Answer: b

This patient had a postpartum hemorrhage, defined as blood loss of more than 500 mL after a vaginal delivery (or > 1000 mL after a cesarean section). The most common cause of postpartum hemorrhage is atony and this patient has the risk factors of grand multiparity and fetal macrosomia. Uterine rupture would typically present with sudden pain during labor and fetal distress. Cervical lacerations can cause rapid postpartum bleeding, but are epidemiologically less likely. Uterine inversion presents with a protruding pelvic mass along with hemorrhage. Vaginal lacerations can cause bleeding, but are less likely to cause this much blood loss, especially in a multiparous patient.

A 17-year-old G1P0 is postoperative 3 days after a cesarean section done for arrest of descent. Her labor course was complicated by chorioamnionitis for which she was given ampicillin and erythromycin in labor and then 24 hours of gentamycin and clindamycin. She develops a fever to 101.5°F. Her examination is notable for bilateral breast engorgement, mild fundal tenderness, and 2+ symmetric lower extremity edema. What is the most likely source of her fever?

a. Breast engorgement
b. Mastitis
c. Endometritis
d. Deep venous thrombosis (DVT)

Answer: c

Endometritis is the most common cause of fever postpartum. This patient has the risk factors of having a cesarean delivery and having chorioamnionitis. On examination, fundal tenderness is the hallmark sign. While her breasts are engorged on examination, this is not typically a cause of a fever as high as 101.5°F. Her breasts are not asymmetric or erythematous and so mastitis is not likely. Finally, 2+ edema is not an uncommon clinical finding postpartum. Given the symmetric and lack of erythema or tenderness, DVT is an unlikely diagnosis.

SECTION IV

Women's Health Issues

CHAPTER 11

Issues in Women's Health

PREVENTATIVE HEALTH

When should screening for cervical cancer begin?

At the age of 21 years.

How frequent should Pap smears be performed?

The general consensus to date is annual or biennial examinations for women less than 30 years old.

For women more than 30 years old, Paps can be done every 3 years IF HPV testing is done in conjunction. The frequency can be reduced to every 2 to 3 years if they have had 3 normal consecutive Pap smears without concurrent HPV testing.

What is the Breast Cancer Risk Assessment Tool (Gail Model)?

It is a tool that allows calculation of a woman's individual risk of developing breast cancer over the next 5 years and lifetime risk beginning at the age of 35 and until the age of 90. It accounts for patient factors such as current age, race, history of breast cancer, ductal carcinoma in situ, lobular carcinoma in situ, number of first degree relatives with breast cancer, number of previous breast biopsies, age at menarche, and age of first live birth.

It does not account for extended family history, breast density and cystic disease and it has not been validated for all ethnicities.

When should routine breast screening with mammography in an average risk woman begin?

Most major North American groups now advocate for screening to begin at the age of 50 years.

For those between the age of 40 and 50 years, it is recommended that the risks and benefits of mammography be discussed. The decision to have mammography should be determined based on the patient's risk and values after an education discussion with their provider.

How frequently should a screening mammography be performed in an average risk woman?

Every 1 to 2 years

What are the recommendations for clinical breast screening (CBE) examinations?

The American Cancer Society recommends CBE every 3 years between the age of 20 and 39 years, and annually thereafter. Clinical breast examinations should not be used alone as a screening tool. ACS also validates self breast examination (SBE), however, the many other guidelines do not.

When should screening for colon cancer begin in an average risk woman?

Screening for colon cancer should begin at the age of 50 years. Common methods of screening include annual FOBTs (3 samples), flexible sigmoidoscopy every 5 years, and colonoscopy every 10 years.

DOMESTIC VIOLENCE

Describe the epidemiology of domestic violence:

When violence occurs within the household, 90% to 95% of the victims are women. Annually, nearly 5 million women are victims of domestic or intimate partner violence and **one-fifth of American women will be abused by an intimate partner within their lifetime.**

Domestic or intimate partner violence perpetuated against women in family or intimate relationships typically follows a predictable cycle. Describe the three stages of the cycle of violence:

The three phases of the cycle include the following:

1. **Tension-building phase:** usually contains intense arguing and blaming
2. **Battering phase:** characterized by verbal threats, physical battering sexual abuse, or assault with weapons
3. **Honeymoon phase:** is characterized by the abuser's attempt to apologize, deny, or offer gift compensation for previous violence. With time, the tension-building phase gets longer and more frequent, and the honeymoon phase gets shorter and less frequent.

What are four major social risk factors for domestic violence?

Although domestic violence spans all socioeconomic groups, the following tend to be highly associated with a history of domestic violence.

1. **Poverty**
2. **Unemployment**
3. **Alcohol**
4. **Substance abuse**

How do battered women often present for medical care?

Women who are being battered present for medical care with a wide variety of complaints, ranging from **sexual dysfunction** (decreased interest or arousal, dyspareunia, etc) and **persistent somatic complaints** (headaches, abdominal pain, sleep, or eating disorders) to **psychiatric illnesses** (depression, posttraumatic stress disorder [PTSD], or multiple personality disorder). Because there is no pathognomonic presentation of domestic violence, many cases go undiagnosed.

Note: Other factors that should trigger practitioners to inquire regarding possible violence in the home include apparent **noncompliance, frequent emergency room visits, or frequently cancelled appointments.**

What screening questions can be asked of all women to increase the likelihood of diagnosing domestic violence despite its various presentations?

Women presenting for routine preventative care or urgent care visits should be routinely screened for domestic violence regardless of their socioeconomic background.

Stage 1 screening should be directed at specific behaviors. Sample questions include:

Has anyone close to you ever threatened to hurt you?

Has anyone ever hit, kicked, choked, or hurt you physically?

Has anyone, even your partner, ever forced you to have sex against your will?

Are you afraid of your partner?

What questions should be asked after violence has been determined to be present in a household?

Stage 2 screening should **assess safety and lethality of violence and develop a safety plan**. Patients who are unsafe at home should be offered shelter.

Has your partner ever threatened to kill you or your children?

Are there weapons in the house?

Does your partner abuse drugs or alcohol?

Is it safe for you to go home?

Are your children safe at home?

What agencies should be utilized in the referral of a patient who is a victim of domestic violence?

Contact information for local police and emergency departments, women's shelters, rape crisis centers, counseling services, self-help, and advocacy agencies should be given to battered women.

SEXUAL ASSAULT

What is sexual assault?

Sexual assault is the performance of genital, anal, or oral penetration by one person on another without the person's consent.

Describe the epidemiology of sexual assault:

Although some authors estimate that less than 50% of sexual assaults are reported, **nearly 1 million women are sexually assaulted annually.**

Furthermore, 20% of adult women, 15% of college-age women, and 12% of adolescents have been sexually assaulted in their lifetime.

Sexual assault can happen under a variety of conditions and relationships. Describe four special variants of sexual assault:

Marital rape is forced sexual acts within a marital relationship without the consent of a partner. **Acquaintance rape** is sexual assault committed by someone known to the victim. **Incest** involves sexual assault perpetuated by a family member. **Date rape** is sexual assault occurring in the context of a dating relationship.

What is statutory rape?

Statutory rape occurs when an adult has intercourse with a minor, whose age makes him or her legally incapable of consenting to sexual intercourse. Many states mandate physician reporting of statutory rape. Legal definitions for a minor, or someone at the age of consent, vary, depending on jurisdiction.

What is child sexual abuse?

Child sexual abuse is any contact between a child and an adult where the child is being used for sexual stimulation of the adult. This type of behavior must be immediately reported to child protection services.

Date rape drugs diminish a woman's ability either to consent to sexual activity or remember an assault. What drugs are considered date rape drugs?

Many of the **benzodiazepines,** because of their sedative/hypnotic properties and their propensity to cause amnesia can be considered to be date rape drugs. Currently, **flunitrazepam (Rohypnol) and gamma-hydroxybutyrate (GHB)** are the two most frequently used date rape drugs; however, ketamine, chloral hydrate, and MDMA (Ecstasy) have the potential to be abused in this manner.

What is the Rape Trauma Syndrome (RTS) and how does it differ from PTSD?	**Rape Trauma Syndrome is a biphasic PTSD-like condition that occurs within hours to days after a sexual assault and can persist for months to years.** In the acute or disorganization stage, which occurs over 2 weeks following a sexual assault and can have a cyclical relapsing-remitting presentation, the victim's coping mechanisms are impaired leading to either an emotionally labile, expressive catharsis or a controlled, emotional detachment. In the late or reorganization phase, minimal symptoms of PTSD emerge, but do not disrupt the victim's life as in PTSD. During this phase, some victims experience nightmares, flashbacks, feelings of alienation and isolation, depression, and anxiety.
After obtaining informed consent to do a careful history and full, chaperoned physical examination, what specimen will be collected from the patient to look for DNA evidence to identify the perpetrator?	Victim's clothing.
	Air-dried swabs and smears from the oropharynx, vagina, and rectum.
	Cervical mucus for a Pap smear.
	Washings from the skin and vagina.
	Combed specimen from scalp and pubic hair with control samples of the victim's hair from each site.
	Fingernail scrapings and clippings.
	Whole blood samples.
	Saliva samples.
	The patient should be counseled regarding the ability to photograph any physical findings. The consent process for taking pictures should include a discussion of the disposition and confidentiality surrounding these photographs.
What substances contained within the collected specimen will be used as evidence of sexual assault and to identify the perpetrator?	Motile and nonmotile sperm and hair to provide evidence of sexual assault and for DNA
	Acid phosphatase to provide evidence of sexual assault

The following are conditions and their prophylactic treatments the victim should receive immediately after verifying the patient's allergy history.

Condition	Treatment
Chlamydia	Azithromycin (1 g PO) or Doxycycline (100 mg, PO, bid × 7 days)
Gonorrhea	Ceftriaxone (125 mg, IM)
Trichomoniasis	Metronidazole (2 g, PO × 1 or 500 mg bid, PO × 7 days)
Hepatitis B	Hepatitis B immune globulin and Hepatitis B vaccine (0, 1, and 6 months)
HIV	Low risk (basic regimen): ZDV (TDF, d4T or ddI) and 3TC or FTC
	High risk: basic regimen and either LPV/RTV, SQV/RTV, NFV, ATV ± RTV, IDV ± RTV, or FPV ± RTV
Pregnancy	Yuzpe (100 mcg ethinyl estradiol, 0.5 mg levonorgestrel): Q12H × 2
	Plan B (0.75 mg levonorgestrel): Q12H × 2 doses
	Mifepristone (RU 486): 600 mg, PO

ZDV, zidovudine; TDF, tenofovir; d4T, stavudine; ddI, didanosine; 3TC, lamivudine; FTC, emtricitabine; LPV, lopinavir; RTV, ritonavir; SQV, saquinavir; NFV, nefinavir; ATV, atazanavir; IDV, indinavir; FPV, fosamprenavir

ETHICS AND LAW

Two forms of advanced directives include the living will and a durable power of attorney for health care. These structures allow patients to state their preferences for future medical treatment in the event of loss of capacity because of medical illness. How does the living will differ from the power of attorney?

The living will offer a competent adult patient a means to express her wishes and offer informed consent governing the use of life-sustaining treatments in writing in advance of a medical condition that leads to incapacity or incompetence. However, in making a power of attorney, the patient appoints a surrogate decision maker to stand in her place and express her wishes or give informed consent in the event of incapacity or incompetence.

The doctrine of informed consent requires physicians to obtain the patient's permission for treatment, operations, or some diagnostic procedures. What conditions need to be met in order to validate the patient's offering of consent?

A valid informed consent must be voluntarily granted by a competent patient who has full comprehension of the risk, benefits, alternatives, and consequences of the relevant, available diagnostic or treatment options.

Under what circumstances is the requirement of informed consent waived?

Informed consent is often not required before administering treatment or performing lifesaving procedures in a medical emergency, preventing suicide, or attending to minors in the absence of a parent.

In general, the information disclosed by a patient during a physician consultation is strictly confidential, and thus should not be revealed without the patient's consent, unless disclosure is required by law. Under what circumstances is the maintenance of strict patient confidentiality not required?

Patient confidentiality can be broken under the following circumstances:

When a patient discloses an intention to inflict serious bodily harm on herself or another person.

In the event of a life-threatening emergency.

When a reportable, communicable disease has been diagnosed.

However, in these and other cases, disclosure is permitted only to those for whom it is medically or legally necessary.

Laws governing malpractice are formed by two mechanisms, from legislative action or from judicial opinion rendered during precedent cases. Under which type of law do most malpractice claims proceed?

Most malpractice claims proceed under the body of law defined by judicial opinion derived from precedent cases, or common law. A dynamic body of law, common law is constantly changing and thus continually redefining the grounds for potential litigation.

What are the four principles that must be proven in order to establish medical liability in a negligence suit?

Medical liability requires the plaintiff to demonstrate the presence of duty, breach of duty, causation, and consequent damages. Causation is defined as the link between the alleged breach of duty and an injury and must be supported by proof of causation. Damages constitute demonstrable injuries and can either be purely economic (eg, lost wages) or noneconomic (eg, pain and suffering).

Identify the elements needed to prove malpractice in a wrongful birth and wrongful conception claim:

In a wrongful birth claim, a clinician interviewing a pregnant couple (duty) omits the family history and fails to recognize a serious disability that has a hereditary or genetic basis (breach of duty). Consequently, a baby with appreciable disabilities is born (damages) to parents who would have sought termination, but for the clinician's failure, which prevented proper counseling. In a wrongful conception claim, a clinician treating a nonpregnant couple (duty) fails to provide histologic evidence of sterilization during a tubal ligation or provides improper contraceptive counseling or techniques (breach of duty).

Consequently, a normal but unwanted child is born (damages) to the couple seeking sterilization or effective contraception.

CLINICAL VIGNETTES

A 36-year-old woman presents to her internist for evaluation of a lump in her right breast. The physician palpates a 2.0 cm by 2.0 cm lump in the upper outer quadrant of the right breast. She has no history of fibrocystic breast disease and no family history of breast cancer. A mammogram is ordered, which comes back normal. What is the next step in appropriate management?

a. Reassure the patient that no further workup is necessary since her mammogram is normal and she has no family history of breast cancer.
b. Repeat mammogram in 6 months.
c. Testing for BRCA-1 and BRCA-2 now.
d. Breast ultrasound now with fine-needle aspiration.

Answer: d

All palpable breast masses need to undergo a full evaluation. Bilateral mammogram is an useful initial imaging test because it may identify other breast abnormalities that are not palpable on examination. It can also help localize the area for biopsy. However, a negative mammogram should not deter a physician from further workup. The false negative rate of a mammogram is 10%. This patient requires further evaluation by breast ultrasonography with fine-needle aspiration (choice d). Reassuring the patient that no further evaluation is unnecessary (choice a) or repeating the mammogram in 6 months (choice b) will miss or delay diagnosis and therefore are incorrect. Testing for a genetic mutation (choice c) is premature at this stage as the mass has not been diagnosed histologically. As well, there is no known family history of breast cancer.

A 16-year-old female comes to you during free clinic hours and tells you that she had unprotected sex the night before. She is concerned about the possibility of pregnancy. She asks if you can give her emergency contraception (Plan B) as well as prescribe oral contraceptive pills (OCPs). She asks you not to tell her mother. What do you do?

a. Tell her you that you are legally obliged to ask for parental consent for Plan B and OCPs before prescribing it to her.
b. Tell her that you are legally obliged to ask for parental consent for OCPs but not Plan B before prescribing it to her.
c. Tell her that you are legally obliged to ask for parental consent for Plan B but not OCPs before prescribing them.
d. Reassure her that you will not break patient confidentiality and prescribe both Plan B and OCPs for the patient.

Answer: d

Typically, parental consent is not required for dispensing contraception, treating sexually transmitted infections, or treating mental health/substance abuse disorders. Reassurance of patient confidentiality is important in developing a therapeutic alliance with the adolescent patient.

CHAPTER 12

Review Questions and Answers

REVIEW QUESTIONS

1. During a first trimester surgical abortion, signs of complete evacuation include all given except which of the following?

   a. Gritty sensation
   b. Contraction around the uterus
   c. Bubbles in the cannula and hose
   d. Bleeding from the os

2. A 62-year-old woman presents to your office with complaints of 6-month history of intense and painful vulvar itching. She also states that she can feel a "small lump." She denies any vaginal bleeding. Her past medical, surgical, and family history are unremarkable. Examination of the vulvar reveals a small fleshy outgrowth on her left labia majora. A biopsy is performed and pathology reveals squamous cell carcinoma in situ. Which of the following statements is most appropriate in the management of this patient?

   a. Postoperative radiation is recommended
   b. Careful observation for the next 6 months to see if the growth enlarges or remains the same is recommended
   c. Colposcopy of the vagina and cervix should be done postoperatively
   d. Total vulvectomy is recommended
   e. Groin dissection is necessary

3. A 45-year-old woman presents to her gynecologist with complaints of amenorrhea for 7 months. She denies any symptoms of vasomotor instability. Her laboratory work reveals a negative BhCG and a decreased LH and FSH. What is the most likely cause of her amenorrhea?

   a. Menopause
   b. Hypothalamic-pituitary dysfunction
   c. Outflow obstruction
   d. Pregnancy

4. Why is there an increase in total T_4 and T_3 concentrations during pregnancy?
    a. Pregnancy is a state of physiologic stress with up regulation all hormones
    b. β-hCG stimulates TSH receptors
    c. Liver production of binding globulins is decreased
    d. Fetal production results in increased maternal concentrations

5. Maternal obesity is a risk factor for all of the fetal complications except which of the following?
    a. Fetal macrosomia
    b. Neural-tube defects
    c. Dizygotic twinning
    d. Stillbirth

6. Your patient presents at 30 weeks with complaints of vaginal bleeding. There is currently no active vaginal bleeding. She is admitted to a labor room for evaluation. A fetal heart strip is obtained and reveals an FHR of 130 bpm with no accelerations or decelerations. An ultrasound is obtained and reveals a partial previa. What is the next step in management?
    a. Observation in L&D
    b. Assessment of fetal lung maturity
    c. Cesarean delivery
    d. Gentle cervical examination to assess dilation and amnionic membrane status

7. What is the most common complication arising from a first trimester surgical pregnancy termination?
    a. Uterine perforation
    b. Cervical trauma
    c. Retained products of conception
    d. Pelvic infection
    e. Vaginal laceration

8. An 18-year-old female with no history of STIs and who has had two sexual partners presents to her gynecologists office for her last dose of her HPV vaccine. She asks how often she needs to have a Pap smear. What is the correct response?
    a. Every 3 years
    b. Every 5 years
    c. Annually
    d. Never again—she is now immune to HPV

9. A 26-year-old woman presents with 8 months of irregular bleeding. Bleeding occurs at markedly irregular intervals and varies in its quantity. A progesterone challenge test demonstrates withdrawal bleeding. Which of the following laboratory work is not indicated for the evaluation of dysfunctional uterine bleeding in this woman?
    a. CBC
    b. Coagulation profile
    c. Endocrine profile (TSH, LH, FSH, prolactin)
    d. Endometrial biopsy

10. All of the following increase during pregnancy except which of the following?
    a. Tidal volume
    b. Minute ventilation
    c. Total lung capacity
    d. Alveolar partial pressure of oxygen

11. Your pregnant patient has mitral stenosis and is New York Heart Association functional class II. Which of the following sets of vaccinations is indicated during her pregnancy?
    a. Influenza, pneumococcal, intrapartum bacterial endocarditis prophylaxis
    b. Influenza, pneumococcal, group B streptococcal vaginal and rectal culture at 36 weeks
    c. Influenza, pneumococcal, intrapartum bacterial endocarditis prophylaxis, group B streptococcal vaginal and rectal culture at 36 weeks
    d. Influenza and pneumococcal vaccine

12. Which of the following lower genital tract organisms is not associated with increased puerperal infection?
    a. *Trichomonas vaginalis*
    b. Group B streptococcus
    c. *Gardnerella vaginalis*
    d. *Mycoplasma hominis*

13. A 41-year-old G3P3 presents to the emergency department with complaints of unrelenting lower abdominal pain. She denies nausea and vomiting but reports subjective fevers. In the emergency department, she is febrile to 100.9°F. Pelvic examination reveals a mobile 12-week-size uterus with point tenderness midline in the lower abdomen, no cervical motion tenderness, no discharge. UA is significant for few white cells with many squamous cells. You obtain an ultrasound which reveals a myomatous uterus with multiple subserosal anterior myoma of 6-cm size with internal components suggestive of calcification and necrosis; adnexal structures are within normal limits. What is this patient's diagnosis?
    a. PID
    b. Cystitis
    c. Degenerating fibroid
    d. Appendicitis

14. A 62-year-old G2P2002 presented for her gynecological visit and was found to have HSIL. A colposcopy was performed and found to be negative; however the SCJ was unable to be visualized. Which is the next appropriate step in management?
    a. Conization
    b. Repeat Pap smear within 3 months
    c. Endocervical curettage
    d. Biopsy of cervical tissue

15. The above patient underwent conization via LEEP which was found to be negative. Which of the following follow-up management is the most appropriate?

  a. Repeat Pap smear in 4 to 6 months
  b. Repeat Pap smear in 1 year
  c. Repeat colposcopy in 6 months
  d. Repeat conization in 6 months

16. A 37-year-old woman is diagnosed with invasive squamous cell carcinoma of the cervix. She is found to have minimal microscopic stromal invasion that is confined to the cervix. She has completed childbearing. What is the most appropriate treatment option?

  a. Simple hysterectomy
  b. Radical hystectomy
  c. Radiotherapy
  d. Combination chemotherapy

17. For a patient with osteoporosis, which of the following laboratory abnormalities would you expect?

  a. High calcium, low phosphorous, low PTH
  b. Low calcium, high phosphorous, high PTH
  c. Low calcium, low phosphorous, low PTH
  d. No laboratory abnormalities

18. According to the World Health Organization (WHO), osteoporosis is defined as which of the following?

  a. Bone mineral density (BMD) between 1.5 to 2.0 standard deviations below the mean for young normal adults (T score)
  b. BMD is between 1.5 to 2.0 standard deviations below the mean for age-matched adults (Z score)
  c. BMD is less than 2.5 standard deviations below the mean for young normal adults (T score)
  d. BMD is less than 2.5 standard deviations below the mean for age-matched adults (Z score)

19. How does progesterone affect various organ systems during pregnancy?

  a. Lowers diastolic blood pressure less than systolic
  b. Increases lower esophageal sphincter tone causing painful spasms
  c. Decreases the central respiratory drive resulting in dyspnea of pregnancy
  d. Reduces ureteral tone, decreases peristalsis, and relaxes the bladder wall

20. Which surgical procedure is most commonly performed in the second trimester?

  a. Ovarian cystectomy
  b. Cholecystectomy
  c. Laparoscopy
  d. Appendectomy

21. During the third stage of labor, your patient's uterus inverts and the placenta becomes detached from the uterus. Which of the following is the next nest step in management?

    a. Prompt oxytocin administration
    b. Attempt to manually replace the uterus
    c. Prompt hysterectomy
    d. Administration of inhalation anesthetics prior to manual replacement

22. Typically, when do postabortal infections present?

    a. Within the first 24 to 36 hours
    b. Within the first 48 to 96 hours
    c. Within the first 6 days
    d. After at least 1 week postprocedure

23. A 65-year-old woman presents to her gynecologist with complaints of progressive vulvar itching and perineal pain. On examination, there is diffuse atrophy with one raised, whitish area on the posterior aspect of the vulva. What is the most appropriate first step in her management?

    a. Trial of low dose corticosteroid cream
    b. Trial of high dose corticosteroid cream
    c. Trial of topical antifungal cream
    d. Vulvar biopsy of the affected area

24. The biopsy results for the above patient demonstrate VIN II. What is the most appropriate treatment for her?

    a. Chemotherapy
    b. Complete local excision
    c. Wide excision with laser ablation
    d. Chemotherapy followed by localized radiation

25. What is the major cause of menopause related bone loss?

    a. Decline in calcium production
    b. Decline in calcium absorption
    c. Decline in estrogen levels
    d. Rise in LH and FSH levels

26. Herniation of the peritoneum between the uterosacral ligaments through the pouch of Douglas into the rectovaginal septum represents which of the following defects?

    a. Uterine prolapse
    b. Rectocele
    c. Enterocele
    d. Urethrocele
    e. Cystocele
    f. Retrodisplacement of the uterus

27. What uterotonic is not appropriate to administer a woman with preeclampsia?
   a. Oxytocin (pitocin)
   b. Carboprost (hemabate)
   c. Methylergonovine (methergine)
   d. Misoprostol (cytotec)

28. All of the following mothers are advised to breastfeed except?
   a. HIV with a low viral count
   b. Fluctuant and indurated mastitis
   c. Current hepatitis A infection
   d. Hepatitis B following infant vaccination and IgG administration

29. When does menstruation begin in a postpartum woman?
   a. Average duration is about 20 weeks postpartum in a breastfeeding woman
   b. Average duration is about 8 weeks postpartum in a breastfeeding woman
   c. Average duration is about 20 weeks in a postpartum nonlactating woman
   d. Average duration is about 8 weeks postpartum in a nonlactating woman

30. During a suction D&C, the surgeons note a midline perforation. If the uterus is not completely evacuated, all of the below options may be indicated except which of the following?
   a. Continue with the same procedure
   b. Exploratory laparotomy
   c. Perform US
   d. Exploratory laparoscopy

31. A 28-year-old woman present to you with symptoms of a leiomyoma. Which set of symptoms is most consistent with a leiomyoma?
   a. Hirsutism, acne, amenorrhea, virulizatio
   b. Pelvic pain, dyspareunia, urinary incontinence, menorrhagia
   c. Dysmenorrhea, dyspareunia, infertility, painful defecation

32. Which of the following sets describes the clinical appearance of lichen sclerosis?
   a. Moist, thick, white, scaly plaques
   b. Nontender ulcerative lesions
   c. White, thin, atrophic appearing plaques
   d. Excoriated, thickened, and erythematous epithelium

33. A 21-year-old woman presents to you complaining of a 1 month history of pyruria and dyspareunia. She is newly married and returned from her honeymoon 2 weeks ago. She is concerned that this will affect her marriage. What is the most likely cause of her discomfort?
   a. Trichomonas
   b. Candida
   c. *Escherichia coli*
   d. Lactobacillus
   e. Inadequate vaginal lubrication

34. An Rh negative mother has just undergone a normal spontaneous vaginal delivery with significant postpartum hemorrhage attributed to atony. What test would assist in determining how much RhoGam should be administered postpartum?
    a. Quantitative titer analysis of maternal circulating antibodies
    b. Flow cytometry to determine which isoforms the mother has developed
    c. Kleihauer-Betke serum stain
    d. Indirect Coombs test

35. A woman with gestational diabetes class A1 and poor glycemic control requests a repeat cesarean deliver. Fetal lung maturity (FLM) at 37 weeks shows a lecithin/sphingomyelin ratio of 2.2/1 and phosphatdylglycerol negative. Following delivery, the infant develops respiratory distress syndrome (RDS). What about the patient's history would suggest that the infant was as risk for RDS?
    a. Two or more types of fetal lung maturity tests should be used when determining the risk of RDS.
    b. Elective cesarean delivery should only take place after 39 weeks.
    c. The amniocentesis was likely contaminated with blood resulting in a false L/S ratio.
    d. Surfactant function and production is adversely affected by increased fetal insulin and maternal diabetes.

36. Which class of gestational diabetes in NOT at increased risk for unexplained stillbirth?
    a. A1
    b. A2
    c. B
    d. C

37. With preexisting diabetes, what fetal malformation is most strongly associated with diabetes?
    a. Neural-tube defects
    b. Congenital heart defects
    c. Caudal regression
    d. Renal agenesis

38. A 21-year-old woman presents to the emergency department stating that she was raped. Which of the medications should be given to her for prevention of STDs?
    a. Ceftriaxone plus azithromycin
    b. Ceftriaxone plus cefixime
    c. Ceftriaxone plus doxycycline
    d. Ceftriaxone plus penicillin

39. A 31-year-old woman presents to you with complaints of intense vaginal itching and frothy discharge with malodorous odor. Pelvic examination reveals greenish-gray discharge with numerous "strawberry like" punctate marks on the cervix. What is the proper treatment for this patient?

    a. Fluconzazole
    b. Estrogen Cream
    c. Metronidazole
    d. Penicillin
    e. Doxcycline

40. Your 23-year-old woman has mild endometriosis. Her symptoms include irregular menses with no pelvic pain. Which of the following is the best treatment for her?

    a. Oral estrogen
    b. GnRH agonists
    c. Danazol
    d. Oral contraceptive pills
    e. Medroxyprogesterone acetate

41. A 34-year-old woman had a colposcopic examination with a negative biopsy result. Her endocervical canal curettage result returned positive. What is the next appropriate step in management?

    a. Observe for the next 4 to 6 months
    b. No follow-up is needed
    c. Repeat colposcopic examination in the next 2 to 3 months
    d. Vaginal hysterectomy
    e. Perform conization of the cervix

42. Which of the following sets contain the most important risk factors for cervical cancer?

    a. The use of oral contraceptives
    b. Family history of cervical cancer
    c. Marriage at an early age and having HSV-1
    d. History of smoking, multiple sex partners, and first intercourse in the adolescent years
    e. Multiparous woman with marriage at a late age

43. A 21-year-old G0 with a history of irregular menses presents for her first gynecologic examination. Pelvic examination reveals fullness in the right adnexa. The examination is otherwise unremarkable. You obtain a transvaginal ultrasound which reveals a thin-walled 4-cm unilocular clear fluid appearing cystic structure in the right ovary. How do you manage this patient?

    a. Send tumor markers
    b. Followup sonogram in 3 to 6 months
    c. Drainage of the cyst via transvaginal approach
    d. Laparoscopy and cystectomy

44. An 18-year-old female presents to the emergency department with acute right sided pain. She reports nausea and vomiting and states that her pain is unrelenting when it is present though it seems to "come and go" over the last few hours. Her examination is significant for involuntary rebound and guarding. You obtain a transvaginal ultrasound, which reveals an adnexal mass consistent with a 7-cm unilocular structure with both hyperechoic and hypoechoic components. How do you manage this patient?

    a. Call general surgery consult for suspected appendicitis
    b. Paracentesis of adnexal structure
    c. Laparscopy and oophorectomy
    d. Laparoscopy and cystectomy

45. A 72-year-old woman presents to her gynecologist with purities and soreness of the vulva. On inspection, there are multiple well-demarcated white hyperkeratotic areas on a bright red background. What is the most likely diagnosis?

    a. Squamous cell carcinoma of the vulva
    b. Basal cell carcinoma of the vulva
    c. Paget's disease of the vulva
    d. Vulvar melanoma

46. A 62-year-old postmenopausal woman presents to your office with episodic vaginal bleeding over the past 3 months. Which of the following is most likely?

    a. Perimenopausal spotting
    b. Adrenal hyperplasia
    c. Cancer
    d. Fibroids

47. A 16-year-old G1P1 presents to her obstetrician 4 weeks postpartum with increased vaginal bleeding. An ultrasound is performed which reveals heterogeneous material in the uterus. Which of the following steps should be used in management?

    a. D&C
    b. Serum BhCG level
    c. CXR
    d. Expectant management

48. What is the most common cause of female sexual dysfunction?

    a. Vaginismus
    b. Inhibited sexual desire
    c. Arousal disorder
    d. Anorgasmia

49. Which antidepressant listed below is the best to avoid sexual dysfunction?

    a. Prozac
    b. Zoloft
    c. Wellbutrin
    d. Effexor

50. A patient with amenorrhea does not have withdrawal bleeding after a progesterone challenge test. What is the next test that is indicated?

    a. An estrogen-progesterone test
    b. Head CT
    c. Hysteroscopy
    d. Laparoscopy

51. When following up on the results of a DEXA scan for one of your postmenopausal patients, you notice her BMD is 1.5 standard deviations below the mean. What is her diagnosis?

    a. Normal age related bone loss
    b. Osteopenia
    c. Osteoporosis
    d. Osteomalacia

52. A 17-year-old female presents to her gynecologist with complaints of cramping lower abdominal pain that begins with menstruation. She also admits to mild nausea and diarrhea around the same time. Her physical examination is unremarkable. What should be used as first-line therapy?

    a. NSAIDS
    b. Oral contraceptive pills
    c. Presacral neurectomy
    d. Antispasmodic agents

53. An 18-year-old female with no prenatal care presents to L&D in labor. After delivery, her neonate infant is found to have sensorineural deafness, cataracts, PDA, hepatosplenomegaly, hyperbilirubinemia, and blue purpura that appear like blueberry muffin. What congenital infection is the most likely culprit?

    a. Toxoplasma
    b. Rubella
    c. Cytomegalovirus
    d. Syphillis

54. Which of the following are modalities of mother-to-child HIV transmission?

    a. Transplacental infection
    b. Peripartum infection
    c. Breast feeding
    d. All of the above

55. A 28-year-old woman presents with increasing pelvic pain with menstruation that is not relieved with NSAIDS. Physical examination reveals some uterine immobility as well as tender nodularities in the posterior cul de sac. What is the most likely diagnosis?

    a. Primary dysmenorrhea
    b. Endometriosis
    c. Leiomyomas
    d. Adenomyosis

56. A 22-year-old G1P0 presents with uterine bleeding at 8 weeks gestation. On physical examination, her cervix is found to be dilated to 2 cm. Vaginal ultrasound reveals products of conception in the uterine cavity. What is her diagnosis?

   a. Complete abortion
   b. Inevitable abortion
   c. Incomplete abortion
   d. Missed abortion

57. A 28-year-old G3P1011 at 10 weeks gestation presents to the emergency department with uterine bleeding. Her cervix is found to be closed and her BhCG is at an appropriate level for the stated gestational age. Ultrasound reveals a nonviable fetus in the uterine cavity. What is her diagnosis?

   a. Complete abortion
   b. Inevitable abortion
   c. Incomplete abortion
   d. Missed abortion

58. A 42-year-old G3P3 presents with 12 weeks of amenorrhea, nausea, vomiting, and mild tremors. Ultrasound reveals a heterogenous intrauterine mass with theca-lutein cysts that appears like a snowstorm. What is the most likely diagnosis?

   a. Early intrauterine pregnancy
   b. Perimenopause
   c. Partial mole
   d. Complete mole

59. A G3P3 female presents 2 months postpartum with irregular vaginal bleeding. Physical examination reveals an enlarged uterus with bilateral ovarian cysts. Ultrasonographic evaluation reveals an enlarging, heterogenous, hypervascular mass in the uterus with areas of hemorrhage and necrosis. What is the most likely diagnosis?

   a. Pregnancy
   b. Partial mole
   c. Complete mole
   d. Choriocarcinoma

60. A 65-year-old menopausal woman presents to your office with complaints of urinary difficulty and discomfort in the vagina. She complains that the feeling in her vagina is like she is "sitting on an egg" and she desires definitive treatment. What is the appropriate therapy?

   a. Remove the foreign body
   b. Vaginal hysterectomy
   c. Pessary placement
   d. Reassurance

61. In evaluating an infertile couple, the postcoital test is performed to assess which of the following?

   a. Interaction of sperm with cervical mucus prior to ovulation
   b. Interaction of sperm with cervical mucus anytime during the cycle
   c. Interaction of sperm with cervical mucus prior to ovulation
   d. Interaction of sperm with cervical in mid-luteal phase

62. All of the following may be direct causes of female infertility except which of the following?

   a. Previous uncomplicated abortion
   b. Endometriosis
   c. Pelvic inflammatory disease (PID)
   d. Hyperprolactinemia
   e. Polycystic ovarian syndrome (PCOS)

63. All of the following cause persistent or increasing levels of β-hCG except?

   a. Retained products of conception
   b. Trophoblastic disease
   c. Choriocarcinoma
   d. Complete spontaneous abortion

Match each of the following terms to their correct description:

64. Prolonged, irregular menstrual bleeding   a. menorrhagia

65. Prolonged, regular menstrual bleeding   b. metrorrhagia

66. Irregular menstrual bleeding   c. menometrorrhagia

67. What is the "gold standard" for the diagnosis of genital herpes virus in adults?

   a. ELISA or serology
   b. DNA probes
   c. Tissue culture
   d. Cytological examination

68. A 29-year-old G1P0 presents to L&D after 3 hours of painful contractions occurring every 3 minutes. Her initial cervical examination on the floor was 5/80%/-2. Two hours later no change in noted. An IUPC is placed and her contractions are found to have 250 Montevideo units over the next 2 hours. What is the most appropriate diagnosis?

   a. Normal latent labor
   b. Arrest of labor
   c. Protraction of labor
   d. Inadequate contractions

69. An ultrasound is preformed at a 28-week prenatal visit, the fetus is found to be in breech presentation with its hips and knees flexed. What type of breech presentation is this?

   a. Frank breech
   b. Complete breech
   c. Footling breech

70. A G2P1001 is in active labor with her last cervical examination two hours prior of 3/90%/-1. You begin to notice decelerations on the monitor. The decelerations rapidly drop approximately 20 bpm below baseline, quickly return to baseline, and appear unrelated to uterine contractions. What causes this type of deceleration?

    a. Fetal scalp compression
    b. Uteroplacental insufficiency
    c. Umbilical cord compression
    d. Fetal acidosis

71. A 21-year-old woman with a history of PID presents to the emergency department with right sided pelvic pain and vaginal bleeding. She is hemodynamically stable. Her LMP was 8 weeks ago and her urine BhCG is positive. What is the next appropriate step in management?

    a. Serum BhCG
    b. Transvaginal ultrasound
    c. Immediate laparoscopy
    d. Immediate laparotomy

72. A 21-year-old G0 with a history of irregular menses presents for her first gynecologic examination. Pelvic examination reveals fullness in the right adnexa. The examination is otherwise unremarkable. You obtain a transvaginal ultrasound which reveals a thin-walled 4 cm unilocular clear fluid appearing cystic structure in the right ovary. How do you manage this patient?

    a. Send tumor markers
    b. Followup sonogram in 3 to 6 months
    c. Drainage of the cyst via transvaginal approach
    d. Laparoscopy and cystectomy

73. A 52-year-old woman has been experiencing signs of menopause, including increasing hot flushes during day and night, difficulty sleeping, emotional lability, and anxiety. She denies any other complaints or medical illnesses. Her last period was approximately 12 months ago. Her vital signs are all within normal range. Her pelvic examination reveals atrophic external genitalia, a small anteverted uterus, and no adnexal masses. The rest of her examination is normal. What is the most effective treatment option for this patient?

    a. Progestin alone
    b. Estrogen alone (ERT)
    c. Antidepressants
    d. Estrogen with progestin (hormone replacement therapy (HRT)

74. Your current patient is pregnant and has a history of DVT in her previous pregnancy. How should she be managed during this pregnancy?

    a. Low dose aspirin
    b. Careful observation
    c. Prophylactic-dose subcutaneous heparin
    d. Full prophylactic dose subcutaneous heparin

75. Your patient is pregnant and is found to be positive for hepatitis C. Which of the following outcomes is associated with hepatitis C?

    a. Abruptio placentae
    b. Fetal growth restriction
    c. Vertical transmission of hepatitis C
    d. Preterm birth

76. At which of the following time periods does zygotic division formation of dichorionic, diamnionic twins occur following fertilization?

    a. More than 264 hours
    b. More than 120 and less than or equal to 240 hours
    c. More than 72 and less than or equal to 120 hours
    d. Less than or equal to 72 hours

77. Which of the following hemodynamic values remains unchanged in pregnancy?

    a. Pulmonary vascular resistance
    b. Colloid osmotic pressure
    c. Pulmonary capillary pressure
    d. Systemic vascular resistance

78. What screening test is listed with the appropriate condition?

    a. Maternal serum alpha fetal protein and neural tube defects
    b. Urine dip and gestational diabetes
    c. Magnetic resonance imaging and cleft lip
    d. Percutaneous umbilical blood sampling and Rh isoimmunization

79. What is the appropriate diagnostic test for the following?

    a. Maternal serum alpha fetal protein and aneuploidies
    b. Amniocentesis and Down syndrome
    c. Glucose challenge test and gestational diabetes.
    d. Biophysical profile and fetal lung maturity

80. A distraught couple presents to your office upset of not being able to conceive after 1 year of regular, unprotected intercourse. The female is a nulligravid, takes no medication, and denies any medical illnesses. The husband reports that he is healthy as well and has never father a child before. What is the most appropriate initial step in the evaluation of this couple?

    a. Basal body temperature charting
    b. Postcoital test
    c. Semen analysis, including sperm antibodies
    d. History and physical examination of both couples
    e. Laparoscopy

81. Which of the following is the most common cause of precocious puberty in females?

    a. Adrenal tumor
    b. Ovarian tumor
    c. Idiopathic
    d. Functional ovarian cyst

82. The amniotic membranes in the above patient are artificially ruptured in order to accelerate labor. The fluid is noted to be clear with a slightly greenish tint. Of what is the fetus at risk?

    a. Renal failure
    b. Conjunctivitis
    c. Toxoplasmosis
    d. Chemical pneumonitis

83. According to the World Health Organization (WHO), how is osteoporosis defined?

    a. Bone mineral density (BMD) between 1.5 to 2.0 standard deviations below the mean for young normal adults (T score)
    b. BMD is between 1.5 to 2.0 standard deviations below the mean for age-matched adults (Z score)
    c. BMD is less than 2.5 standard deviations below the mean for young normal adults (T score)
    d. BMD is less than 2.5 standard deviations below the mean for age-matched adults (Z score)

84. How is zero station determined on sterile vaginal examination?

    a. The leading fetal edge is flush with the introitus
    b. The leading fetal edge is parallel with the maternal ischial spines
    c. The leading fetal edge is engaged in the maternal pelvis
    d. The leading fetal edge is engaged in a fully dilated cervix

85. A pregnant patient presents with symptoms and signs of thyrotoxic storm. All of the below medications are indicated except which of the following?

    a. Potassium iodide
    b. Magnesium sulfate
    c. Dexamethasone
    d. Propylthiouracil

86. A 36-year-old woman has heavy, painless bleeding every 4 to 5 months. She comes to your office asking for contraceptives. An examination of her cervix is normal and her Pap smear is NIL. What is the most appropriate procedure?

    a. Oral estrogen only
    b. Bilateral-salpingo-oophorectomy
    c. Cyclic oral contraceptive agents
    d. Fractional dilation and curettage (d and c)
    e. Conization of the cervix

87. A 44-year-old woman is diagnosed with epithelial ovarian cancer. She is found to have cancer that is limited to one ovary with extension to the uterus and fallopian tubes. What ovarian cancer stage should be assigned to this patient?

    a. Stage 1
    b. Stage IIA
    c. Stage IIB
    d. Stage IIC
    e. Stage III

88. Tubal patency or "pelvic factor" in evaluation of infertility is best accomplished by which of the following?

    a. Hysterosalpingogram (HSG)
    b. Hysteroscopy
    c. Pelvic magnetic resonance imaging (MRI)
    d. Transvaginal ultrasound
    e. Pelvic CT scan

89. Through chromosome analysis, you find that your patient has a sex genotype of XO. What is the proper therapeutic regimen for this patient?

    a. Androgens and cortisol
    b. Cortisol and human growth hormone
    c. Small doses of estrogen in early childhood
    d. Progesterone, estrogen, and cortisol
    e. Androgens, human growth hormones, small doses of estrogen, and later progesterone

90. What is the gold standard for the diagnosis of osteoporosis?

    a. Plain x-ray of the thoracic spine
    b. Qualitative ultrasound densitometry
    c. Peripheral DXA
    d. Central DXA
    e. A QCT

91. Your patient has a history of epilepsy and is also found to be pregnant. She refuses to take antiepileptic medications. Of which of the following complications are fetuses at an increased risk?

    a. Fetal growth restriction
    b. Congenital malformation
    c. Seizure disorder
    d. Perinatal death

92. All of the following drugs can be used for the treatment of migraine headaches during pregnancy except?

    a. Propanolol
    b. Meperidine
    c. Amitriptyline
    d. Ergonovine

93. What is the best treatment for syphilis in a penicillin-allergic patient during pregnancy?

    a. Penicillin desensitization
    b. Tetracycline
    c. Ceftriaxone
    d. Erythromycin

94. Which of the following is increased in pregnancies complicated by sickle-cell trait?

    a. UTI
    b. Low birthweight
    c. Perinatal mortality
    d. Spontaneous abortion

95. A multigravid mother has a history of previous GBS negative pregnancies, a GBS+ urinary tract infection during the current pregnancy, and a negative GBS culture at 36 weeks. She presents to labor and delivery with spontaneous rupture of membranes and contractions every 5 minutes. Which of the following is indicated?

    a. Immediate urine analysis for signs of current infection
    b. Immediate urine culture and rectal swab for identification of GBS status
    c. Empiric treatment for unknown GBS status
    d. Antibiotics immediately due to history of GBS colonization

96. What is the difference between gestational hypertension and preeclampsia?

    a. Proteinuria is present in preeclampsia, and it is absent in gestational hypertension.
    b. Patient has a history of hypertension in gestational hypertension
    c. Patient exhibits sustained elevated blood pressures in preeclampsia
    d. Patient reports lower extremity pitting edema

97. What is the cure for preeclampsia?

    a. Magnesium sulfate
    b. Delivery
    c. Nifedipine
    d. Diazepam

98. What is not a complication of placenta previa?

    a. Maternal hemorrhage
    b. Placenta accrete
    c. Gestational diabetes
    d. Preterm premature rupture of the membranes (PPROM)

99. What intrapartum obstetrical maneuvers are used to treat a shoulder dystocia?

    a. McRoberts maneuver
    b. Fundal pressure
    c. Decreasing anesthesia so to facilitate maternal effort
    d. Placing the mother in the left lateral decubitus position

100. A 29-year-old G1P0 presents to L&D at 33 weeks gestation in preterm labor. Her GBS status is unknown and she has no known drug allergies. What is the best management for this patient?

    a. Penicillin
    b. Clindamycin
    c. Erythromycin
    d. No antibiotics are required

101. A 23-year-old G1P0 at 39 weeks gestation presents to L&D with painful contractions every 3 minutes. She has a history of HSV-2 and on sterile speculum examination she is found to have an active lesion on the right labia. Which of the following is an appropriate next step in management?
    a. Cesarean section
    b. Treatment with acyclovir
    c. Careful delivery with pediatrics present at birth
    d. All of the above

102. The "double-bubble" sign is an ultrasonographic finding of which of the following anomalies?
    a. Aqueductal stenosis
    b. Cystic hygroma
    c. Duodenal atresia
    d. Two-vessel umbilical cord

103. An obese 38-year-old with chronic hypertension and type II diabetes is found to be 6 weeks pregnant. Her medications include: an ACE inhibitor, beta blocker, thiazide diuretic, metformin, folic acid and a multivitamin. Which of the following regiments is safe in pregnancy?
    a. Insulin, glyburide, beta blocker, methyldopa
    b. Insulin, lispro, beta blocker, ACE inhibitor
    c. Insulin, metformin, beta blocker, thiazide
    d. Glargine, insulin, calcium channel blocker, thiazide

Review Answers

1. d	2. c	3. b
4. b	5. c	6. a
7. d	8. c	9. d
10. c	11. b	12. a
13. c	14. a	15. a
16. b	17. d	18. c
19. d	20. d	21. b
22. b	23. d	24. b
25. c	26. b	27. c
28. a	29. d	30. a
31. b	32. c	33. c
34. c	35. d	36. a
37. c	38. a	39. c
40. d	41. e	42. d
43. b	44. d	45. c
46. c	47. a	48. b
49. c	50. a	51. b
52. a	53. b	54. d
55. b	56. b	57. d
58. d	59. d	60. b
61. a	62. a	63. d
64. c	65. a	66. b
67. d	68. b	69. b
70. c	71. b	72. b
73. d	74. c	75. c
76. d	77. d	78. a
79. b	80. d	81. c
82. d	83. c	84. b
85. b	86. d	87. c
88. a	89. e	90. d
91. c	92. d	93. a
94. a	95. d	96. a
97. b	98. c	99. a
100. a	101. a	102. b
103. d		

Suggested Reading

Beckmann CRB, Ling FW, Smith RP, Barzansky BM, Herbert W, and Laube DW. *Obstetrics and Gynecology*. 6th ed. Philadelphia, PA: Lippincott Williams & Wilkins; 2009.

Berek JS. *Berek and Novak's Gynecology (Novak's Textbook Gynecology)*. 14th ed. Philadelphia, PA: Lippincott Williams & Wilkins; 2006.

Carlson KJ, Eisenstat SA, Frigoletto Jr. FD, Schiff I. *Primary Care of Women*. 2nd ed. St. Louis, MO: Mosby-Year Book; 2002.

Centers for Disease Control and Prevention. http://www.cdc.gov. Accessed January 26, 2011.

Cunningham FG, Leveno KJ, Bloom SL, Hauth JC, Rouse DJ, Spong CY. *Williams Obstetrics*. 23rd ed. New York, NY: McGraw-Hill; 2009.

Decherney AH, Nathan L, Goodwin TM, Laufer N. *Current Diagnosis & Treatment*. 10th ed. New York, NY: McGraw-Hill; 2007.

Menopause Practice: A Clinician's Guide. 3rd Edition. Cleveland, OH: The North American Menopause Society; 2007.

The American Congress of Obstetrician and Gynecologists. http://www.acog.org. Accessed January 26, 2011.

U.S. Department of Health & Human Services. Agency for Healthcare Research and Quality. U.S. Preventive Services Task Force (USPSTF). http://www.uspstf.gov/clinic/uspstfix.htm. Accessed January 26, 2011.

UpToDate. http://www.UpToDate.com. Accessed January 26, 2011.

Index

Note: Page numbers followed by *f* denote figures; page numbers followed by *t* denote tables.